Soft Tissue Management:
The Restorative Perspective
Putting Concepts into Practice

Soft Tissue Management
THE RESTORATIVE PERSPECTIVE

Putting Concepts into Practice

Ariel J. Raigrodski, DMD, MS
Professor
Department of Restorative Dentistry
School of Dentistry
University of Washington
Seattle, Washington
Private Practice
Kenmore, Washington

Quintessence Publishing Co, Inc

Chicago, Berlin, Tokyo, London, Paris, Milan, Barcelona, Istanbul, Moscow, New Delhi, Prague, São Paulo, Seoul, and Warsaw

Dedication

To my parents, Noa and Pinchas Raigrodski, who gave me the love and foundation to be who I am.
To my wife, Dana, for her endless love, patience, understanding, and unconditional support.
To my children—Daphne, Tal, and Maya—who make it all worthwhile.
And to all my teachers—past, present, and future.

Library of Congress Cataloging-in-Publication Data

Raigrodski, Ariel J., author.
Soft tissue management : the restorative perspective : putting concepts into practice / Ariel J. Raigrodski.
p. ; cm.
Includes bibliographical references and index.
ISBN 978-0-86715-691-1
I. Title.
[DNLM: 1. Dental Implantation. 2. Dental Prosthesis. 3. Guided Tissue Regeneration, Periodontal. 4. Periodontium. 5. Technology, Dental. WU 640]
RK667.I45
617.6'9--dc23

201404616

quintessence books

Quintessence Publishing Co, Inc
4350 Chandler Drive
Hanover Park, IL 60133
www.quintpub.com

5 4 3 2 1

Editor: Leah Huffman
Design: Ted Pereda
Production: Kaye Clemens

Printed in China

Contents

Foreword

What is the definition of a "true" teacher? The answer lies in understanding what the underlying goals and objectives are in conveying knowledge. A "true" teacher shares the gift of wisdom and experience without the expectation of receiving anything in return. It is this act of sharing in itself that yields fulfillment.

In a dental world filled with both academic and clinical rivalry, it is unusual today to find a teacher who is not driven solely by the need to "self-promote" and to continually create opportunities to showcase his or her most successful treatment outcomes. It is with this in mind that Dr Raigrodski has written a book for our profession in which he teaches with no other reason than to share his knowledge with dentists who will greatly benefit from its content.

This book is dedicated to providing a better understanding of the soft tissue–restorative interface and its influence on the final restorative result. It provides a simplified, well-organized, evidence-based, step-by-step approach to achieving esthetically pleasing restorative outcomes.

To achieve a predictable soft tissue outcome around natural teeth or dental implants requires not only strict discipline in the clinical protocol but also a keen understanding and control of tooth contour and emergence profile. As this text illustrates—with superb detail and interdisciplinary treatment—the ultimate challenge lies in all of the fine details and nuances of crafting the provisional restorations as well as the definitive ones.

As with all experienced teachers, Ariel has recognized the value of collaboration on a project of this magnitude. As you make your way through this textbook, you will begin to appreciate the level of commitment that the University of Washington graduate students have made with their own teaching contribution to the profession. There was great sensitivity to presenting information in a way that would be clearly understandable and most user-friendly.

Soft Tissue Management: The Restorative Perspective will provide substantial and tangible tools to restorative dentists, which will subsequently help them become more "complete" clinicians to their patients. As dentists become more capable of controlling the "soft tissue frame," they will better be able to meet or exceed their patient's ever-demanding expectations.

Gerard J. Chiche
Augusta, Georgia

Michael Cohen
Seattle, Washington

Preface

Ten years ago, I was invited to give a lecture on how to manage soft tissue from the perspective of the restorative dentist. The request came from a group of dental practitioners who had been working comprehensively in an interdisciplinary manner to provide better care for their patients. However, many times they were frustrated with the definitive treatment outcome in terms of how the restorations blended with the soft tissue. I carefully developed the lecture, and with time it grew into a program, with inspiration from my graduate students, colleagues, and mentors as well as my experience in private practice. It has culminated in this book.

Soft tissue management from the restorative perspective is a topic that is fundamental for success in providing patients with esthetic and functional restorations and for improved patient care. This is where the beautiful artistic work of the dental technician meets with the finish line of the tooth preparation and with the dentogingival complex at the soft tissue–restorative interface. Creating and managing the soft tissue frame is the essence of restorative dentistry, and it is a constant challenge for clinicians, regardless of the type of restoration (tooth borne or implant supported) being provided. In every step of restorative therapy, the soft tissue may be susceptible to trauma that may or may not be reversible and may adversely affect the desired esthetic outcome.

Much has already been written on this topic from both research and clinical perspectives. The vision for this book, however, is to provide clinicians with evidence-based concepts that will guide them as technologies and materials in dentistry continue to evolve. The goal is to demystify clinical restorative procedures and help restorative dentists ensure better control of the soft tissue frame (also known as the *pink esthetics*) during all clinical steps of restorative therapy while enhancing a healthy and esthetic treatment outcome. Therefore, the book offers a simplified approach for soft tissue management during restorative therapy and practical tools that restorative dentists may apply in their daily practice.

Writing this book provided me with a great opportunity to learn more and augment my knowledge and clinical skills. I can only hope that this book similarly provides restorative dentists with practical, tangible, and valuable tools based on sound scientific concepts that will help them in their everyday practice.

Acknowledgments

First, I would like to thank all the contributors to this book as well as all the faculty members at the University of Washington, especially Deans Martha J. Somerman, Timothy A. DeRouen, and Joel H. Berg. In addition, this book would not be possible without the inspiration and collaboration of my graduate students in the Graduate Prosthodontics program. I am also in debt to all the clinicians and dental technicians (including Kimiyo Sawyer and her team from Cusp Dental Laboratory) whose excellent work is depicted in the cases presented in this book (see page x).

Carole Green and Jeff Meadows from the Graduate Prosthodontics clinic and my office manager, Paige Moody, have offered me significant support and assistance, for which I am grateful. Many thanks as well to Heather Bright from the Seattle Study Club and Michelle Butcher from the Graduate Prosthodontics program.

I am also grateful for the education I received at the Hebrew University School of Dental Medicine in Jerusalem, Israel, and at Louisiana State University School of Dentistry.

My deepest appreciation and gratitude go to my program director, Israel M. Finger, and my master research mentor, Shawky E. Mohamed, for their wisdom and guidance. Finally, I must express my eternal gratitude to Gerard J. Chiche, who continues to inspire me as an excellent teacher, superior clinician, and a genuine human being, and Michael Cohen, who has inspired me to write this book and continues to be a mentor, a friend, and a family.

Contributors

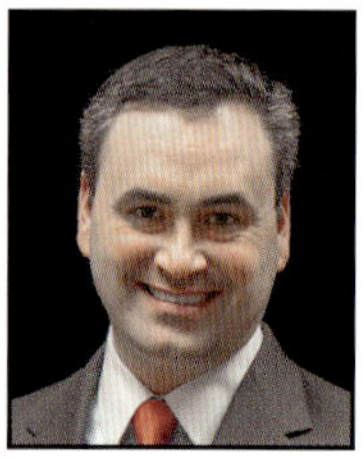

Matthew R. Anderson, DMD, MSD, earned his DMD degree from the University of Pennsylvania School of Dental Medicine, after which he completed specialty training in prosthodontics at the University of Washington School of Dentistry, where he earned his certificate and MSD degree. While there, Dr Anderson was named the David L. Wands Fellow and also received a fellowship from the American Dental Association & Dentsply International. His research during his residency earned him a Tylman Grant and award from the American Academy of Fixed Prosthodontics. Dr Anderson maintains a private practice in Santa Rosa, California.

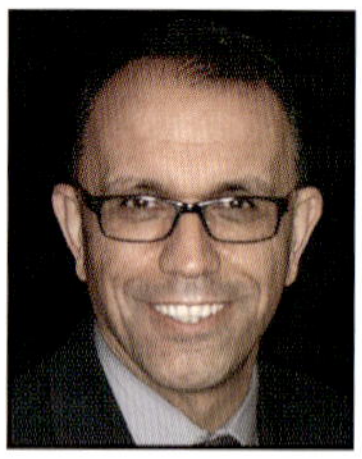

Sami Dogan, DDS, Dr med dent, received his dental degrees from the University of Ankara, Turkey, and from the School of Dentistry at the University of Hannover, Germany. He completed his postgraduate training in the Department of Restorative Dentistry at the University of Washington. He is currently an assistant professor at the University of Washington in Seattle, where he teaches dental and graduate students. Dr Dogan's research includes clinical and in vitro studies and focuses on remineralization of teeth and the quality assessment of dental materials. He has published extensively in peer-reviewed journals and holds an intramural practice limited to prosthodontics at the University of Washington.

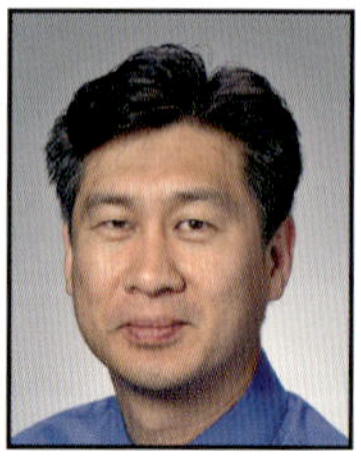

Sul-Ki Hong, DDS, received his dental degree from the University of São Paulo, Brazil, where he then entered the postgraduate program in prosthodontics and taught both prosthodontics and periodontics. He received his certificate in periodontics from Nova Southeastern University in Florida and is a Diplomate of the American Board of Periodontology. Currently, he is a clinical assistant professor in the Department of Periodontics at the University of Washington. He also maintains a private practice limited to periodontics in Bellevue, Washington.

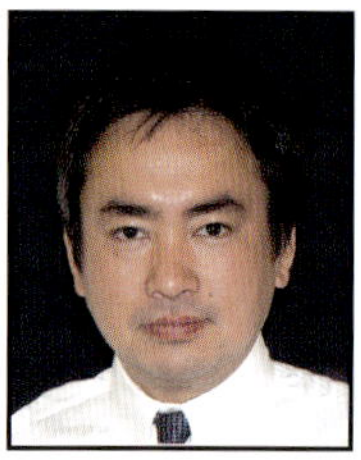

Motoaki Ishibe, DDS, MSD, received his DDS degree from Nihon University School of Dentistry in Tokyo, Japan, where he also completed a 1-year residency in general dentistry and served as a resident in oral and maxillofacial surgery. He further pursued his postgraduate training in prosthodontics at the University of Washington, where he received his specialty certificate in prosthodontics and MSD degree. He is currently an affiliate assistant professor in the Department of Restorative Dentistry at the University of Washington. He also maintains a private practice in Kofu, Yamanashi, Japan.

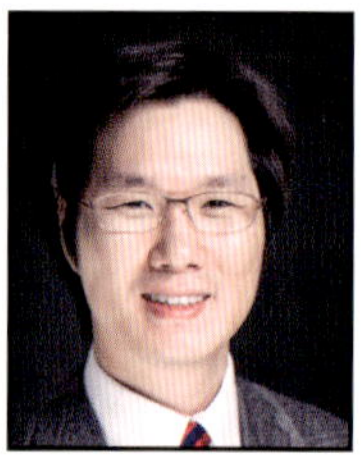

Jae Seon Kim, DDS, MSD, received his DDS degree from Yonsei University College of Dentistry in Seoul, Korea, and his MSD degree and certificate in prosthodontics from the University of Washington School of Dentistry. He is currently an assistant professor in the Oral Rehabilitation Department at Georgia Regents University College of Dental Medicine in Augusta, Georgia. He is also part of the esthetic team in the Ronald Goldstein Center for Esthetic and Implant Dentistry. Dr Kim is a Diplomate of the American Board of Prosthodontics and a Fellow of the American College of Prosthodontists.

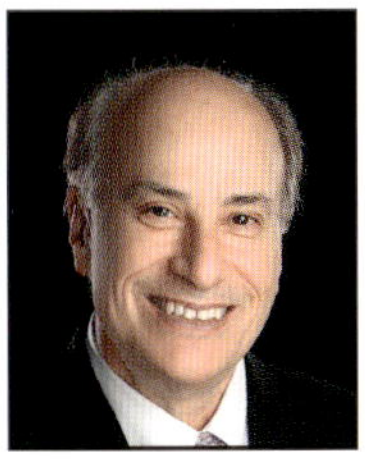

Robert M. London, DDS, received his dental degree from the University of California–Los Angeles School of Dentistry and his certificate in periodontics from the University of Washington in Seattle. He has held previous appointments at Nova Southeastern University and the University of Southern California School of Dentistry. Dr London is currently a clinical professor of postdoctoral periodontics at the University of Washington. He is a member of the editorial review boards for the *International Journal of Oral & Maxillofacial Implants*, the *Journal of Periodontology*, and *Clinical Advances in Periodontics* as well as a consultant for the Washington State Department of Health. A Diplomate of the American Board of Periodontology, Dr London has researched bone grafting, guided tissue regeneration, physiology of implant surface–bone interactions, and implant therapy, including esthetic and tissue responses to custom CAD/CAM abutments. He has also published several book chapters and scientific articles in peer-reviewed journals and lectures extensively both nationally and internationally.

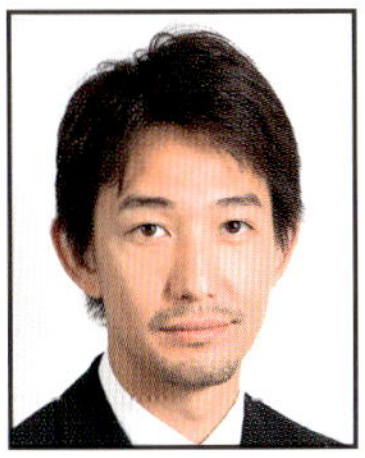

Takafumi Otani, DDS, PhD, MSD, received his DDS degree from Osaka University School of Dentistry in Japan, where he continued his studies in the Graduate Fixed Prosthodontics program, receiving his PhD. After maintaining a private practice in Japan and teaching at Osaka University for 3 years, he enrolled in the Graduate Prosthodontics program at the University of Washington, where he received his certificate in prosthodontics and MSD degree. Dr Otani is currently an affiliate assistant professor in the Department of Restorative Dentistry at the University of Washington and maintains a private practice in Seattle. He also lectures both nationally and internationally.

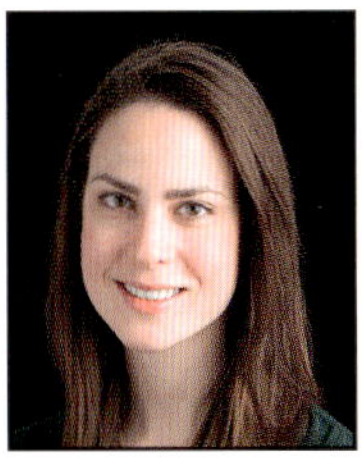

Tijana Stijacic, DMD, MSD, earned her DMD degree from the University of Manitoba, where she graduated at the top of her class. After practicing as a general dentist in Winnipeg, Canada, she earned her certificate in prosthodontics and MSD degree from the University of Washington. Dr Stijacic is a recipient of multiple awards within the dental community and maintains a private practice limited to prosthodontics in Houston, Texas. She is also a part-time clinical assistant professor at the University of Texas Health Science Center at Houston, where she continues her involvement in dental research.

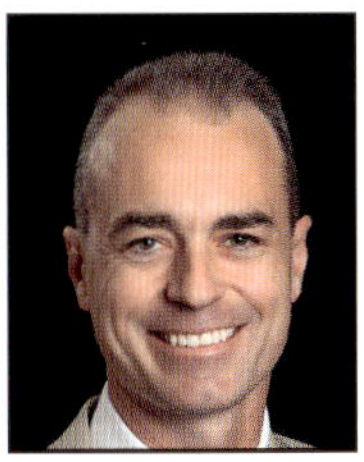

Robert D. Walter, DDS, MSD, received his DDS degree from Loma Linda University School of Dentistry in California. Ten years later, he completed a 3-year graduate program in prosthodontics and earned his MSD degree at the University of Washington. He is currently an associate professor in the Department of Restorative Dentistry at Loma Linda University School of Dentistry, a Diplomate of the American Board of Prosthodontics, and a Fellow of the American College of Prosthodontists.

List of Cases and Treating Clinicians

The cases in this book are presented continuously from chapter to chapter, with each chapter focusing on a specific aspect of the restorative treatment sequence. Therefore, a given case may leave off in one chapter and pick up again in the following chapter or a few chapters later to illustrate a later stage of treatment. Each case is identified with a uniquely colored, lettered icon to help the reader follow along. Each case presentation is labeled with this icon, and the corresponding icon appears in the margins of the text to indicate when the case is referenced.

Case A

Prosthodontists: Takafumi Otani and Ariel J. Raigrodski; Periodontist: Kimberly Marshall; Dental technicians: Nori Kajita and Masayuki Saito

Case B

Prosthodontist: Ariel J. Raigrodski; Periodontist: Michael Cohen; Orthodontist: Mark E. Simons; Dental technicians: Nori Kajita and Masayuki Saito

Case C*

Prosthodontist: Ariel J. Raigrodski; Periodontist: Michael Cohen; Dental technician: Sang Jun

Case D

Prosthodontist: Ariel J. Raigrodski; Dental technician: Harald Heindl; Coping design: Bob Williams

Case E†

Prosthodontist: Ariel J. Raigrodski; Dental technicians: Nori Kajita and Masayuki Saito

Case F

Prosthodontists: Robert D. Walter and Ariel J. Raigrodski; Periodontist: Traelach P. Tuohy; Dental technicians: Nori Kajita and Hiro Tokutomi

Case G

Prosthodontists: Satoshi Go and Ariel J. Raigrodski; Periodontist: Bradley Weinstein; Dental technicians: Nori Kajita and Masayuki Saito

Case H

Prosthodontist: Ariel J. Raigrodski; Periodontist: Sul-Ki Hong; Dental technicians: Nori Kajita and Masayuki Saito

Case I*

Prosthodontist: Ariel J. Raigrodski; Endodontist: Matthew A. Mandel; Dental technician: Harald Heindl

Case J

Prosthodontist: Ariel J. Raigrodski; Dental technician: Harald Heindl; Coping design: Bob Williams

Case K‡

Prosthodontists: Motoaki Ishibe and Ariel J. Raigrodski; Periodontist: Victor Mak; Dental technicians: Nori Kajita and Hiro Tokutomi

Case L

Prosthodontists: Satoshi Go and Ariel J. Raigrodski; Dental technicians: Nori Kajita and Masayuki Saito

Case M§

Prosthodontists: Ariel J. Raigrodski and Jennifer Emerson; Periodontists: Caroline Herron, Robert M. London, and Michael Chiully; Dental technicians: Nori Kajita and Hiro Tokutomi; Mandibular abutments: Issaquah Dental Laboratory

Case N

Prosthodontist: Ariel J. Raigrodski; Dental technicians: Nori Kajita and Hiro Tokutomi

Case O

Prosthodontists: Robert D. Walter and Ariel J. Raigrodski; Periodontists: Traelach P. Tuohy and Robert M. London; Dental technicians: Nori Kajita and Hiro Tokutomi

Case P

Prosthodontists: Matthew R. Anderson, Tijana Stijacic, and Ariel J. Raigrodski; Periodontists: Jaden Erwin and Robert M. London; Dental technician: Manfred Pornbacher

**Select images previously published in J Cosmet Dent 2013;28(4):46–58.*

†Select images previously published in J Cosmet Dent 2014;30(2):40–52.

‡Select images previously published in Seattle Study Club J 2010;15(1):19–24 and Seattle Study Club J 2011;15(2):10–15.

§Select images previously published in J Prosthet Dent 2014;111:154–158.

Fundamental Concepts of Periodontal Tissues

1

Robert M. London | Sul-Ki Hong | Ariel J. Raigrodski

Periodontal tissues are vital and responsive to their environment. They develop and differentiate as teeth erupt into the oral cavity, and once in function, they change and adapt to environmental stimuli. Restorative dentistry is a major source of environmental stimuli. By developing a strong understanding of the underlying tissues and how they are impacted by our clinical procedures, clinicians can execute a restorative plan that maximizes health and esthetics at the soft tissue–restorative interface.

Periodontal tissues can be defined in simple terms: epithelium, connective tissue, and bone. Of course, there is a vascular component and a component comprised of immune cells—neutrophils, macrophages, T and B lymphocytes, and plasma cells. From a clinical perspective, an understanding of the epithelium and connective tissues, together with their health parameters, gives a good foundation for facilitating and optimizing patient care.

Epithelium is the fast-moving tissue responsible for maintaining a seal between the body and the oral cavity, and it is quick to repair when injured.[1] When a tooth first erupts, the epithelium remains attached to the enamel coronal to the cementoenamel junction (CEJ). As the patient matures into adulthood and the tooth continues to function, the junctional epithelium (the epithelium actually forming the attachment to the tooth) moves apically. Initially adhering to the enamel, the junctional epithelium will eventually lie on the most coronal portion of the tooth root. It adheres via a hemidesmosomal attachment[2]; the epithelial cells adhere directly to the root structure at a strength similar to that of cell-cell connections.

Gingival connective tissue forms the durable attachment around teeth. During the time of development and calcification of the cementum and bone, gingival fibers become embedded, suspending the tooth in its socket. These fibers, known as *Sharpey's fibers*, are functionally oriented and form the periodontal ligament of the socket. Above the bone crest, the Sharpey's fibers extend from the cementum perpendicularly outward into the surrounding gingival connective tissue, anchoring it to the tooth.[3] This fibrous attachment is deemed stronger and more resistant to trauma than epithelial attachment.

Biologic Width and Teeth

In order to maintain appropriate function, the tooth requires a minimal distance from the crest of bone moving coronally to the base of the gingival sulcus. This allows for supracrestal connective tissue attachment and epithelial attachment to the tooth above the bone. The sum of these attachments is defined as the *biologic width*.[4] Biologic width can vary significantly from patient to patient and even from tooth to tooth in the same patient.[5,6] In areas where the

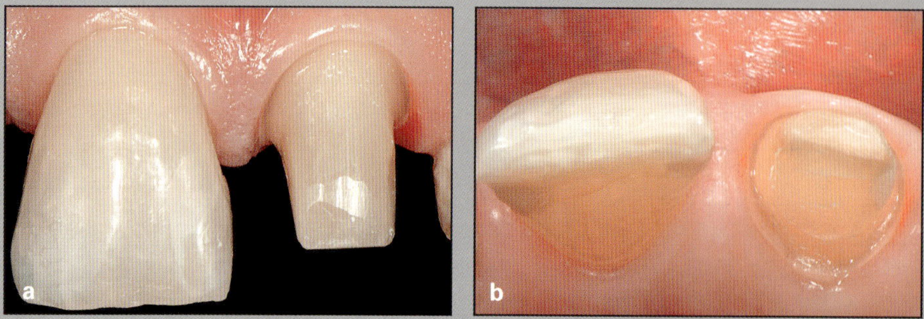

Fig 1-1 *(a and b)* A crown preparation for a ceramic crown with the finish line placed 0.5 to 1.0 mm below the free gingival margins on the facial and interproximal aspects. Note the equigingival and supragingival finish line placement on the palatal aspect and the general gingival health.

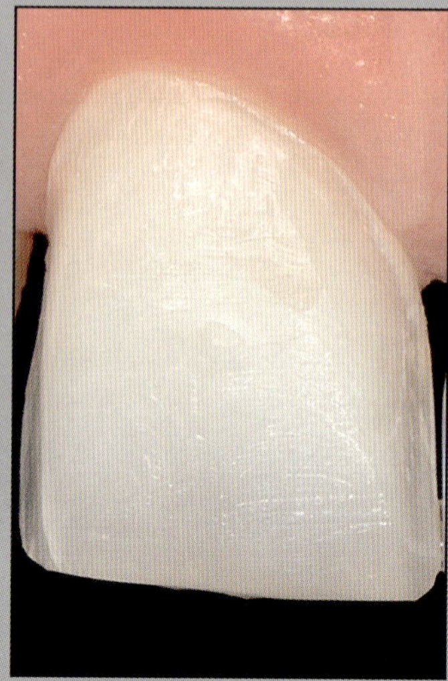

Fig 1-2 Facial view of a tooth preparation for a ceramic veneer with supragingival finish line placement on the facial aspect. Note the excellent gingival health.

root is prominent and the bone is dehisced, the width of the soft tissue attachment can be many millimeters greater than the mean values. In other situations, particularly if a tooth has not completely erupted, this width can be quite narrow.

In a classic cadaver study, Gargiulo et al[5] demonstrated an average sulcus depth of 0.69 mm, an average epithelial attachment width of 0.97 mm, and an average connective tissue attachment width of 1.07 mm. While these numbers are often quoted, the article demonstrated significant variability within these three different components. In a later study by Vacek et al,[6] very similar averages were seen with a somewhat narrower but still highly variable range. From a clinical perspective, most practitioners have accepted an average distance of about 3 mm between the free gingival margin and the crest of the facial bone. This distance consists of 1 mm of sulcular depth followed by an attachment consisting of 1 mm of junctional epithelium and 1 mm of connective tissue attachment.

Biologic width and finish line placement for complete-coverage restorations

Periodontal tissue response and the esthetic outcome may be affected by several factors, including location of the crown margin, type of restorative material, selection of implant abutment and/or restorative implant components, presence of bone and keratinized gingiva, the implant-abutment interface (microgap), and oral hygiene.[7–15] The finish line of a tooth preparation for a complete-coverage restoration can be placed supragingivally, equigingivally, or subgingivally. In clinical practice, subgingival placement of the finish line may be required to hide the tooth-restorative interface for esthetics, to address dental caries or a preexisting restoration, to manage a coronal endodontic perforation, to manage crown or coronal root fracture, and for retention and resistance purposes. Ideally, in such clinical scenarios, the finish line is placed 0.5 to 1.0 mm below the free gingival margin (Fig 1-1). Theoretically, any level above the base of the sulcus is acceptable. Consequently, the finish line must not intrude further into the periodontal attachment apparatus, because this can lead to violation of the biologic width.[16]

Subgingival finish line placement may, however, result in more gingival inflammation, loss of attachment, and gingival recession compared with equigingival or supragingival finish line placement.[7,8,17,18] This is more evident in patients with poor plaque control.[19] The tissue is certainly the healthiest when the margins of the restoration are kept away from it (Fig 1-2). Similarly, when esthetics dictates that restorative materials must be hidden below the free gingival margin, the likelihood of inflammation is increased. In addition to bacterially induced inflammation, physical encroachment on the epithelial or even connective tissue attachment may occur. This mechanical invasion may initiate its own inflammatory remodeling of soft tissue and bone. Additionally, because luting cements flow initially as liquids[20] away from the crown margin, inaccessible restoration margins may increase the challenge of removing excess cement. This can occur around tooth-borne restorations and particularly around cement-retained implant-supported restorations. The resultant tissue inflammation in response to the cement can subsequently lead to inflammatory bone loss.[21,22]

If the zone of biologic width is invaded, this biologic seal (ie, the periodontal tissues) must adapt and reconstruct itself. Thus, if a tooth preparation finish line is placed into the attachment, the inflammatory response may resorb bone until there is adequate distance for the various attachment layers. Sometimes this resorption can go undetected, such as on the facial aspect of a restoration, where bone loss cannot be detected radiographically. In other circumstances, the inflammatory process may occur with slow remodeling, resulting in erythematous tissue color changes.

Clinicians must be prudent during patient evaluation prior to surgical and restorative procedures and must ensure that adequate periodontal health is achieved prior to a definitive assessment of the dentogingival complex. Periodontal probing may overestimate the available sulcus depth when the gingiva is not healthy. In a series of studies summarized in 1980,[23–25] Listgarten evaluated where a probe stops in the sulcus. In healthy tissues, the probe penetrated partially through the junctional epithelium. In inflamed and diseased tissue, the probe penetrated through the epithelium into the underlying connective tissue.[26] These measurement inaccuracies worsened with disease.[27] Thus, prior to commencing restorative procedures, one might think that there is adequate sulcus to avoid impinging on the attachment when, in reality, the sulcus may be overestimated by over 1 mm.

The zone of keratinized gingival tissue can also influence the extent and severity of gingival inflammation around restorations with subgingival margins. Sites with a narrow zone of keratinization (≤ 2 mm) showed more noticeable gingival inflammation when compared with sites with a wide band of gingiva. A total of 5 mm of keratinized gingiva—2 mm of free gingiva and 3 mm of attached gingiva—is recommended for gingival health around teeth with subgingival finish line placement.[16,28] Furthermore, ill-fitting margins can contribute to the progression of periodontal disease by facilitating plaque accumulation and shift of the subgingival flora to a more pathogenic one.[29,30]

Kois[31] has coined three categories of biologic width based on sulcus depth and total attachment width. Referring to the bone level, he called these *normal crest*, *high crest*, and *low crest*. *Crest* refers to the facial height of bone as detected by a periodontal probe sounding to the bone through the sulcus. A normal crest is defined as 3 mm from the free gingival margin to the bone crest on the facial aspect of the tooth and 3.0 to 4.5 mm at the interproximal areas. A lesser number indicates a high crest, suggesting that bone is closer to the CEJ than normal. A low crest is farther away from the free gingival margin, indicating a larger total width of the dentogingival complex and the possibility of resecting gingiva without encroaching on a normal biologic width. Later Kois[32] described preparation guidelines related to respecting the biologic width. For the normal crest dentogingival complex, the finish line on the facial aspect should be placed 0.5 to 1.0 mm below the free gingival margin.

When bone is lost in an uncontrolled fashion, the periodontal damage may result in either increased pocket depth or gingival recession. Because satisfactory esthetics requires a healthy and adequately contoured gingival frame surrounding the restoration, the stability of bone and attachment levels is essential. Just as bone supports the soft tissue to create the attractive, scalloped appearance of healthy gingiva, lost bone will typically translate to negative esthetic gingival changes.

Biologic width management and correction

If the restoration margin infringes on the biologic width, the natural width can be reestablished only by creating adequate distance between the free gingival margin and the bone crest. Such an infringement may be prevented by keeping the finish line of the tooth preparation and subsequently the margin of the restoration more coronal during tooth preparation. However, when it is necessary to extend the finish line apically, one of two courses of treatment may be selected. The first and most common choice is crown lengthening osseous surgery—resecting bone to restore a proper biologic width and positioning tissue in a manner that will maintain health and viable esthetics. The alternative is to consider orthodontic extrusion of the tooth, thus moving the margin in a coronal direction. Bone tends to follow the tooth movement, resulting in no net change in the attachment width; to prevent bone from following, fiberotomy is used during orthodontics,[33–35] or limited crown lengthening surgery can be performed once orthodontics is complete. The authors concur with Berglundh et al[36] that fiberotomy may not yield the complete desired lengthening, because the tissue continues to follow the tooth movement but to a lesser degree than without fiberotomy. In such cases, extrusion should be followed by additional surgery to establish biologic width and balance the esthetics.

The gingival attachment repairs itself after injury. With a clean injury, as in surgery, if all the tissue components remain, the connective tissue will reattach, and the epithelium will re-form its hemidesmosomal junction coronal to that connective tissue attachment. In primate models, this repair takes over 6 weeks.[37] In humans, repair and remodeling can go on for much longer, ranging from 6 to 12 months.[38] Lanning et al[39] found that a normal biologic width and gingival dimension was restored after 6 months of healing. This was referenced to the new, more apical bone crest. Ganji et al[40] found that biologic width is reestablished by 3 months after either osseous resective surgery or gingivectomy, although the osseous procedure was more effective for stability of clinical crown lengthening. To avoid confusion, the term *osseous resective crown lengthening* should be used.[41]

Gingivectomy addresses only the soft tissue component of the dentogingival complex. Because it does not change the level of bone and thus cannot relocate the level of the biologic attachment, gingivectomy risks encroachment on the

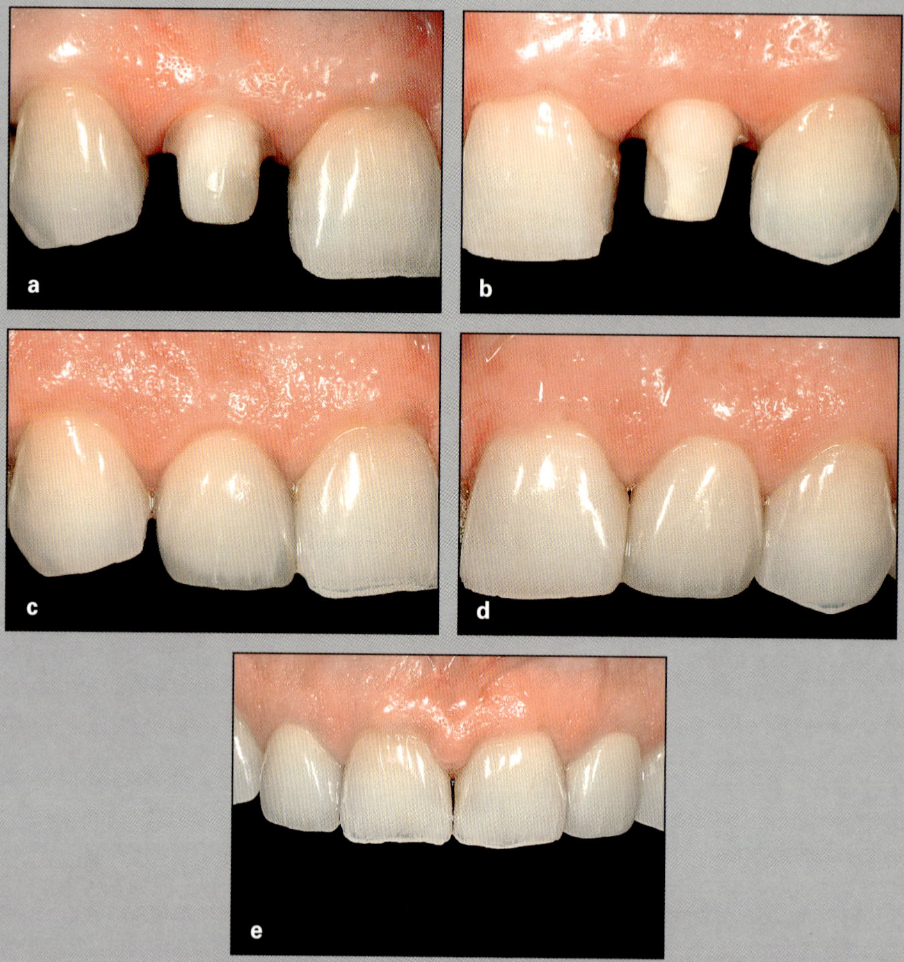

Fig 1-3 *(a and b)* Facial views of teeth prepared for zirconia-based ceramic crowns with minimal trauma to the soft tissue. *(c and d)* Facial views of the zirconia-based ceramic crowns 1 year after delivery, demonstrating that the trauma to the soft tissue has been reversible. *(e)* Facial view of the crowns 4 years after delivery, demonstrating soft tissue stability around the crowns. (Ceramics: Andreas Saltzer.)

healthy biologic width. As mentioned above, the periodontal probe extends partially into the attachment, resulting in a perception that the sulcus is deeper than it is biologically.[24] Gingivectomy should only be considered if the tissue depth from the proposed free gingival margin to the level of the attachment is at least 3.0 mm, allowing for biologic width without bone resection. Regardless of choice of instrumentation, a residual sulcus of at least 1.5 mm should remain after soft tissue resection, or an osseous resective crown lengthening surgery should be performed.

When the soft tissue is placed apically to expose more coronal tooth structure, the tissue may remain stable where apically positioned, or it may rebound coronally, covering some of the previously exposed tooth structure and increasing the subgingival location of the crown margin. This too can be explained by the concept of biologic width. Flaps placed at the bone crest may not have room apically for a normal width. They may proliferate coronally until a normal width has occurred, as evidenced from greater rebound when positioned at the crest.[42] This coronal migration is also more prevalent in patients with a thicker tissue type.[41] Six months would be prudent to allow stable healing after osseous resective crown lengthening surgery, recognizing that minor further changes may occur for up to 12 months.[43] Prior to commencing or continuing with definitive restorative procedures, clinicians should wait at least 3 months for healing after minor gingivectomy procedures and 6 to 12 months after osseous resective crown lengthening surgery.

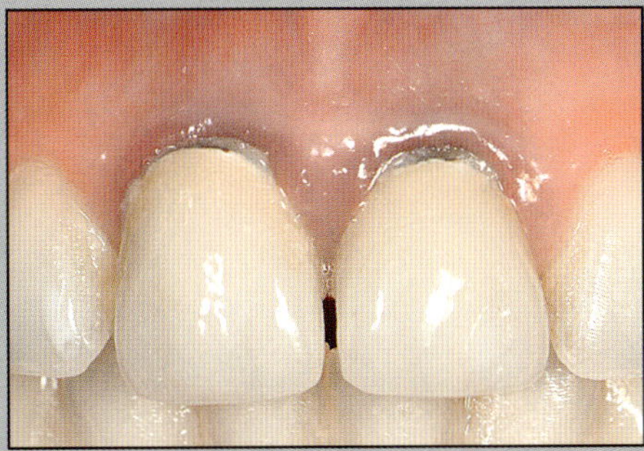

Fig 1-4 Facial view of failing metal-ceramic crowns. Note the questionable marginal adaptation that fosters plaque accumulation, resulting in increased inflammation as compared with the adjacent teeth.

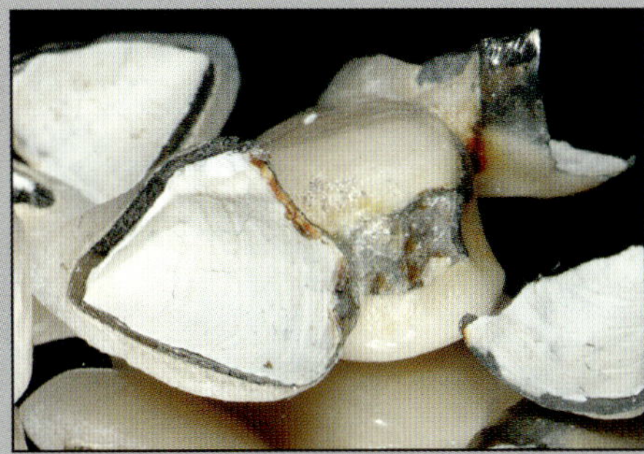

Fig 1-5 Removed restoration with a pontic that is inadequately designed. Note the concave ridge lap design and the rough intaglio surface, which may adversely affect the ability of the patient to clean as well as subsequently compromise the health of the pontic site.

Impact of restorations on gingival attachment

Both the restorative process and the resulting restorations have an impact on the gingival tissues. Preparation, provisionalization procedures, retraction and impression procedures, and delivery (conventional luting and adhesive cementation) procedures all irritate the tissue. Epithelium is typically disrupted or even removed by the aforementioned routine procedures. Emphasis should be placed on trying to accomplish the treatment with minimal irritation to the tissue and then allowing repair to begin (Fig 1-3). Cumulative irritation from repeated attempts to perform such procedures may result in longer duration of inflammation and greater remodeling of the attachment level.

Marginal adaptation, cement line exposure, and restorative contours all influence future tissue health. Any contours or gaps that foster plaque accumulation increase the likelihood of inflammation. Inadequate preparation design in terms of axial reduction and finish line width may result in an overcontoured restoration. This is especially true at the facial aspect, where adequate thickness of restorative materials is necessary to provide adequate translucency and esthetics (Fig 1-4). Such overcontoured restorations may mechanically encourage tissue change, such as recession, as well as trap plaque. In animal model studies, overcontouring was found to increase plaque retention and contributed to higher loss of clinical attachment levels compared with normally contoured controls. Crowns that are comparably contoured to the original tooth form provided the highest levels of periodontal health. Despite greater attachment loss in overcontoured groups, carefully instituted hygiene procedures mitigated the damage to only slightly worse conditions than the controls.[44]

Many studying the effects of crown contour on tissue health have concluded that undercontouring is equal to a natural contour or an improvement in terms of gingival health. This has been evaluated in animal models and in humans, discrediting the idea of a protective function of a supragingival bulge. In fact, more plaque accumulates with a larger contour, whereas flatter contours favor gingival health.[45–48]

Ovate Pontic Sites

Ovate pontics are considered optimal for esthetics and for cleansability. Being smooth and convex, such pontics support the edentulous space while providing appropriate facial and interproximal contours (Figs 1-5 to 1-7). Procedures to enhance the tissue ridge to accommodate such pontics have been proposed.[49] The design and fabrication for close adaptation of the pontic to the pontic site require special techniques,[50] which are discussed in the following chapters.

The question arises as to tissue response to materials intimately adapted to these structures. There are many materials that can be used for restorations in contact with tissue. Ovate pontics provide an opportunity to assess tissue response to various metal alloys, polymers (ie, acrylic resins and composite resins), and ceramics. With proper home care and a daily flossing regimen, no real differences are seen among a wide variety of materials.[14] This can perhaps be explained by the repeated and frequent separation of the epithelial interface from the restorative material. Flossing this area completely is principally possible under such convex pontics. During initial healing following placement of the pontics, tissue responses may indeed vary. Low-fusing ceramic may be favored over acrylic resins.[51] Edentulous spaces in contact with ovate pontics do not show clinical and histologic signs of inflammation in the presence of adequate oral hygiene measures (Fig 1-8). Histologically, this style of pontic is associated with a thinner keratin layer and

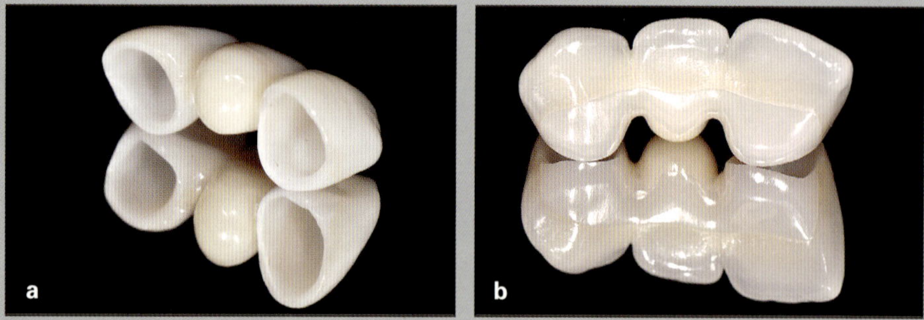

Fig 1-6 *(a)* View of the intaglio surface of an ovate pontic. *(b)* Being smooth and convex, such pontics support the edentulous space while providing appropriate facial and interproximal contours and allowing the patient to maintain adequate oral hygiene. (Ceramics: Masayuki Saito.)

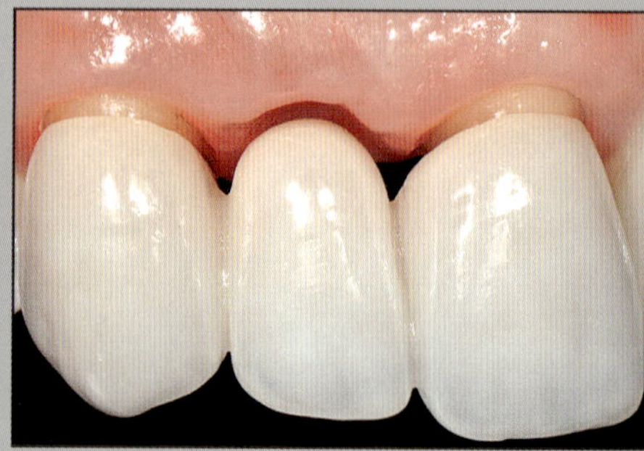

Fig 1-7 Facial view of the try-in of a ceramic zirconia-based fixed dental prosthesis with an ovate pontic. A cautious and delicate approach is applied during the provisional phase to facilitate an adequate design and a close adaptation of the pontic to the pontic site.

mild changes in the composition of the adjacent connective tissue, in comparison with tissues not in contact with the pontic.[52] Despite a lack of specific research, the tissue is presumed healed by 6 weeks and mature by 12 weeks.

When plaque accumulation and severity of gingival inflammation were evaluated underneath pontic sites fabricated with different dental materials (gold alloys, silver-palladium, cobalt-chromium, nickel-chromium, feldspathic porcelain, and composite resin), high levels of plaque control were associated with healthy gingival tissue irrespective of the pontic material used. Inadequate plaque control was associated with the development of gingival inflammation and increases in the amount of bacterial plaque underneath and around the pontic site.[14,15]

Biologic Width and Implants

General concepts

Lessons learned from the biologic width of natural teeth have parallels when working with dental implants. Like teeth, implants also display a zone of epithelial attachment and a zone of connective tissue apical to that. The connective tissue has different characteristics but occupies the same location as around natural teeth. Unlike teeth with perpendicularly oriented Sharpey's fibers, with implants, connective tissue fibers display an orientation mostly parallel or oblique to the implant surface.[53,54] When titanium abutments are placed at the time of surgery and are never removed, epithelium and connective tissue can attach themselves to the abutment itself.[55] This has been evidenced in human cadavers.[56] The result is a wider band of total attachment than that seen on natural teeth or when implant components are removed and replaced. In a dog model, when similar abutments were removed and replaced repeatedly, epithelial attachment was found to be positioned more apically on the abutment. More bone resorption was also observed when the zone of connective tissue was more apically positioned. It would appear that bone resorbs to allow for an appropriate reestablishment of biologic width even around implants.[57] The degree of resorption was similar in a human study comparing abutments placed at the time of surgery with abutments removed and replaced twice.[58]

Similarly to what is seen with crown lengthening procedures when the tissue is positioned very close to the bone crest, implants also appear to need enough tissue height to form the biologic width to avoid bone resorption. When implants are placed with excessively thinned flap tissues, biologic width has to be re-formed. Loss of crestal bone height is seen in both animal[59] and human[60] models. It is recommended that flaps placed around implants be coronally positioned adequately to allow for over 2 mm of vertical tissue thickness in order to ensure that biologic width is established without bone resorption.

From a structural point of view, Moon et al[61] described the nature of the biologic attachment around dental implants in a beagle dog model. In evaluating the connective tissue zone, they observed one zone of 40 µm close to the implant surface and one more distant zone of 160 µm. While the zones were continuous with one another, they had different characteristics. The zone against the implant was characterized by an absence of blood vessels and an abundance of fibroblasts. The fibroblasts were interposed between thin collagen fibers. The zone farther from the implant contained fewer fibroblasts but more collagen fibers and blood vessels. They speculated that the more fibroblast-rich region plays a role in maintenance of a proper seal to the titanium between the oral environment and the peri-implant bone.

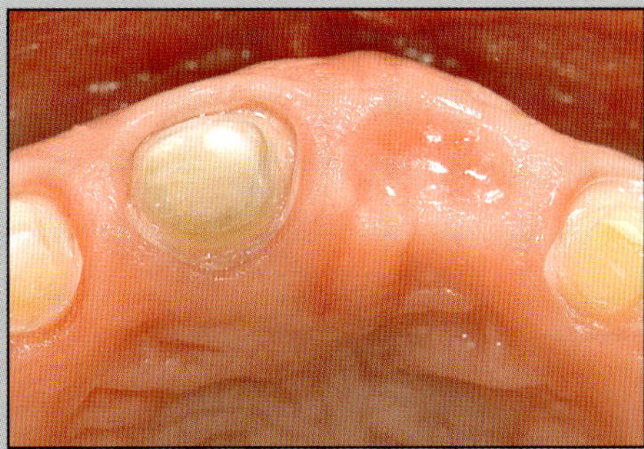

Fig 1-8 Occlusal view of an ovate pontic site demonstrating no clinical signs of inflammation.

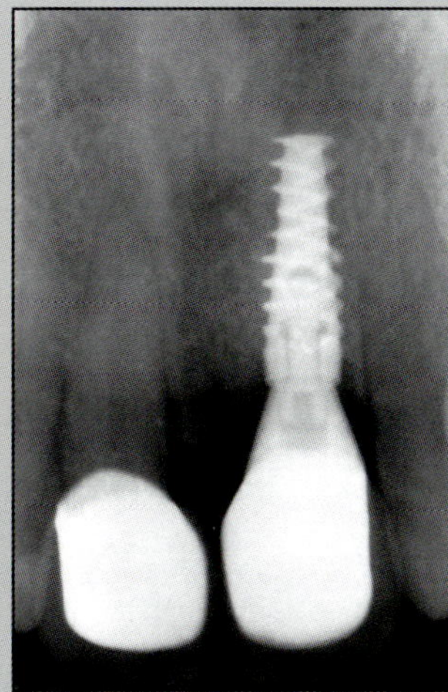

Fig 1-9 Periapical radiograph demonstrating the platform switching approach. Note that the implant abutment is smaller in diameter at the platform level.

In another beagle dog study, Abrahamsson et al[62] examined the nature of attachment to different dental materials used on implant abutments. In observations on titanium, densely sintered high-purity alumina, gold alloy, and feldspathic porcelain (for metal-ceramic restorations), they found that titanium and alumina allowed formation of attachment that included a normal epithelial and connective tissue band totaling approximately 3.5 mm. In contrast, when gold alloy or feldspathic porcelain was used, no attachment was formed on the abutments. The free gingival margin receded and bone resorption occurred, causing the biologic width to reform apical to the materials. This pattern has been repeated in a dog model in which zirconia and titanium maintained attachment while gold alloy lost attachment and adjacent bone over 5 months.[63]

Biologic width and implant platform switching

A proposed way to preserve marginal bone around implants is to utilize an implant abutment that is smaller in diameter than the head/platform of the implant, a technique called *platform switching*. In this manner, an inward horizontal offset at the top of the implant is accomplished (Fig 1-9). Because this moves the implant-abutment interface away from bone, it increases the distance available for biologic width. Much has been made of this phenomenon, with designs that incorporate an offset considered superior by the manufacturers.

Two-piece implants are designed for placement of the implant at the level of the bone crest, followed by connection of the implant abutment. The microscopic space between the parts is known as the *microgap* or the *implant-abutment interface*. Proximity to the alveolar bone crest implicates this interface as being responsible for remodeling of bone at the time of abutment connection, inflammation of peri-implant mucosa, and peri-implantitis.[12,13,64,65] The implant-abutment interface may favor bacterial colonization. The dimension of the interface space is about 10 μm, while the mean diameter of bacteria is less than 2.0 μm.[66,67] This microbial leakage may be the main culprit for the presence of chronic inflammatory infiltrate and crestal bone resorption. Occlusal loading of the abutment may result in additional opening of the interface, increasing the level of bacterial penetration.[12,66,68–75] The mere presence and contamination of the microgap by periodontal pathogens, however, may not necessarily result in inflammation of the peri-implant mucosa or peri-implantitis.[66,75]

Many studies have evaluated the effect of platform switching. Some take place in the form of cohort clinical studies (without controls), while others are in the form of randomized controlled trials. Results of such trials have been inconsistent. Generally speaking, platform switching results in a small but statistically significant difference at 1 year after the restoration delivery compared with implants restored with abutments matching the implant platform diameter. Studies demonstrate a difference ranging from 0.25 to 0.37 mm of bone preserved by platform switching.[76,77] However, some studies showed no difference at 1 year.[78] In a systematic review, the authors concluded that there may be about 0.5 mm of bone preservation with platform-switched

Table 1-1 Features of thin and thick gingival phenotypes*

	Thin phenotype	Thick phenotype
Gingival thickness	< 1 mm	≥ 1 mm
Gingival tissue	Delicate and friable	Dense and fibrotic
Keratinized gingiva	Narrow band	Wide band
Soft tissue architecture	Scalloped	Flat
Underlying bony architecture	Thin or minimal	Thick
Crown form	Tapered	Square
Cervical convexity	Subtle	Distinct
Proximal contact area	Located near the incisal edge	Located more apically

*Data compiled from multiple studies.[86–93]

implants.[79] In the same review, however, caution was emphasized because heterogeneity of data and publication bias were noted. No systematic reviews showed a difference in implant survival rates between the two types of restorative design.[77,79] Enkling et al[80] performed a randomized clinical trial and concluded that at the 3-year follow-up there was no significant difference in bone height, with a mean intra-individual difference of 0.05 mm between the platform switching and the traditional implant/abutment approaches. In a 5-year follow-up study, Vigolo and Givani[81] showed a similar 1-year difference of 0.3 mm, favoring bone levels on platform-switched abutments. No changes were noted from that point out to 5 years.

The smaller abutment diameter would seem to be unfavorable to load, but this may depend on the design of the implant-abutment interface. In an in vitro study, Leutert et al[82] found that internally connected abutments with a smaller diameter than the implant platform showed significantly higher bending moments compared with abutments of the same diameter. The small offset does present an obstacle to probing and periodontal maintenance curetting in cases where there is implant disease. In larger teeth, it may also create a larger size mismatch, negatively affecting tissue emergence profile angle.

Based on the available research evidence, it seems reasonable to conclude that platform switching results in a slightly (approximately 0.4 mm) better maintenance of crestal bone height around the implant at 1 year. This does not appear to make a clinically significant difference in patient outcomes; thus, at present, it seems reasonable to choose either a platform-switched or conventional equal-diameter restorative solution based on other parameters. Such parameters might include contour matched to the proposed restoration, availability of a specific custom abutment modality, and desired placement of restorative margins.[83] The exception to this may be when adjacent implants must be placed in close proximity.[84,85] It remains to be seen in longer-term studies if there is a difference in incidence of peri-implant disease based on abutment diameter at the implant platform.

Tissue Phenotype

General concepts

In 1969, Ochsenbein and Ross[86] reported two main types of gingival morphology: flat and scalloped. The flat gingival morphology was closely related to a square tooth form with a minimal distance between the buccal gingival margin and interdental gingival levels. The scalloped gingival morphology was associated with a tapered tooth form and considerable height—about 5 to 6 mm—between the buccal gingival margin and interdental gingival levels. They also indicated that the gingival contours mimic and follow the contours of the underlying bone. Later, the term *periodontal biotype* was proposed by Seibert and Lindhe,[87] classifying the gingiva into two distinct types of gingival morphology: thin (less than 1 mm) and scalloped, or thick (more than 1 mm) and flat. This term has been frequently used clinically to describe the faciolingual thickness of the facial gingiva around teeth (synonymous with gingival thickness), relating it to papilla height. The thin and scalloped gingival type is associated with a tooth with tapered crown form, subtle cervical convexity, small proximal contact areas located near the incisal edge of the tooth, shallow probing depths, a narrow zone of keratinized gingiva, and thin alveolar bone. The thick and flat type corresponds to a tooth with squared facial form, distinct cervical convexity, relatively large and more apically located contact areas, a wide zone of keratinized gingiva, and thicker alveolar bone[88] (Table 1-1). In a study assessing different morphologic characteristics of the gingiva, Müller and Eger[94] proposed the use of the term *phenotype* instead of *biotype* as the correct term in describing features of the marginal periodontium that are influenced by both genetic and environmental factors.

However, not all patients will fit the molds of thin scalloped or thick flat gingival morphology. There are certainly variations and combinations of the morphologic characteristics from the basic two gingival phenotypes. De Rouck et al[89] identified and confirmed through a cluster analysis the existence of three different gingival types around the maxil-

Table 1-2 Clinical implications of gingival phenotype*

	Thin phenotype	Thick phenotype
Inflammation		
Soft tissue	Gingival recession without pocket formation	Marginal inflammation with pocket formation, bleeding on probing, and edema
Hard tissue	Loss of the thin vestibular bone plate	Formation of intrabony defects
Surgical procedures		
Osseous surgery	More susceptible to gingival recession	Marginal periodontal tissue shows a tendency to grow in a coronal direction
Mucogingival surgeries	Associated with partial root coverage	Associated with complete root coverage
Guided tissue regeneration	Greater postoperative recession	Less postoperative recession
Orthodontic treatment	Greater risk of developing soft tissue recession	Prevents or minimizes soft tissue recession
Implant therapy	More susceptible to marginal bone loss, angular bone defects, and recession	Maintains stable crestal bone and is less prone to recession
Restorative procedures	Restoration may be slightly visible through the thin soft tissue	May mask discoloration from metal-ceramic restorations with metal collars and disappearing margins, metal implant abutments, and discolored roots
Extractions	Extensive ridge resorption	Minimal ridge resorption

*Data compiled from multiple studies.[41,59,90,92,93,100–107]

lary central incisors in a sample of 100 participants: cluster A1, slender tooth form and thin gingiva; cluster A2, slender tooth form and thick gingiva; and cluster B, quadratic tooth form with thick gingiva. Cluster A1 corresponds to the thin scalloped phenotype, while cluster B represents the thick flat phenotype. The participants from cluster A2 differed significantly from the other clusters, showing a definitive thick gingiva but slender teeth. Thin gingiva was found in one-third, mainly female participants, while thick gingiva was found in two-thirds of the participants and was predominantly a male trait.

Patients will frequently present with both thick and thin periodontium in the same dentition. Canines and mesiobuccal roots of maxillary molars tend to have a thin periodontium due to their position in the dental arch. Central incisors are usually associated with thick periodontium. As a general rule, the prevalence of thick periodontium is more common in males than in females, in younger patients than in older patients, in the maxilla than in the mandible, and in white patients (72% to 88%) than in patients of Asian descent (< 40%). These differences are due to intra- and interindividual variations in conjunction with tooth type, tooth shape, tooth position, and genetic determinants.[90,94–99]

The thick phenotype is commonly associated with periodontal durability and health. It is characterized by dense fibrotic gingival tissue, a wide band of keratinized tissue, and flat soft tissue with thick underlying bony architecture. The thin phenotype is usually associated with delicate and friable gingiva that is almost translucent in appearance, a narrow band of keratinized tissue, and highly scalloped soft tissue with thin or minimal underlying buccal bony thickness[86–93] (see Table 1-1).

Clinical implications of tissue phenotype

The clinician should be able to correctly identify and categorize these two distinct gingival phenotypes. Differences in gingival and osseous architecture have been shown to have a significant impact on treatment outcomes. Accordingly, thin and thick phenotypes behave differently when subjected to inflammation, tooth extraction, and surgical trauma[93] (Table 1-2). They also respond differently to restorative, periodontal, implant, and orthodontic therapy.[41,60,86,89,90,92,93,97,100–107]

Gingival recession

A major clinical challenge is gingival recession around ceramic veneers and complete-coverage restorations when the finish line is placed subgingivally. Many etiologic factors have been proposed as the cause for recession. Faulty restorative margins, mechanical and chemical irritants from impression procedures, overcontoured restorations, incomplete removal of excess cement, violation of biologic width, or adverse gingival reactions to alloys used in the oral cavity have all been implicated.[92] Patients with thin gingival phenotype are more susceptible to such recession. Gingival grafting should be considered prior to restoration to modify the phenotype to a thicker state.

Gingival inflammation

The thin phenotype reacts to insult by initial gingival inflammation followed by gingival recession, while the thick phenotype responds by tissue proliferation and eventual formation of a periodontal pocket. This is probably due to the fact that a thick periodontium has a greater volume of soft tissue than the thin periodontium, with attachment loss leading to development of a periodontal pocket instead of recession.[92]

Surgical periodontal therapy

During the healing stages following osseous resective crown lengthening surgery, the marginal periodontal tissue shows a tendency to grow in a coronal direction. This pattern of coronal displacement of the gingival margin is more pronounced in patients with a thick periodontium compared with those with a thin periodontium phenotype.[41] In the context of osseous surgery, it is extremely important to make a distinction presurgically between flat and scalloped gingival architecture. Usually, markedly scalloped soft tissue architecture would be more challenging in terms of pocket recurrence than flat architecture in the interproximal area. This is especially true if the gingiva takes on a scalloped architecture while the underlying osseous tissue does not follow the same scalloped pattern, resulting in greater distance between the tip of the papilla and the crest of the bone, leading to the formation of interproximal pocket depth.[86]

For mucogingival surgery such as the coronally positioned flap, it has been shown that greater initial thickness of gingival tissues (> 0.8 to 1.1 mm) is positively associated with complete root coverage. The probabilities of obtaining better root coverage outcomes are strongly related to the marginal tissue thickness.[108,109] Tissue thickness is also an important factor to be considered during regenerative procedures around teeth. Tissue thickness greater than 1 mm led to less postoperative recession at 6 months compared with thin tissue (0.6 vs 2.1 mm).[102]

Orthodontic therapy

The development of gingival recession during orthodontic treatment is a major concern as well. Alterations of the mucogingival complex are inevitable during orthodontic therapy, but the important factors to consider are the direction of the tooth movement and the thickness of the buccal gingival tissue. Movement of the tooth in the lingual direction will result in increased thickness of the gingival tissue on the facial aspect. It will also result in coronal migration of the free gingival margin. Movement of the tooth in the facial direction will result in reduced tissue thickness and migration of tissue apically, resulting in increased crown height. The thickness of the soft tissue correlates to the prevention of soft tissue recession. The risk of developing recession is increased in the presence of thin tissue when the tooth is being moved out of the alveolar bone housing. If mucogingival surgery is considered in order to prevent or reduce the risk of developing recession, it should be aimed at increasing the thickness of marginal soft tissue rather than only the width of keratinized gingiva.[103]

Implant therapy

In the case of dental implants, there is evidence indicating that the tissue phenotype is a key element for predictable and successful esthetic outcomes. Thin gingival tissues are more susceptible to marginal bone loss, angular bone defects, and recession, while thick gingival tissue results in the maintenance of stable crestal bone and is less prone to recession around dental implants.[59,104,105]

Restorative procedures

A thick periodontium reduces the risk of gingival recession when the finish line of the crown preparation for a ceramic crown or a porcelain laminate veneer is placed subgingivally for esthetics. It can mask and eliminate the grayish discoloration from metal-ceramic restorations with metal collars or disappearing margins. The placement of retraction cord can be accomplished with a reduced risk of inducing recession, which may lead to disparate gingival levels and compromise the esthetic outcome.[106] With thin tissue phenotypes, the risk of inducing recession is increased, mainly during impression procedures. Clinicians may opt to use metal-free restorations such as ceramic crowns and fixed dental prostheses. When the finish line is placed subgingivally, it is placed more conservatively than with metal-ceramic restorations. Therefore, the likelihood of trauma to the tissue is diminished, and the color of the soft tissue, mainly in terms of brightness, will be uncompromised even though the restoration may be slightly visible through the thin soft tissue.[107]

In summary, an accurate evaluation of the soft tissue morphology and phenotype not only helps clinicians predict therapeutic outcomes but also helps them determine the most appropriate periodontal and restorative management, leading to more favorable and predictable treatment outcomes.[97,100]

Gingival phenotype assessment

Many different methods are available for gingival phenotype assessment. An ideal method should be simple to use, accurate, reproducible, and noninvasive. It should allow clinicians to predict risks in terms of soft tissue treatment complications and enhance the customization of therapy for each patient. The gingival thickness can be evaluated by invasive methods such as transgingival probing as well as by noninvasive methods such as visual evaluation of the gingiva, periodontal probing, direct measurement with a caliper immediately postextraction, and cone beam computed tomography (CBCT), if indicated.[91,95–97,110]

Visual evaluation of the gingiva

Visual evaluation was one of the first methods used to evaluate tissue phenotype.[86,87] Because of its simplicity, it is widely used in clinical practice settings to identify high-risk patients. While simple, this method may lack accuracy.

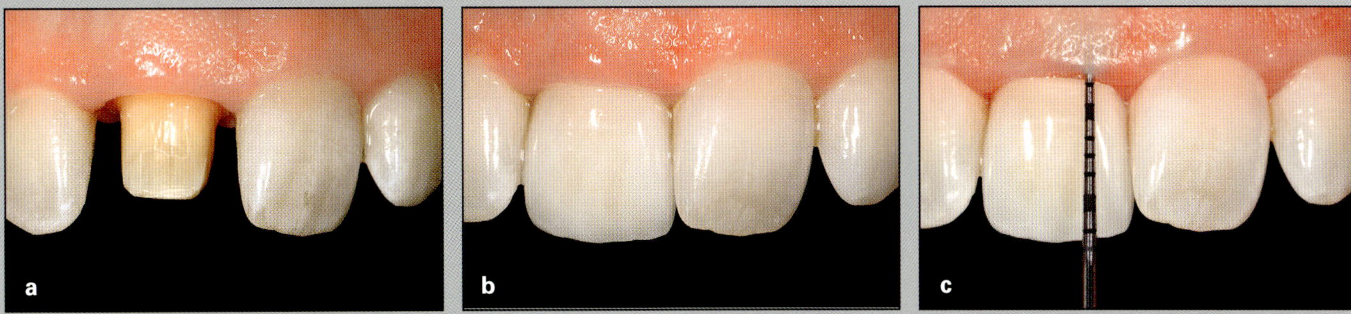

Fig 1-10 *(a)* Facial view of a tooth prepared for a zirconia-based ceramic crown. *(b)* Crown at the 4-year recall. Note the visual appearance of the tissue, looking relatively flat and thick. *(c)* The outline of a periodontal probe positioned into the sulcus is visible through the gingiva, demonstrating that the tissue is thin and translucent. (Ceramics: Andreas Saltzer.)

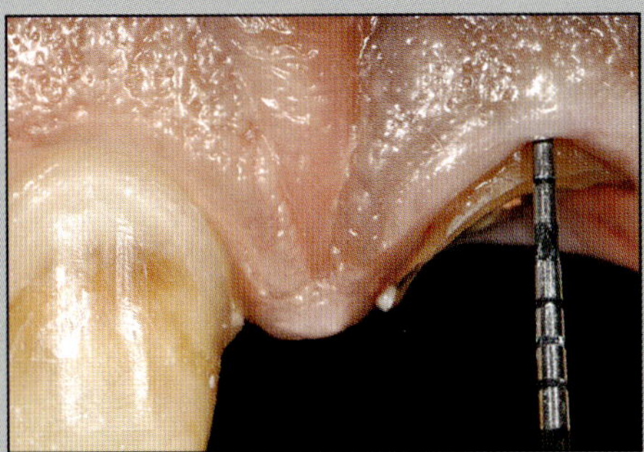

Fig 1-11 Facial view of a failing tooth planned to be restored with an implant-supported restoration. The outline of a periodontal probe positioned into the sulcus is not visible through the gingiva, demonstrating that the tissue is thick and opaque.

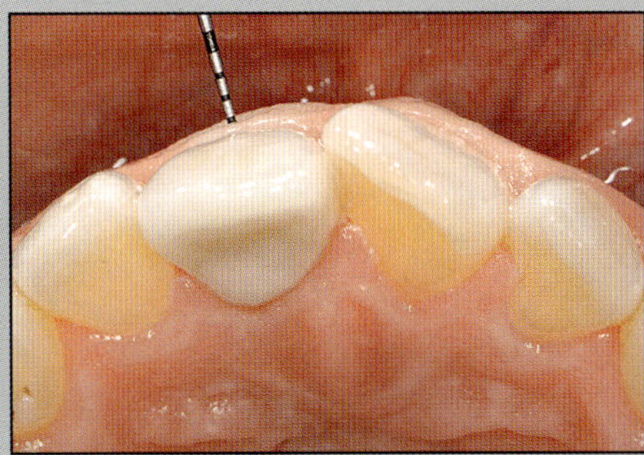

Fig 1-12 Transgingival probing of less than 1 mm at a point 2 mm apical to the facial free gingival margins confirms that the tissue is thin, as demonstrated in Fig 1-10c. (Ceramics: Andreas Saltzer.)

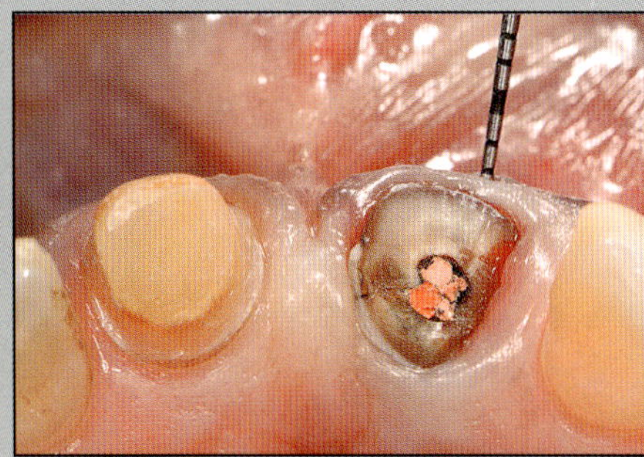

Fig 1-13 Transgingival probing of just less than 2 mm at a point 2 mm apical to the facial free gingival margins confirms that the tissue is thick, as demonstrated in Fig 1-11.

Accuracy of a visual inspection method for identification of three different groups of patients (thin scalloped, thick flat, thick scalloped) was evaluated based on clinical photographic slides.[111] The thick flat phenotype was relatively easily identified, but about half of the thin scalloped cases were misidentified. Precise identification of different phenotypes by means of visual evaluation was not reliable, as half of the patients at high risk were overlooked. In a similar study, 124 clinicians were asked to assign each of 53 patients to one of three phenotypes: thin scalloped, thick flat, or thick scalloped.[97] The results showed that visual evaluation was not very effective in identifying different phenotypes, with less than 50% probability of identifying the correct cluster.

Periodontal probing

The gingival tissue around teeth and implants can be classified as thick or thin by assessing tissue translucency. A periodontal probe is positioned into the sulcus, and the clinician assesses whether or not the underlying periodontal probe can be seen through the tissue. If the outline of the probe is visible through the gingiva, the tissue is considered to be thin.[91,112] This method is extremely simple, minimally invasive, reliable, objective, and reproducible[89,97,112,113] (Figs 1-10 and 1-11).

Transgingival probing

This is a very simple method in which a periodontal probe or endodontic file is used to measure the gingival thickness, usually at a point 2 mm apical to the gingival margin. However, this method is limited by the precision of the probe, which is usually rounded to the nearest 0.5 mm; the angulation of the probe penetration through the soft tissue; distortion of the tissue during the probing; a need for anesthesia; and the invasive nature of this tissue-penetrating procedure[112–114] (Figs 1-12 and 1-13). Alternatively, the use of an endodontic file with a stop has been advocated as well.

Direct measurement with a caliper

This method is limited for tissue assessment prior to immediate implant placement. A comparison was made among three different methods of evaluation of gingival phenotype around maxillary anterior teeth scheduled for extraction and immediate implant placement. A statistically significant dif-

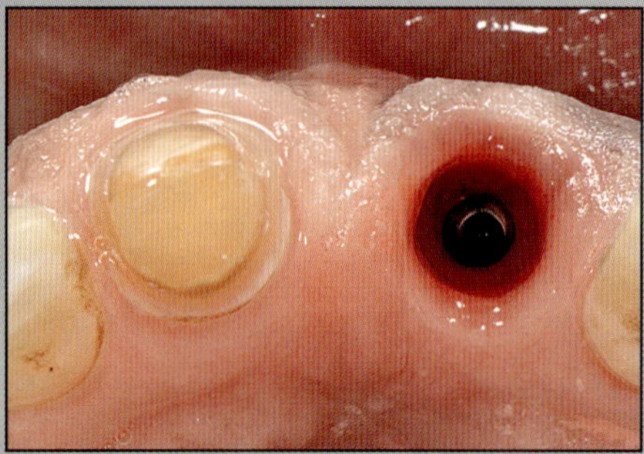

Fig 1-14 Occlusal view of an implant prior to impression making, demonstrating thick tissue on the facial aspect.

ference was noted between visual inspection and both periodontal probing and the direct caliper measurement method. However, no significant difference was noted between periodontal probing and direct caliper measurement.[91] The only drawback of the caliper method is that it cannot be used for presurgical evaluation, because it can only be used at the time of tooth extraction.[112,115,116]

CBCT scans of tissue thickness

CBCT scans are used extensively for three-dimensional imaging of hard tissue for orthodontics, endodontics, extractions, and especially for implant-related procedures.[117] Another useful novel application of CBCT scans is to measure the thickness of soft tissues.[97,110,111,118] One study used a caliper for clinical measurement of facial gingival thickness and compared this to CBCT measurements.[119] There was no significant difference between the clinical and CBCT measurements. Due to radiation concerns, this method can only be applied to patients requiring a diagnostic evaluation and visualization of the anatomical structures and/or underlying bone prior to treatment.

Strategies for Managing Soft Tissue Phenotype with Implant-Supported Restorations

Management strategies to maintain or improve existing soft and hard tissue architecture revolve around a goal of thick bone and thick soft tissue. A thick periodontium can optimize esthetics around implant-supported restorations. It can reduce the amount of gingival recession and create a better, more stable restorative environment[93,120,121] (Fig 1-14). Periodontal plastic surgery and osseous regenerative procedures are available to convert a thin phenotype into a thick phenotype, which is easier and more predictable to manage for the restorative dentist.[93,120,121] This has been examined with immediate and delayed implant placement protocols.

Immediate implant placement

Esthetic advantages of using subepithelial connective tissue grafts around dental implants have been reported. The change in the buccolingual width of the ridge around immediate implants has been evaluated with and without connective tissue grafts. After 6 months of healing, a loss of 1.063 mm of labial tissue was noted in a horizontal dimension in the nongrafted sites, while the grafted sites had a gain of 0.34 mm of labial tissue. Nine out of 12 nongrafted sites were considered to have compromised esthetics, with a "disturbing shadow" appearance, while no compromised esthetics were seen in the grafted sites.[120]

A successful conversion of a thin to a thick phenotype around immediate implants was demonstrated by subepithelial connective tissue graft placement in 20 patients. A thick phenotype was presented by 8 patients and thin phenotype by 12 patients prior to surgery. After a mean follow-up of 2 years, the mean facial free gingival margin change for the thick phenotype patients was +0.23 mm, whereas for the thin phenotype patients it was +0.06 mm. All the treated implant sites exhibited a thick phenotype.[122] Thus, the enhanced facial free gingival margins can be maintained at appropriate levels regardless of the initial gingival phenotype presented by the patient.

Subepithelial connective tissue grafts should have large dimensions with a vertical height of 9 mm and a horizontal width equal to the mesiodistal extent of the recipient site. A minimal thickness of 1.5 mm is used to prevent shrinkage following surgery.[123] Evaluation of long-term efficacy reveals a very predictable approach for achieving favorable functional and esthetic results around implant-supported crowns.[124] Therefore, additional soft tissue volume needed in esthetically demanding areas must be established surgically.[121]

Delayed implant placement

Bone regeneration and soft tissue grafting procedures in conjunction with delayed implant placement has also been described.[121,125,126] One clinical study reported on dimensional changes of peri-implant tissues by comparing pre- and posttreatment soft tissue dimensions. Placement of implants with simultaneous bone regenerative efforts and connective tissue grafting was successful in increasing the tissue volume. A 1.3-mm gain of buccal thickness and only 0.2 mm of recession (from crown delivery to 1 year postfunction) indicated stability of peri-implant tissues at 1 year.[125]

Successful esthetic outcomes can be achieved utilizing guided bone regeneration and soft tissue grafting in sites with missing facial bone. In one clinical study, implants were positioned in deficient sites followed by simultaneous horizontal and vertical augmentation. Six months later, at the time of membrane removal, connective tissue grafts were placed. The average bone gain was 3.75 ± 0.47 mm horizontally and 6.5 ± 0.81 mm vertically. The surgical procedure was able to provide predictable esthetic outcomes in deficient sites with favorable long-term soft tissue contour.[126]

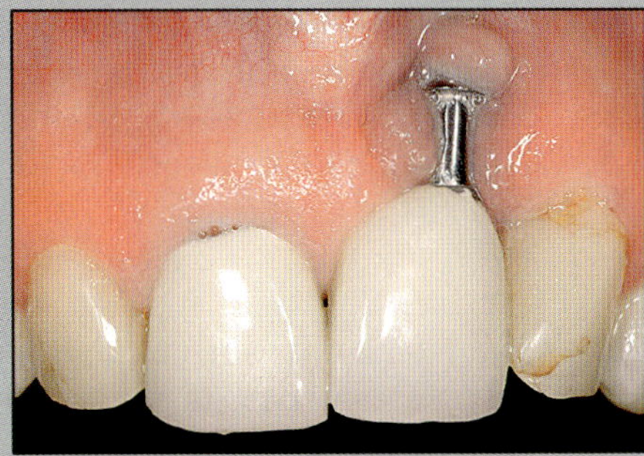

Fig 1-15 Facial view of a failing implant-supported restoration, which may be the result of multiple factors including less than ideal implant positioning in every dimension.

Enhancing Existing Peri-implant Soft Tissues

Malpositioned implants may cause esthetic and maintenance complications (Fig 1-15). Improper soft tissue management may create a defect complicated by the malposition, and inadequate initial hard and soft tissue volume prior to implant placement can be extremely difficult to correct once the implant is positioned. There may be a need to repair an unesthetic situation and/or regain pre-extraction ridge contours.[93] Treatment options such as implant removal, recontouring of the abutment, and soft tissue grafting should be considered. Several studies have shown improvement in cases of adverse esthetics around dental implants by means of connective tissue grafting and/or use of allogeneic bone grafts.[127–130]

Gingival phenotype again contributes to the amount and prevalence of gingival recession. One clinical study analyzing the esthetic outcomes of 42 single implant-supported restorations (mean time in function, 18.9 months) reported a mean recession of 0.9 mm. Patients with the thin phenotype had slightly greater recession compared with patients with the thick phenotype. That finding was further supported by another similar study reporting that recession was more prevalent in thin phenotype sites. Recession was present at 6 of 25 thin phenotype sites compared with 2 of 19 thick phenotype sites.[105,131]

Recession around implant-supported restorations

A dental prosthesis with soft tissue that truly mimics the soft tissue of the adjacent dentition and blends with the natural adjacent teeth is a challenging goal.[132,133] Various studies report the apparently inevitable occurrence of marginal gingival recession around dental implants leading to adverse esthetic outcomes. Long clinical crowns, grayish appearance through the thin peri-implant tissue, and exposure of crown margins, abutments, or even implant threads are not uncommon.[105,121,131,134–136]

Several factors have been implicated in the etiology of marginal gingival recession. These include implant position,[105,131,137–141] tissue phenotype,[104,105,131,136,139] integrity and thickness of the facial bone,[60,136,140,142,143] surgical approach (conventional vs flapless),[136,144] and presence or lack of immediate provisionalization.[144–146]

Implant position within the alveolar bony housing is considered to be one of the most important contributing factors for gingival recession. Recession is more pronounced for implants placed facially compared with those implants placed lingually within the extraction socket. In addition, facially positioned implants showed three times more recession than implants positioned lingually (1.8 vs 0.6 mm).[105,131] Undoubtedly, excessive lingual positioning may create unnatural buccal emergence angles or unmaintainable contours. Optimal placement is a balance of these issues.

Peri-implant soft tissue recession can be improved by employing a combination of coronally advanced flaps and connective tissue grafts. In one study,[129] significant improvement was achieved in 10 patients from baseline, but complete coverage could not be achieved. Significant shrinkage (66%) at 6 months followed coronal advancement of the flap. Alternatively, a prosthetic-surgical method has been proposed to correct the peri-implant soft tissue dehiscence around single implants. After the existing crown is removed, the abutment is modified, and a coronally advanced flap in conjunction with a connective tissue graft is performed. A year after delivery of the definitive restoration, the mean coverage of the dehiscence was about 96%, with complete coverage in 75% of the cases. Facial tissue thickness was increased an average of 1.54 ± 0.21 mm with a significant esthetic improvement.[130]

Esthetic improvement in clinical scenarios of suboptimal implant placement can also be achieved by means of a pediculated connective tissue graft. The existing crown and abutment are removed, and the soft tissue is allowed to naturally "self-cover." Approximately 3 months later, the implant is exposed, followed by placement of a 2-mm-tall healing abutment. A pediculated connective tissue graft is rotated from the palate, then flipped over the implant/healing abutment and secured with sutures. The second-stage surgery is performed in 4 months, followed by restorative procedures. This technique is able to increase the volume of soft tissue, resolving the initial esthetic complications.[127]

Acellular dermal matrix grafting in conjunction with coronally advanced peri-implant tissue has also been shown to improve implant esthetics. This technique was reported in a patient presenting with deficient esthetics, thin peri-implant tissue, and 3 mm of recession. Results of the case showed great esthetic improvement with partial coverage, thicker peri-implant tissue, no bleeding on probing, and no significant probing depths. This procedure demonstrated an alternative to harvesting tissue from the patient's palate.[128]

Integrity and thickness of facial bone

The presence and volume of bone is one of the most critical anatomical factors to be considered for achieving an esthetic outcome. Once the implant is positioned, a circumferential moatlike bone remodeling of approximately 1.4-mm width occurs.[147] At least 2 mm of buccal bone thickness is proposed to avoid loss of buccal crestal bone in a vertical direction. Moreover, additional bone grafting around implant sites with dehiscence or inadequate bone volume is strongly recommended. A lack of bone volume may jeopardize the esthetic outcome due to considerable risk of soft tissue recession.[140]

Evidence indicates that the placement of bone graft material in the gap between the implant surface and facial bone has positive effects in animal and human studies. The bone graft can counteract, or at least reduce, the inevitable bone remodeling process around implants immediately placed in fresh extraction sockets. When a bone graft of porcine origin was used to fill the gap in test sites with a resorbable membrane covering the entire extraction socket, test sites showed a stable bone level and even some bone gain. Extensive bone remodeling was observed in the control sites.[148] In a similar study comparing immediate implant sites with and without placement of xenogeneic graft material, the test sites (with bone graft) had *(1)* a peri-implant bone level located 1 mm more coronally, *(2)* thicker facial tissue (1 ± 0.3 mm versus 0.4 ± 0.4 mm), *(3)* facial bone located more coronally on the implant (0.1 ± 0.5 mm versus 1.3 ± 0.7 mm), and *(4)* thicker facial bone (1.1 ± 0.5 mm versus 0.1 ± 0.2 mm at 1 mm apical to the implant platform).[149]

In a case series with 10 patients, a "trimodal" approach (immediate implant placement, flapless approach, and immediate provisionalization) was employed. Xenograft was placed in the gap between the facial bone and the implant surface, and a subepithelial connective tissue graft was interposed onto the facial bone. Favorable implant success and peri-implant tissue were achieved with a mean marginal bone and facial free gingival level change of +0.10 mm and −0.05 mm, respectively. The authors concluded that the facial free gingival margin could be maintained without any further recession when immediate implants are treated with a subepithelial connective tissue graft, ideal three-dimensional positioning of the implant, and the use of graft material to fill the gap between the facial bone and the implant surface.[150] Therefore, placement of bone graft material in the gap can be beneficial in minimizing the bone remodeling process, resulting in more favorable hard and soft tissue status around the implant.[151]

Immediate implants have a similar survival and success rate compared with implants placed into healed sites. The advantages of immediate placement include decreased treatment time, a reduction in the number of surgical interventions, and the potential for immediate provisionalization. This may allow preservation of existing soft tissue and osseous architecture.[152–154] When clinicians are considering immediate implant placement in patients with a thin phenotype, careful and detailed evaluation of both the soft tissue and the underlying bony architecture should be carried out. In certain cases, a delayed approach may be the most appropriate treatment when very thin tissue or bone is present. When the possibility of significant recession is expected, hard and soft tissue augmentation should precede implant placement.[93] It should be assumed that thin facial bone is present.

Minimally invasive or flapless surgery may be possible and selected as a means to minimize disruption of blood supply to the surrounding hard and soft tissue components. Once the implant is positioned toward the palatal aspect, bone graft is used to fill the gap between the facial bone and implant surface. Where a flap must be elevated to assess structures and surgical landmarks, a subepithelial connective tissue graft should be harvested from the palate and secured over the facial bone. If an implant-supported provisional restoration is provided, it should initially have a concave subgingival profile on the facial aspect to reduce the risk of apical migration of the free gingival margin.[104,155]

Preserving thin facial bone plates

The mean thickness of facial bone for the maxillary anterior teeth (from canine to canine) is about 0.8 mm, with 87% of sites having a facial bone thickness ≤ 1.0 mm. Measurement of the facial bone thickness of anterior teeth in the maxilla by means of CBCT scans showed that the majority of all teeth examined had ≤ 1.0 mm of bone thickness. Nearly 50% of sites had bone thickness that was ≤ 0.5 mm. Most extraction sites in the maxilla will therefore experience extensive ridge alteration, demanding additional grafting procedures to achieve a minimal width of bone. At least 1 to 2 mm of buccal bone is required for stability of hard and soft tissues.[140,156,157]

Vertical bone loss is marked after immediate implant placement. A mean vertical bone loss of 0.7 to 1.3 mm on the facial and lingual aspects and a 0.4-mm reduction in the thickness of facial bone at the time of abutment connection can be expected. An exaggerated pattern of vertical bone remodeling around immediate implants was confirmed in an animal study.[148] Reference measurements were made from the implant platform to the bone crest and to the bone contacting the implant within the remodeling zone. The distance between the abutment-implant junction and the first bone-to-implant contact was 4.11 ± 1.9 mm, and the distance to the crest of bone was 1.23 ± 0.48 mm for immediate implant sites. In comparison, the mean distances were 2.02 ± 0.78 mm and 0.46 ± 0.51 mm, respectively, for the delayed implant sites.[158]

Tissue effects of tooth extraction

Tooth extractions performed on patients with thick flat gingival architecture may result in minimal dimensional changes to the surrounding gingiva and bone. Extractions performed on patients with thin scalloped gingival architecture, associated with thin bone, dehiscences, and fenestrations, may result in obvious dimensional tissue changes causing significant esthetic concerns.[159] For patients with a thin periodontium, atraumatic and very precise surgical techniques should be applied during the extraction to minimize adverse effects on the bone remodeling process.[93,160] Ideally, minimal flap elevation or a flapless approach should be used to limit the disruption of blood supply. An animal study compared tooth extraction with and without flap elevation and its effect on the bone remodeling process. The results demonstrated significantly less bone resorption for the flapless group than the flapped group.[160] Atraumatic extraction can be accomplished with controlled and steady application of forces on the interproximal areas, limiting any leveraging forces on the thin facial bone. Sectioning of the roots, careful use of periotomes to luxate and expand the periodontal ligament space, and use of controlled extraction devices can also assist in facilitating a satisfactory outcome with minimal hard and soft tissue complications.[93] Controlled extraction devices are mechanical devices that lift from a special post placed in the root canal of a crownless tooth. Adjacent teeth support them while they smoothly apply vertical extraction forces.

Ridge preservation procedures

Once the tooth is removed, it is critical to limit the bone remodeling process, especially in patients with the thin tissue phenotype.[60,142,143] The goal of preserving an adequate amount of bone volume for future implant placement can be met by socket grafting or ridge augmentation procedures.[93] Various surgical approaches and materials for ridge preservation have been described. As a general rule, ridge preservation involves the use of a bone graft material placed into the extraction socket. This may be in conjunction with the use of absorbable collagen matrices or nonabsorbable barrier membranes secured with sutures on top of the bone graft.[161–167]

Several human and animal studies have documented the effectiveness of ridge preservation procedures. These procedures limit, but may not totally prevent, the ridge alterations in both horizontal and vertical dimensions. Lekovic et al[161] evaluated alterations in ridge dimensions in 10 subjects by covering the experimental sites with expanded polytetrafluoroethylene barrier membranes with primary closure. Control sites remained ungrafted. The clinical measurements demonstrated increased remodeling in the control group of 0.7 mm vertically and 2.6 mm horizontally compared with the test group. Another clinical study compared a ridge preservation approach using mineralized freeze-dried bone allograft and resorbable collagen membranes without primary closure.[167] The horizontal width changed from 9.2 ± 1.2 mm to 8.0 ± 1.4 mm for the test group and 9.1 ± 1.0 mm to 6.4 ± 2.2 mm for the extraction-only control group. The difference horizontally was 1.6 mm between the groups. In vertical change, the test group had a gain of 1.3 ± 2.0 mm while the control group lost 0.9 ± 1.6 mm, for a vertical difference of 2.2 mm between the groups.

Fu et al[168] proposed increasing the soft tissue thickness around dental implants by means of a method they called PDP, which stands for implant **p**osition, implant **d**iameter, and **p**rosthetic design. The authors advocated three steps: *(1)* a more palatal and apical positioning of the implant platform so more soft tissue volume is present on the facial aspect; *(2)* use of smaller-diameter or platform-switched implants to maintain an adequate amount of bone thickness, thus limiting the amount of gingival recession; and *(3)* use of concave subgingival contours for the abutments or crowns to allow ingrowth of peri-implant soft tissue. This article highlights the importance of not only the surgical methods but also the prosthetic methods or combinations thereof when it comes to soft tissue management.

Soft tissue–bone relationship

For proper decision-making, it is critical for the clinician to predict how different gingival phenotypes respond differently to implant-related therapy. If the soft tissue morphology and the underlying bony architecture differ from one another, the clinician should employ different management strategies (ie, for thin vs thick phenotypes). *Bundle bone* is the alveolar bone that receives the Sharpey's fibers of the periodontal ligament. After extraction, the function of the bundle bone is no longer needed, usually resulting in substantial horizontal and vertical bone reduction. Following the removal of teeth, the bundle bone has minimal potential for remodeling and is therefore lost. Where bone is thinner, there is no capacity for this bone to be regenerated.[169]

There is evidence of a positive relationship between the gingival phenotype and the thickness of facial bone. Patients with thin phenotype are associated with thinner facial bone thickness, a narrow band of keratinized tissue, substantial distance from the CEJ to the alveolar bone crest, and a high prevalence of dehiscence and fenestration.[159,170]

The thickness of the facial bone is one of the most important clinical parameters in achieving predictable esthetic outcomes with dental implants. Facial bone thickness of 1 to 2 mm has been suggested to provide adequate soft tissue support and to prevent or minimize the amount of bone resorption. This minimizes the risk of soft tissue recession around implant-supported restorations.[121,171–173] Around immediate dental implants, substantial bone fill was observed when the thickness of buccal bone was greater than 1 mm.[141]

Several animal and clinical studies demonstrate the correlation between soft tissue thickness and crestal bone remodeling following implant placement. In histologic studies conducted in dogs, thin tissue around dental implants consistently resulted in more bone resorption following abutment connection. There was also a tendency to form angular bony defects, whereas thick tissues tended to maintain more stable crestal bone.[59,174] Similar results were reported in human studies. Implants placed in naturally thick soft tissue resulted in minor remodeling of bone, while implants placed in naturally thin soft tissues resulted in more bone remodeling with crestal bone loss of up to 1.45 mm.[60,142,143] It is interesting to note that implants restored with a platform switching design were not able to preserve the crestal bone when compared with conventional matched-abutment implants in the presence of thin soft tissue.[175]

Presence of keratinized gingiva

The presence of keratinized gingiva is considered to be beneficial for the stability of peri-implant soft tissue because of its ability to form a microbial barrier. It plays an important role in the long-term maintenance and survival of dental implants.[176]

The relationship between keratinized gingiva and health status of the peri-implant mucosa was evaluated around implant-supported overdentures. The absence of adequate width of keratinized tissue (less than 2 mm) resulted in higher gingival and plaque index scores, a higher tendency for bleeding, and more radiographic bone loss.[177] In a 5-year clinical study, even when patients were performing good oral hygiene and received regular maintenance therapy, buccal soft tissue recession, more bleeding, and plaque accumulation was noted at sites with less than 2 mm of keratinized gingiva.[178,179]

Interdental Papillae

The papillae between natural teeth fill the space under the proximal contacts. They have vertical, facial, and lingual surfaces, with a gingival col under the contact. With bone loss, the distance from the bone to the apical portion of the contact increases. Having a limited height range, the papilla may no longer reach the contact, resulting in a dark space between the teeth. The distance from the contact point to the crest of bone is a major factor in the esthetic adequacy of the papilla. Papillae are present around natural teeth 100% of the time when the distance from the contact point to the crest of bone is ≤ 5 mm. If the distance is 6 mm, the papilla is present only 56% of the time, and the papilla is present less than 27% of the time if that distance is ≥ 7 mm.[101] After complete denudation of the interproximal bone, a mean distance of 4.33 mm between the location of the interproximal papilla tip and the contact had developed 3 years post-treatment, demonstrating the body's tendency to return to a normal level.[180]

Single implants

The presence of normal interdental papillae is a key part of achieving optimal esthetics around implant-supported restorations. Papillae can be influenced by several factors. Tissue phenotype, implant-implant or implant-tooth distance, and level of interproximal bone crest of the adjacent teeth can all affect bone healing at the interproximal area and subsequently the presence or absence of a papilla. The space between the interproximal contact point of the definitive restoration and underlying interdental bone crest forms the interproximal gingival embrasure. As with natural dentition, the distance between the apical aspect of the interproximal contact and the interdental bone crest predicts the fill of the gingival embrasure space. Consequently, the presence or absence of an unfilled gingival embrasure space is dependent on both the surgical and prosthetic phases of the implant therapy.[100,131,139,181–184]

Single implants and phenotype

The complete fill of the interdental space by the papilla around natural teeth and implants can be influenced by the gingival phenotype of the patient. In a study evaluating the presence of papillae around natural teeth, the thin phenotype presented a significantly higher presence of papillae (71.1%) than did the thick phenotype group (59.6%).[100] The papilla was considered present when there was no visible space apical to the contact point. The high prevalence of interproximal papilla fill around natural teeth for the thin phenotype may be explained by gingival architecture characteristics, because subjects with thin tissue also have accentuated tissue scalloping with a tendency for taller papillae. However, these subjects are also more susceptible to loss of gingival tissue following surgical procedures or tooth removal.

In evaluating the presence or absence of interproximal papillae around single implants, it was noted that the presence of the papilla was strongly associated with the thick tissue phenotype (84% of cases vs 42% for the thin phenotype).[181] The high prevalence of interproximal papilla fill around implants with the thick phenotype may be due to greater total dimension of the peri-implant mucosa.[184] In a study assessing the dimensions of peri-implant mucosa around anterior single implant-supported restorations in individuals with thick versus thin tissue phenotype, the peri-implant tissue heights were approximately 4.5 mm for the thick phenotype and 3.8 mm for the thin phenotype. Apparently, papilla heights up to 4.5 mm from the underlying bone can be maintained or re-created around sites with thick phenotype. For the thin phenotype, less than 4.0 mm of papilla height from the underlying bone is expected.[184]

Distance to bone

The distance between the apical aspect of the interproximal contact and the interdental bone crest and its relationship with papilla height between a single implant and its adjacent natural tooth has also been examined. When the distance from the contact point to the crest of bone was ≤ 5 mm, the papilla was present 100% of the time. However, when the distance was ≥ 6 mm, the papilla was present in only 50% or fewer of the cases.[185] These results are very similar to the previous study evaluating papillae height around natural dentition,[101] indicating that the bone crest of the adjacent teeth determines the papilla level around single implant-supported crowns.[139,184] These studies highlight the importance of maintaining and preserving the interproximal crestal bone of adjacent teeth next to the single implant to maintain optimal papilla levels.

According to a recent systematic review, the distance from the contact point to the underlying interproximal bone was the most significant factor associated with papilla fill.[139] The sites with complete papilla fill had a mean distance of 4.7 ± 0.9 mm from contact point to the underlying interproximal bone. Therefore, re-creation of the "full" papilla around single implants is predictable when the distance from the contact point to the bone crest is ≤ 5 mm.[184,185]

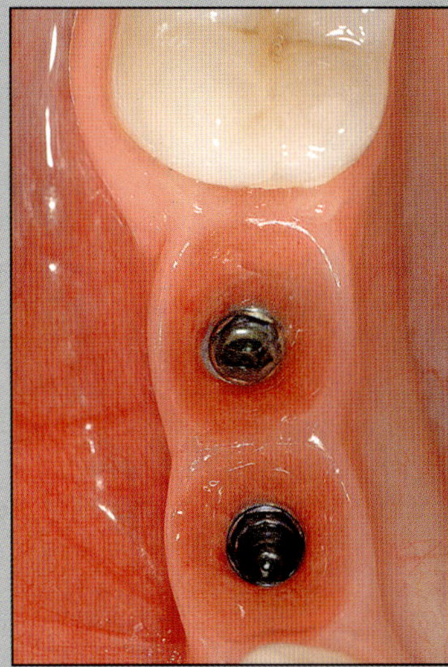

Fig 1-16 Occlusal view of adjacent implants replacing mandibular premolars and the corresponding soft tissue contours, demonstrating the challenge of creating an ideal interproximal papilla between the implants.

Distance to teeth

With regard to implant-tooth distance, the presence of papillae filling the entire proximal space was strongly related to an implant-tooth distance of 2.5 to 4.0 mm.[181] Based on Tarnow et al's finding of 1.4 mm of lateral bone remodeling, a minimal distance of 1.5 to 2.0 mm is desirable from the implant to the adjacent root surface for an acceptable presence of the papilla, because the bone crest of the adjacent teeth determines the papilla level around single implant-supported crowns.[147]

Jemt proposed a papilla index evaluating the degree of papilla fill in the interproximal embrasure space formed between single implant-supported restorations and adjacent natural teeth.[186] It consists of five different categories: score 0, no papilla present; score 1, less than half the height of the papilla is present; score 2, at least half the height of the papilla is present; score 3, the entire embrasure space is occupied by papilla and in good harmony with adjacent papillae; score 4, hyperplastic papilla.

Spontaneous regeneration of the papilla can occur after restoration of the implant, with significant esthetic improvement possible over time.[182,186–188] An early study reporting on the natural regeneration of the papilla over a mean 1.5 years of follow-up from the time of crown delivery showed an improvement of the Jemt score. The score improved from about 1.5 to about 2.5, indicating substantially more gingival embrasure fill. Moreover, significant improvement over time was noted in regard to complete papilla fill. A score of 3 was only assigned to 10% of the papillae at the time of crown placement, but after several years' follow-up, a score of 3 was seen for 58% of the papillae.[186] Papilla fill adjacent to implants receiving conventional healing abutments or provisional restorations has been evaluated as well. Prior to delivery of the definitive crown, the provisional crown may restore the soft tissue volume faster than the healing abutment. However, a similar volume of soft tissue was noted after 2 years in function. Given time, there was no significant difference between the two single-implant groups.[188]

Papillae between adjacent implants

Developing a normal interdental papilla between two adjacent implants for an implant-supported restoration is significantly more challenging than developing one around a single implant-supported restoration adjacent to natural teeth. Similarly to the papilla around a single implant-supported restoration, it can be influenced by several factors such as the distance between the crest of bone and the contact point, the interimplant distance, and the definitive crown shape (Fig 1-16).

Distance from the crest of the bone to the contact point

The mean average distance from the tip of the papilla to the crest of bone between two adjacent implants was 3.4 mm. The most common recordings were 3 mm (35.3%) or 4 mm (37.5%).[189] A distance of 3 to 4 mm (and never more than 6 mm) from the contact point to the bone crest is recommended to facilitate esthetic success, defined as a score of 2 or 3 according to the Jemt index[186] (at least half to full height of the proximal area occupied by soft tissue).[182]

When two adjacent teeth must be replaced in the esthetic zone, careful evaluation should precede implant placement. Many treatment strategies have been proposed to address this esthetic challenge, and treatment modification may be needed. This challenge is amplified when the site to be restored is adjacent to the facial midline. This may result in an accentuated sagittal asymmetry of the patient's anterior dentogingival complex, especially for a patient with a high smile line. One suggestion is to perform vertical bone augmentation prior to implant placement. The implants are then placed at least 3 mm apart to maintain the vertical bone height. Another choice is to place only one implant, incorporating an ovate cantilever pontic on the adjacent site. Simultaneous soft tissue augmentation may allow better simulation of the interproximal papilla.[189] Another variation is to harvest soft tissue from the tuberosity, which is then positioned in the area of soft tissue deficiency at the time of abutment connection for re-creation of the papilla.[190]

Interimplant distance

Careful planning of the interimplant and implant-tooth distance is an important strategy to achieve ideal papilla height. Vertical bone remodeling around the implants with expected loss of 1.5 to 2.0 mm in the first year after implant placement is very well established.[191] Bone loss around implants also occurs in a radiographically horizontal direction (1.34 mm for the mesial and 1.4 mm for the distal surface of the implant). This is actually circumferential change. When adjacent defects meet, crestal vertical bone loss occurs. Crestal bone loss of 1.04 mm was noted if the interimplant distance was $\leq$ 3 mm, while bone loss of 0.45 mm occurred when the distance was greater than 3 mm. The greater the crestal bone loss, the greater the distance from the contact point to the crest of the bone. This finding has led several authors to recommend a minimal distance of 3 mm when placing adjacent implants to maintain papilla fill.[147]

Similar results were observed in an animal study in which two adjacent implants were placed 2 or 3 mm apart. The contiguous implants were restored, and the mean distance from the contact point to the bone crest was 6 mm and from the papilla tip to the bone crest 3.3 mm.[192] The authors concluded that these distances were similar in both groups. Therefore, the ideal distance from the contact point to the bone crest should be less than 5 mm. At least 3 to 4 mm may compensate for crestal bone remodeling and establishment of desirable papilla fill between two adjacent implants.

This minimum distance may be influenced by different implant designs. One clinical study evaluated vertical and horizontal bone remodeling around two adjacent platform-switched implants placed less than 3 mm (2.23 $\pm$ 0.55 mm) apart. These had been restored for 6 to 24 months. The peri-implant crestal bone peak was preserved in 64% of sites and was lost in 36% of sites. A significant improvement was observed with platform-switched implants compared with conventional non–platform-switched implants, with a mean vertical bone loss of 2 mm compared with 0.62 mm and a mean horizontal bone loss of 1.4 mm compared with 0.60 mm, respectively. Consequently, platform-switched designs may be more suitable in narrow mesiodistal spaces where less than 3 mm of bone is available between the implants. Such an approach may minimize the loss of the critical peak of interproximal bone.[84]

Crown shape

The crown shape influences the esthetics around implant-supported crowns. Tooth shapes can be categorized as square, ovoid, or triangular. The portion of the tooth coronal to the free gingival margin will influence the volume and height of the gingival embrasure, while the portion apical to the free gingival margin will support the soft tissue facially and interproximally. Triangular-shaped embrasure forms are at great risk for "black triangles" because they create large embrasure spaces that require greater volume of soft tissue to fill. Square-shaped crowns, due to their longer proximal contact, are at lower risk. A restorative modification of the crown shape may be preferred to achieve improved esthetic results.[104]

Additional Implant-Related Considerations

Implant position

Ideal three-dimensional placement of the implant results in optimal support and stability of the hard and soft tissues. This, in turn, will allow for an esthetically pleasing implant-supported restoration. In regard to the buccolingual position of the implant, the buccal extent of the implant platform should be positioned 1 to 2 mm lingual to the proposed free gingival margin. Alternative references can be lingual to an imaginary line connecting the emergence profile of the adjacent teeth or 1 to 2 mm lingual to the labial position of the proposed CEJ of the future restoration. It should be no more than 2 mm lingual to that point of reference.[137,153,193]

Free gingival margin position

Evaluation of the initial level of the free gingival margin prior to immediate implant placement allows for prediction of the future gingival symmetry. Sites with free gingival margins coronal to the contralateral tooth resulted in similar gingival levels after the therapy. However, sites in which gingival levels were initially leveled or apically positioned in relation to the contralateral tooth failed to achieve gingival symmetry following therapy.[105]

Flapless surgical approach

Patients presenting with intact facial bone and a thick gingival phenotype are less prone to advanced recession (> 1 mm) when treated by flapless implant surgery and an immediate implant crown.[136] One study evaluated peri-implant soft tissue alterations following immediate and conventional implant placement in 39 patients with intact socket walls and a thick gingival phenotype. The impact of a flapless versus a flapped approach was analyzed. It was shown that a flapless approach had less soft tissue recession compared with a flapped approach, with a mean difference of 0.89 mm at 52 weeks.[194]

Immediate provisionalization and soft tissue

In addition to providing instant esthetics and comfort for the patient, one of the greatest benefits of implant-supported provisional restorations delivered at the time of implant placement is the preservation of soft tissue architecture.[146] In immediately placed implants, recession around a delayed provisional restoration was 2.5 to 3 times higher than those with immediate provisionalization (1.16 vs 0.41 mm, respectively). For both immediate and delayed implant placement protocols, placement of an immediate fixed provisional restoration at the time of implant placement had a positive impact on the maintenance of the soft tissue architecture. It preserved 1 mm more facial gingival tissue for the immediate group compared with the delayed group.[145] The fabrication of an immediate provisional restoration is recommended to limit the amount of marginal soft tissue recession in cases where good primary stability of the implant is achieved.[144]

Clinicians should expect about 1 mm of soft tissue recession, with the majority of recession occurring within 3 to 6 months.[121,122,135,154] One study suggested to wait at least 3 months prior to making a master impression and/or selecting a definitive implant abutment,[135] while another study recommended use of an implant-supported provisional restoration for at least 6 months prior to placing the definitive restoration.[121] Some studies report longer evaluation periods (1 to 3 years) of peri-implant soft tissue. They demonstrate continuing remodeling of soft tissue in certain patients, up to 1.7 mm after placement of the definitive restoration. These findings suggest potential esthetic complications over time, as there is a certain subset of patients who experience recession. This should be taken into account when treatment planning for esthetic outcomes with implant-supported restorations, particularly when initial recession is seen.[158,195,196]

Materials Biocompatibility

General concepts

Adhesion of bacteria in the mouth to different hard surfaces—teeth, restorative material, and dental prostheses—is one of the mechanisms for accumulation of bacterial plaque. It is influenced by two material-related factors: surface roughness and surface free energy. Surface roughness tends to promote formation and maturation of the bacterial plaque. Surface free energy (wettability) is related to how strongly the bacteria and the surface of the restorative material can bond. For the supragingival environment, it is desirable to have a smooth surface with low levels of surface free energy to prevent or minimize supragingival plaque formation. In the subgingival environment, the influence of surface roughness is negligible and of minor importance when comparing two different types of implant abutments (machined titanium vs highly polished ceramic). This is due to the ability of bacteria to prosper in that subgingival environment.[197–199]

Type of restorative material

Soft tissue health may also be related to the biocompatibility of the material at the margins of crowns and fixed dental prostheses when the finish line is placed at or below the free gingival margins. Various types of ceramics and noble and high-noble dental alloys are considered safe for use in the oral environment from a biocompatibility perspective.[200,201] Several types of ceramics have demonstrated different levels of cytotoxicity,[202] and different types of metal alloys demonstrated continuous corrosion.[200] Little is known on the specific effects of metal alloys and ceramic materials on the gingiva. One study demonstrated severe gingival histologic reaction to copper-based alloy compared with gold-based alloy crowns.[203] Inclusion of several elements was detected in histologic sections of gingiva in contact with casting alloys.[204]

One clinical study evaluated the relationship between periodontal health and three different subgingival restorations (amalgam, glass-ionomer cement, and composite resin). At the 1-year follow-up, the clinical parameters were similar among the experimental groups, but the bacterial count and the shift in subgingival flora to more gram-negative microbiota were noted in the composite resin group. Restorations made of this type of composite resin (and perhaps others) may have a negative impact on the quality of subgingival plaque.[205]

The implant abutment material can influence the stability of the peri-implant seal, characterized by the presence or absence of alveolar bone loss and/or peri-implant mucosa recession.[206] For abutments made of titanium and alumina-based ceramics, the mucosal healing was similar for both materials, with a formation of 2.0 mm of epithelial attachment and 1.0 to 1.5 mm of connective tissue attachment. In contrast, no proper attachment formed around gold or feldspathic porcelain abutments, resulting in recession and bone resorption.[62] Histologic evaluation of healing between 2 and 5 months revealed formation of a stable dimension of soft tissue barrier around titanium and zirconia abutments. Apical migration of the junctional epithelium and marginal bone was noted around gold alloy abutments. Lesser amounts of collagen, fewer fibroblasts, and large numbers of inflammatory cells were noted in the connective tissue around gold alloy abutments. This suggests better soft tissue response to titanium and zirconia abutments.[63] Titanium and the once-used alumina ceramic are highly biocompatible. These materials are stable and resistant to corrosion in living tissue with direct and strong adhesion to the surrounding tissues.[62] More importantly, no effects on cell morphology and growth in epithelial cells and fibroblasts were reported.[207,208]

Titanium abutments are considered the gold standard due to their mechanical strength, stability, and high survival rates.[209] However, one shortcoming is the gray color that shows through the soft tissue, resulting in compromised esthetic outcomes. Titanium abutments may be treated to create a gold-colored titanium nitride surface for better esthetics. In a human study, titanium nitride–coated surfaces demonstrated reduced colonization of bacteria as compared with standard machined titanium.[210] Zirconia abutments are esthetically pleasing with similar biologic integration,[63,211–217] but the material strength is inferior to that of titanium abutments.[209]

Several clinical and histologic studies compare titanium and zirconia abutments. Peri-implant mucosa response was evaluated in subjects via gingival biopsy from around titanium and zirconia healing caps. Titanium healing caps showed a high degree of gingival inflammation when compared with zirconia samples, indicating better biocompatibility of the zirconia.[217] A 3-year randomized clinical study compared titanium and zirconia abutments for single implant-supported crowns around canines and posterior tooth sites. Periodontal parameters—probing depth, plaque control, bleeding upon probing, and bone loss—were similar for both abutments. Interestingly, in this study both zirconia and titanium abutments caused similar peri-implant mucosal discoloration compared with the gingiva around natural teeth.[218] A meta-analysis of 5-year survival rates and incidences of complications associated with ceramic (mostly zirconia) and metal abutments was performed.[209] The survival rates were 99% and 97.4% for ceramic and metal abutments, respectively. Abutment screw loosening was the most common technical problem, with incidence of 6.9% for ceramic and 15.9% for metal abutments. Esthetic problems were more frequent for metal abutments. Biologic complications were 5.2% for ceramic abutments and 7.7% for metal abutments. Overall, however, the survival rates and technical and biologic complications were similar for both the ceramic and metal abutments.[209]

Oral Hygiene

A classic study by Loe et al in 1965 demonstrated a cause and effect relationship between bacterial plaque and gingival inflammation.[219] When nine participants abstained from all measures of oral hygiene, gingival inflammation developed within 10 to 21 days. Once oral hygiene was resumed, the gingival inflammation resolved in all participants within a week. It was concluded that bacterial plaque was essential in the production of gingival inflammation. The same cause and effect relationship between plaque accumulation and development of peri-implant mucositis around dental implants was demonstrated when patients were asked to abstain from all oral hygiene practices for 3 weeks.[220]

The microflora around dental implants originates from the oral cavity with similar microbial composition to that surrounding the natural teeth in health. The microflora of failing implants is similar to that of periodontal disease. This may be the result of contamination of the peri-implant sites by periodontal pathogens residing in periodontal pockets.[221–223] Effective plaque control performed by the patient and professional periodontal supportive therapy around natural teeth and dental implants are vital to prevent development and progression of periodontal disease.[224–226]

Adequate plaque control to ensure periodontal stability can be achieved by means of mechanical cleansing devices such as manual or electric toothbrushes, floss, interdental brushes, oral irrigators, and mouthwashes. Toothbrushes are the most commonly used mechanical cleansing device used by patients and recommended by dental professionals. When electric toothbrushes were compared with manual toothbrushes, there was no statistically significant difference in regard to efficacy in plaque removal and gingival health.[227–230] Plaque removal in interproximal sites can be accomplished by means of dental floss and interdental brushes. Interdental brushes are more effective in removing bacterial plaque and should be indicated in patients with open interproximal spaces, while dental floss should be indicated in patients with closed interproximal sites.[226,227]

Chlorhexidine is an effective antiplaque agent that is mainly used as a mouthwash. It is usually indicated for short-term use for presurgical or healing phases of periodontal or implant-related surgery or for intermittent use for patients with high caries risk or extensive prosthetic reconstructions.[231] Long-term use is not indicated due to adverse effects, including staining of the teeth and tongue, bitter aftertaste, taste alterations, and increased calculus formation.[232–234]

Home care around dental implants is not much different from that around natural teeth. Traditional mechanical cleansing devices such as manual or electric toothbrushes, interdental brushes, conventional floss (with or without a threader as needed), and Super Floss (Oral-B) are usually recommended around dental implants. However, there is not enough evidence in the literature to indicate which is the most effective oral home care instrument to maintain healthy tissues around dental implants. Electric toothbrushes are effective and safe around implants, but their efficacy is comparable to that of manual tooth brushing around implant-supported restorations.[235–237]

It is extremely important to establish a scheduled maintenance program for patients with dental implants. They must be evaluated at regular intervals for clinical parameters, and the areas surrounding the implants must be debrided. Customized supportive periodontal therapy should be performed and tailored to each patient, with recall intervals ranging from 1 to 6 months (average of 3 months) based on the level of oral hygiene, calculus formation, periodontal status, and various host factors.[238–242]

At each evaluation, clinical parameters such as probing depth, clinical attachment level, bleeding, mobility, and plaque control should be recorded. Radiographic images should be obtained periodically to assess bone levels and proper fit of the abutment.[243] Cautious debridement around dental implants is imperative to prevent damage to the implant surface. Scratches on the titanium surface may favor plaque accumulation and corrosion of the titanium as well as decreases in cell adhesion and attachment.[244,245] In vitro and animal studies evaluated the ideal instruments to clean around titanium abutments. Interdental brushes, soft toothbrushes, plastic scalers, and rubber cups without paste resulted in clean surfaces with roughness comparable to that of an untreated abutment. Air polishing, metal scalers, and ultrasonic tips resulted in roughened titanium surfaces.[246–248]

The authors recommend a cautious, conservative maintenance approach for implant patients. Recall intervals should begin at 3-month intervals, increasing by 1-month increments as the absence of clinical inflammation signs indicates. All sites should be probed using a metal probe for accuracy, and all changes should be recorded. All negative changes from healed site baselines should dictate more aggressive care. Home care efficacy should be monitored and should influence the recall interval as well. All teeth and implants should be debrided. Plastic curettes, plastic-covered ultrasonic tips, and plain rubber cups should be the only items used on titanium surfaces. With this approach, health can be maintained, and negative trends can be intercepted early.

References

1. Wikesjö UM, Nilvéus RE, Selvig KA. Significance of early healing events on periodontal repair: A review. J Periodontol 1992; 63:158–165.
2. Fiorellini JP, Kao DWK, Kim DM, Uzel NG. Anatomy of the periodontium. In: Newman MG, Takei HH, Klokkevold PR, Carranza FA (eds). Carranza's Clinical Periodontology, ed 11. Philadelphia: Saunders Elsevier, 2012:11–27.
3. Sicher H, Bhaskar SN. Cementum. In: Orban's Oral Histology and Embryology, ed 7. St Louis: CV Mosby, 1972:160–181.
4. Ingber JS, Rose LF, Coslet JG. The "biologic width"—A concept in periodontics and restorative dentistry. Alpha Omegan 1977; 70:62–65.
5. Gargiulo AW, Wentz FM, Orban B. Dimensions and relations of the dentogingival junction in humans. J Periodontol 1961;32:261–267.
6. Vacek JS, Gher ME, Assad DA, Richardson AC, Giambarresi LI. The dimensions of the human dentogingival junction. Int J Periodontics Restorative Dent 1994;14:154–165.
7. Valderhaug J, Birkeland JM. Periodontal conditions in patients 5 years following insertion of fixed prostheses. Pocket depth and loss of attachment. J Oral Rehabil 1976;3:237–243.
8. Valderhaug J. Periodontal conditions and carious lesions following the insertion of fixed prostheses: A 10-year follow-up study. Int Dent J 1980;30:296–304.
9. Watkin A, Kerstein RB. Improving darkened anterior peri-implant tissue color with zirconia custom implant abutments. Compend Contin Educ Dent 2008;29:238–240,242.
10. Wennström JL, Bengazi F, Lekholm U. The influence of the masticatory mucosa on the peri-implant soft tissue condition. Clin Oral Implants Res 1994;5:1–8.
11. Bengazi F, Wennström JL, Lekholm U. Recession of the soft tissue margin at oral implants. A 2-year longitudinal prospective study. Clin Oral Implants Res 1996;7:303–310.
12. Hermann JS, Schoolfield JD, Schenk RK, Buser D, Cochran DL. Influence of the size of the microgap on crestal bone changes around titanium implants. A histometric evaluation of unloaded non-submerged implants in the canine mandible. J Periodontol 2001; 72:1372–1383.
13. King GN, Hermann JS, Schoolfield JD, Buser D, Cochran DL. Influence of the size of the microgap on crestal bone levels in non-submerged dental implants: A radiographic study in the canine mandible. J Periodontol 2002;73:1111–1117.
14. Tolboe H, Isidor F, Budtz-Jørgensen E, Kaaber S. Influence of pontic material on alveolar mucosal conditions. Scand J Dent Res 1988;96:442–447.
15. Tolboe H, Isidor F, Budtz-Jørgensen E, Kaaber S. Influence of oral hygiene on the mucosal conditions beneath bridge pontics. Scand J Dent Res 1987;95:475–482.
16. Maynard JG, Wilson RD. Physiologic dimensions of the periodontium significant to the restorative dentist. J Periodontol 1979;50:170–174.
17. Ericsson I, Lindhe J. Recession in sites with inadequate width of the keratinized gingiva. An experimental study in the dog. J Clin Periodontol 1984;11:95–103.
18. Günay H, Seeger A, Tschernitschek H, Geurtsen W. Placement of the preparation line and periodontal health—A prospective 2-year clinical study. Int J Periodontics Restorative Dent 2000;20:171–181.
19. Reitemeier B, Hänsel K, Walter MH, Kastner C, Toutenburg H. Effect of posterior crown margin placement on gingival health. J Prosthet Dent 2002;87:167–172.
20. Tsukada G, Tanaka T, Kajihara T, Torii M, Inoue K. Film thickness and fluidity of various luting cements determined using a trial indentation meter. Dent Mater 2006;22:183–188.
21. Wilson T. The positive relationship between excess cement and peri-implant disease: A prospective clinical endoscopic study. J Periodontol 2009;80:1388–1392.
22. Pauletto N, Lahiffe BJ, Walton JN. Complications associated with excess cement around crowns on osseointegrated implants: A clinical report. Int J Oral Maxillofac Implants 1999;14:865–868.
23. Listgarten MA. Periodontal probing: What does it mean? J Clin Periodontol 1980;7:165–176.
24. Listgarten MA, Mao R, Robinson PJ. Periodontal probing and the relationship of the probe tip to periodontal tissues. J Periodontol 1976;47:511–513.
25. Magnusson I, Listgarten MA. Histological evaluation of probing depth following periodontal treatment. J Clin Periodontol 1980;7:26–31.

26. Hancock EB, Wirthlin MR. The location of the periodontal probe tip in health and disease. J Periodontol 1981;52:124–129.
27. Greenstein G. Contemporary interpretation of probing depth assessments: Diagnostic and therapeutic implications. A literature review. J Periodontol 1997;68:1194–1205.
28. Stetler KJ, Bissada NF. Significance of the width of keratinized gingiva on the periodontal status of teeth with submarginal restorations. J Periodontol 1987;58:696–700.
29. Brunsvold MA, Lane J. The prevalence of overhanging dental restorations and their relationship to periodontal disease. J Clin Periodontol 1990;17:67–72.
30. Lang NP, Kiel RA, Anderhalden K. Clinical and microbiological effects of subgingival restorations with overhanging or clinically perfect margins. J Clin Periodontol 1983;10:563–578.
31. Kois JC. Altering gingival levels: The restorative connection. Part I: Biologic variables. J Esthet Dent 1994;6:3–9.
32. Kois JC. New paradigms for anterior tooth preparation. Rationale and technique. Oral Health 1998;88:19–22,25–27,29–30.
33. Carvalho CV, Bauer FP, Romito GA, Pannuti CM, De Micheli G. Orthodontic extrusion with or without circumferential supracrestal fiberotomy and root planing. Int J Periodontics Restorative Dent 2006;26:87–93.
34. Schwimer CW, Rosenberg ES, Schwimer DH. Rapid extrusion with fiberotomy. J Esthet Dent 1990;2:82–88.
35. Kozlovsky A, Tal H, Lieberman M. Forced eruption combined with gingival fiberotomy. A technique for clinical crown lengthening. J Clin Periodontol 1988;15:534–538.
36. Berglundh T, Marinello CP, Lindhe J, Thilander B, Liljenberg B. Periodontal tissue reactions to orthodontic extrusion. An experimental study in the dog. J Clin Periodontol 1991;18:330–336.
37. Caton J, Nyman S, Zander H. Histometric evaluation of periodontal surgery. II. Connective tissue attachment levels after four regenerative procedures. J Clin Periodontol 1980;7:224–231.
38. Carnevale G, Kaldahl WB. Osseous resective surgery. Periodontol 2000 2000;22:59–87.
39. Lanning SK, Waldrop TC, Gunsolley JC, Maynard JG. Surgical crown lengthening: Evaluation of the biological width. J Periodontol 2003;74:468–474.
40. Ganji KK, Patil VA, John J. A comparative evaluation for biologic width following surgical crown lengthening using gingivectomy and ostectomy procedure. Int J Dent 2012;2012:479241.
41. Pontoriero R, Carnevale G. Surgical crown lengthening: A 12-month clinical wound healing study. J Periodontol 2001;72:841–848.
42. Deas DE, Moritz AJ, McDonnell HT, Powell CA, Mealey BL. Osseous surgery for crown lengthening: A 6-month clinical study. J Periodontol 2004;75:1288–1294.
43. Hempton TJ, Dominici JT. Contemporary crown-lengthening therapy: A review. J Am Dent Assoc 2010;141:647–655.
44. Kohal RJ, Gerds T, Strub JR. Effect of different crown contours on periodontal health in dogs. Clinical results. J Dent 2003;31:407–413.
45. Perel M. Axial crown contours. J Prosthet Dent 1971;25:642–649.
46. Yuodelis R, Weaver J, Sapkos S. Facial and lingual contours of artificial complete crown restorations and their effect on the periodontium. J Prosthet Dent 1973;29:61–66.
47. Ramfjord S. Periodontal aspects of restorative dentistry. J Oral Rehabil 1974;1:107–126.
48. Becker CM, Kaldahl WB. Current theories of crown contour, margin placement, and pontic design. J Prosthet Dent 1981;45:268–277.
49. Abrams L. Augmentation of the deformed residual edentulous ridge for fixed prosthesis. Compend Contin Educ Gen Dent 1980;1:205–213.
50. Dylina TJ. Contour determination for ovate pontics. J Prosthet Dent 1999;82:136–142.
51. Orsini G, Murmura G, Artese L, Piattelli A, Piccirilli M, Caputi S. Tissue healing under provisional restorations with ovate pontics: A pilot human histological study. J Prosthet Dent 2006;94:252–257.
52. Zitzmann NU, Marinello CP, Berglundh T. The ovate pontic design: A histologic observation in humans. J Prosthet Dent 2002;88:375–380.
53. Tetè S, Mastrangelo F, Bianchi A, Zizzari V, Scarano A. Collagen fiber orientation around machined titanium and zirconia dental implant necks: An animal study. Int J Oral Maxillofac Implants 2009;24:52–58.
54. Comut AA, Weber HP, Shortkroff S, Cui FZ, Spector M. Connective tissue orientation around dental implants in a canine model. Clin Oral Implants Res 2001;12:433–440.
55. Delgado-Ruiz RA, Calvo-Guirado JL, Abboud M, et al. Connective tissue characteristics around healing abutments of different geometries: New methodological technique under circularly polarized light [epub ahead of print 10 October 2013]. Clin Implant Dent Relat Res doi:10.1111/cid.12161.
56. Romanos GE, Traini T, Johansson CB, Piattelli A. Biologic width and morphologic characteristics of soft tissues around immediately loaded implants: Studies performed on human autopsy specimens. J Periodontol 2010;81:70–78.
57. Abrahamsson I, Berglundh T, Lindhe J. The mucosal barrier following abutment dis/reconnection. An experimental study in dogs. J Clin Periodontol 1997;24:568–572.
58. Koutouzis T, Koutouzis G, Gadalla H, Neiva R. The effect of healing abutment reconnection and disconnection on soft and hard peri-implant tissues: A short-term randomized controlled clinical trial. Int J Oral Maxillofac Implants 2013;28:807–814.
59. Berglundh T, Lindhe J. Dimension of the periimplant mucosa. Biological width revisited. J Clin Periodontol 1996;23:971–973.
60. Linkevicius T, Apse P, Grybauskas S, Puisys A. The influence of soft tissue thickness on crestal bone changes around implants: A 1-year prospective controlled clinical trial. Int J Oral Maxillofac Implants 2009;24:712–719.
61. Moon IS, Berglundh T, Abrahamsson I, Linder E, Lindhe J. The barrier between the keratinized mucosa and the dental implant. An experimental study in the dog. J Clin Periodontol 1999;26:658–663.
62. Abrahamsson I, Berglundh T, Glantz PO, Lindhe J. The mucosal attachment at different abutments. An experimental study in dogs. J Clin Periodontol 1998;25:721–727.
63. Welander M, Abrahamsson I, Berglundh T. The mucosal barrier at implant abutments of different materials. Clin Oral Implants Res 2008;19:635–641.
64. Hermann JS, Cochran DL, Nummikoski PV, Buser D. Crestal bone changes around titanium implants: A radiographic evaluation of unloaded nonsubmerged and submerged implants in the canine mandible. J Periodontol 1997;68:1117–1130.
65. Piatelli A, Vrespa G, Petrone G, Iezzi G, Annibali S, Scarano A. Role of the microgap between implant and abutment: A retrospective histologic evaluation of monkeys. J Periodontol 2003;74:346–352.
66. Callan D, Cobb C, Williams K. DNA probe identification of bacteria colonizing internal surfaces of the implant-abutment interface: A preliminary study. J Periodontol 2005;76:115–120.
67. Piatelli A, Scarano A, Paolantonio M, et al. Fluids and microbial penetration in the internal part of cement-retained versus screw-retained implant abutment connections. J Periodontol 2001;72:1146–1150.
68. Quirynen M, Bollen CML, Eyssen H, Van Steeberghe D. Microbial penetration along the implant components of the Brånemark system. An in-vitro study. Clin Oral Implants Res 1994;5:239–244.
69. Quirynen M, Van Steeberghe D. Bacterial colonization of the internal part of two-stage implants. An in vivo study. Clin Oral Implant Res 1993;4:158–161.
70. Jansen VK, Conrads G, Richter EJ. Microbial leakage and marginal fit of the implant-abutment interface. Int J Oral Maxillofac Implants 1997;12:527–540.
71. Ericsson I, Persson LG, Berglundh T, Marinello CP, Lindhe J, Klinge B. Different types of inflammatory reactions in peri-implant soft tissues. J Clin Periodontol 1995;2:255–261.
72. Broggini N, McManus LM, Hermann JS, et al. Persistent acute inflammation at the implant-abutment interface. J Dent Res 2003; 82:232–237.

73. Besimo CE, Guindy JS, Lewetag D, Meyer J. Prevention of bacterial leakage into and from prefabricated screw-retained crowns on implants in vitro. Int J Oral Maxillofac Implants 1999;14:654–660.
74. Steinebrunner L, Wolfart S, Bossmann K, Kern M. In vitro evaluation of bacterial leakage along the implant-abutment interface of different implant systems. Int J Oral Maxillofac Implants 2005;20:875–881.
75. Riondini L, Marin C, Brunella F, Fini M. Internal contamination of a 2-component implant system after occlusal loading and provisionally luted reconstruction with or without a washer device. J Periodontol 2001;72:1652–1657.
76. Telleman G, Raghoebar GM, Vissink A, Meijer HJ. Impact of platform switching on inter-proximal bone levels around short implants in the posterior region, 1-year results from a randomized clinical trial. J Clin Periodontol 2012;39:688–697.
77. Atieh MA, Ibrahim HM, Atieh AH. Platform switching for marginal bone preservation around dental implants: A systematic review and meta-analysis. J Periodontol 2010;81:1350–1366.
78. Enkling N, Jöhren P, Klimberg V, Bayer S, Mericske-Stern R, Jepsen S. Effect of platform switching on peri-implant bone levels: A randomized clinical trial. Clin Oral Implants Res 2011;22:1185–1192.
79. Annibali S, Bignozzi I, Cristalli MP, Graziani F, La Monaca G, Polimeni A. Peri-implant marginal bone level: A systematic review and meta-analysis of studies comparing platform switching versus conventionally restored implants. J Clin Periodontol 2012;39:1097–1113.
80. Enkling N, Jöhren P, Katsoulis J, et al. Influence of platform switching on bone-level alterations: A three-year randomized clinical trial. J Dent Res 2013;92(12 suppl):139S–145S.
81. Vigolo P, Givani A. Platform-switched restorations on wide-diameter implants: A 5-year clinical prospective study. Int J Oral Maxillofac Implants 2009;24:103–109.
82. Leutert CR, Stawarczyk B, Truninger TC, Hämmerle CH, Sailer I. Bending moments and types of failure of zirconia and titanium abutments with internal implant abutment connections: A laboratory study. Int J Oral Maxillofac Implants 2012;27:505–512.
83. Stafford GL. Evidence supporting platform-switching to preserve marginal bone levels not definitive. Evid Based Dent 2012;13:56–57.
84. Rodríguez-Ciurana X, Vela-Nebot X, Segalà-Torres M, et al. The effect of interimplant distance on the height of the interimplant bone crest when using platform-switched implants. Int J Periodontics Restorative Dent 2009;29:141–151.
85. Elian N, Bloom M, Dard M, Cho SC, Trushkowsky RD, Tarnow D. Effect of interimplant distance (2 and 3 mm) on the height of interimplant bone crest: A histomorphometric evaluation. J Periodontol 2011;82:1749–1756.
86. Ochsenbein C, Ross S. A reevaluation of osseous surgery. Dent Clin North Am 1969;13:87–102.
87. Seibert JL, Lindhe J. Esthetics and periodontal therapy. In: Lindhe J (ed). Textbook of Clinical Periodontology, ed 2. Copenhagen: Munksgaard, 1989:477–514.
88. Olsson M, Lindhe J, Marinello CP. On the relationship between crown form and clinical features of the gingiva in adolescents. J Clin Periodontol 1993;20:570–577.
89. De Rouck T, Eghbali R, Collys K, De Bruyn H, Cosyn J. The gingival biotype revisited: Transparency of the periodontal probe through the gingival margin as a method to discriminate thin from thick gingiva. J Clin Periodontol 2009;36:428–433.
90. Kao RT, Pasquinelli K. Thick vs. thin gingival tissue: A key determinant in tissue response to disease and restorative treatment. J Calif Dent Assoc 2002;30:521–526.
91. Kan JY, Morimoto T, Rungcharassaeng K, Roe P, Smith DH. Gingival biotype assessment in the esthetic zone: Visual versus direct measurement. Int J Periodontics Restorative Dent 2010;30:237–243.
92. Weisgold A. Contours of the full crown restoration. Alpha Omegan 1977;70:77–89.
93. Kao RT, Fagan MC, Conte GJ. Thick vs. thin gingival biotypes: A key determinant in treatment planning for dental implants. J Calif Dent Assoc 2008;36:193–198.
94. Müller HP, Eger T. Gingival phenotypes in young male adults. J Clin Periodontol 1997;24:65–71.
95. Vandana KL, Savitha B. Thickness of gingiva in association with age, gender and dental arch location. J Clin Periodontol 2005;32:828–830.
96. Müller HP, Könönen E. Variance components of gingival thickness. J Periodontal Res 2005;40:239–244.
97. Cuny-Houchmand M, Renaudin S, Leroul M, Planche L, Guehennec LL, Soueidan A. Gingival biotype assessement: Visual inspection relevance and maxillary versus mandibular comparison. Open Dent J 2013;7:1–6.
98. Eger T, Müller HP, Heinecke A. Ultrasonic determination of gingival thickness. Subject variation and influence of tooth type and clinical features. J Clin Periodontol 1996;23:839–845.
99. Lee SA, Kim AC, Prusa LA Jr, Kao RT. Characterization of dental anatomy and gingival biotype in Asian populations. J Calif Dent Assoc 2013;41:31–33,36–39.
100. De Lemos AB, Kahn S, Rodrigues WJ, Barceleiro MO. Influence of periodontal biotype on the presence of interdental papillae. Gen Dent 2013;61:20–24.
101. Tarnow DP, Magner AW, Fletcher P. The effect of the distance from the contact point to the crest of bone on the presence or absence of the interproximal dental papilla. J Periodontol 1992;63:995–996.
102. Anderegg CR, Metzler DG, Nicoll BK. Gingiva thickness in guided tissue regeneration and associated recession at facial furcation defects. J Periodontol 1995;66:397–402.
103. Wennström JL. Mucogingival considerations in orthodontic treatment. Semin Orthod 1996;2:46–54.
104. Kois JC. Predictable single-tooth peri-implant esthetics: Five diagnostic keys. Compend Contin Educ Dent 2004;25:895–896,898,900.
105. Chen ST, Darby IB, Reynolds EC, Clement JG. Immediate implant placement postextraction without flap elevation. J Periodontol 2009;80:163–172.
106. Nagaraj KR, Savadi RC, Savadi AR, et al. Gingival biotype—Prosthodontic perspective. J Indian Prosthodont Soc 2010;10:27–30.
107. Jung RE, Holderegger C, Sailer I, Khraisat A, Suter A, Hämmerle CH. The effect of all-ceramic and porcelain-fused-to-metal restorations on marginal peri-implant soft tissue color: A randomized controlled clinical trial. Int J Periodontics Restorative Dent 2008;28:357–365.
108. Baldi C, Pini-Prato G, Pagliaro U, et al. Coronally advanced flap procedure for root coverage. Is flap thickness relevant predictor to achieve root coverage? A 19-case series. J Periodontol 1999;70:1077–1084.
109. Hwang D, Wang HL. Flap thickness as a predictor of root coverage: A systematic review. J Periodontol 2006;77:1625–1634.
110. Januário AL, Barriviera M, Duarte WR. Soft tissue cone-beam computed tomography: A novel method for the measurement of gingival tissue and the dimensions of the dentogingival unit. J Esthet Restor Dent 2008;20:366–374.
111. Eghbali A, De Rouck T, De Bruyn H, Cosyn J. The gingival biotype assessed by experienced and inexperienced clinicians. J Clin Periodontol 2009;36:958–963.
112. Fu JH, Lee A, Wang HL. Influence of tissue biotype on implant esthetics. Int J Oral Maxillofac Implants 2011;26:499–508.
113. Fu JH, Yeh CY, Chan HL, Tatarakis N, Leong DJ, Wang HL. Tissue biotype and its relation to the underlying bone morphology. J Periodontol 2010;81:569–574.
114. Claffey N, Shanley D. Relationship of gingival thickness and bleeding to loss of probing attachment in shallow sites following nonsurgical periodontal therapy. J Clin Periodontol 1986;13:654–657.
115. Arora R, Narula SC, Sharma RK, Tewari S. Supracrestal gingival tissue: Assessing relation with periodontal biotypes in a healthy periodontium. Int J Periodontics Restorative Dent 2013;33:763–771.
116. Esfahrood ZR, Kadkhodazadeh M, Talebi Ardakani MR. Gingival biotype: A review. Gen Dent 2013;61:14–17.
117. Benavides E, Rios HF, Ganz SD, et al. Use of cone beam computed tomography in implant dentistry: The International Congress of Oral Implantologists consensus report. Implant Dent 2012;21:78–86.

118. Song JE, Um YJ, Kim CS, et al. Thickness of posterior palatal masticatory mucosa: The use of computerized tomography. J Periodontol 2008;79:406–412.
119. La Rocca AP, Alemany AS, Levi P Jr, Juan MV, Molina JN, Weisgold AS. Anterior maxillary and mandibular biotype: Relationship between gingival thickness and width with respect to underlying bone thickness. Implant Dent 2012;21:507–515.
120. Grunder U. Crestal ridge width changes when placing implants at the time of tooth extraction with and without soft tissue augmentation after a healing period of 6 months: Report of 24 consecutive cases. Int J Periodontics Restorative Dent 2011;31:9–17.
121. Grunder U. Stability of the mucosal topography around single-tooth implants and adjacent teeth: 1-year results. Int J Periodontics Restorative Dent 2000;20:11–17.
122. Kan JY, Rungcharassaeng K, Morimoto T, Lozada J. Facial gingival tissue stability after connective tissue graft with single immediate tooth replacement in the esthetic zone: Consecutive case report. J Oral Maxillofac Surg 2009;67(11 suppl):40–48.
123. Kan JY, Rungcharassaeng K, Lozada JL. Bilaminar subepithelial connective tissue grafts for immediate implant placement and provisionalization in the esthetic zone. J Calif Dent Assoc 2005;33:865–871.
124. Bianchi AE, Sanfilippo F. Single-tooth replacement by immediate implant and connective tissue graft: A 1-9-year clinical evaluation. Clin Oral Implants Res 2004;15:269–277.
125. Schneider D, Grunder U, Ender A, Hämmerle CH, Jung RE. Volume gain and stability of peri-implant tissue following bone and soft tissue augmentation: 1-year results from a prospective cohort study. Clin Oral Implants Res 2011;22:28–37.
126. Grunder U, Wenz B, Schüpbach P. Guided bone regeneration around single-tooth implants in the esthetic zone: A case series. Int J Periodontics Restorative Dent 2011;31:613–620.
127. Mathews DP. The pediculated connective tissue graft: A technique for improving unaesthetic implant restorations. Pract Proced Aesthet Dent 2002;14:719–724.
128. Mareque-Bueno S. A novel surgical procedure for coronally repositioning of the buccal implant mucosa using acellular dermal matrix: A case report. J Periodontol 2011;82:151–156.
129. Burkhardt R, Joss A, Lang NP. Soft tissue dehiscence coverage around endosseous implants: A prospective cohort study. Clin Oral Implants Res 2008;19:451–457.
130. Zucchelli G, Mazzotti C, Mounssif I, Mele M, Stefanini M, Montebugnoli L. A novel surgical-prosthetic approach for soft tissue dehiscence coverage around single implant. Clin Oral Implants Res 2013;24:957–962.
131. Evans CD, Chen ST. Esthetic outcomes of immediate implant placements. Clin Oral Implants Res 2008;19:73–80.
132. Belser U, Buser D, Higginbottom F. Consensus statements and recommended clinical procedures regarding esthetics in implant dentistry. Int J Oral Maxillofacial Implants 2004;19(suppl):73–74.
133. Chang M, Wennström JL, Odman P, Andersson B. Implant-supported single-tooth replacements compared to contralateral natural teeth. Crowns and soft tissue dimensions. Clin Oral Implants Res 1999;10:185–194.
134. Chen ST, Buser D. Clinical and esthetic outcomes of implants placed in postextraction sites. Int J Oral Maxillofac Implants 2009;24(suppl):186–217.
135. Small PN, Tarnow DP. Gingival recession around implants: A 1-year longitudinal prospective study. Int J Oral Maxillofac Implants 2000;15:527–532.
136. Cosyn J, Hooghe N, De Bruyn H. A systematic review on the frequency of advanced recession following single immediate implant treatment. J Clin Periodontol 2012;39:582–589.
137. Buser D, Martin W, Belser UC. Optimizing esthetics for implant restorations in the anterior maxilla: Anatomic and surgical considerations. Int J Oral Maxillofac Implants 2004;19(suppl):43–61.
138. Cosyn J, Sabzevar MM, De Bruyn H. Predictors of inter-proximal and midfacial recession following single implant treatment in the anterior maxilla: A multivariate analysis. J Clin Periodontol 2012;39:895–903.
139. Nisapakultorn K, Suphanantachat S, Silkosessak O, Rattanamongkolgul S. Factors affecting soft tissue level around anterior maxillary single-tooth implants. Clin Oral Implants Res 2010;21:662–670.
140. Grunder U, Gracis S, Capelli M. Influence of the 3-D bone-to-implant relationship on esthetics. Int J Periodontics Restorative Dent 2005;25:113–119.
141. Ferrus J, Cecchinato D, Pjetursson EB, Lang NP, Sanz M, Lindhe J. Factors influencing ridge alterations following immediate implant placement into extraction sockets. Clin Oral Implants Res 2010;21:22–29.
142. Linkevicius T, Puisys A, Linkeviciene L, Peciuliene V, Schlee M. Crestal bone stability around implants with horizontally matching connection after soft tissue thickening: A prospective clinical trial [epub ahead of print 17 September 2013]. Clin Implant Dent Relat Res doi:10.1111/cid.12155.
143. Puisys A, Linkevicius T. The influence of mucosal tissue thickening on crestal bone stability around bone-level implants. A prospective controlled clinical trial. Clin Oral Implants Res 2015;26:123–129.
144. De Rouck T, Collys K, Wyn I, Cosyn J. Instant provisionalization of immediate single-tooth implants is essential to optimize esthetic treatment outcome. Clin Oral Implants Res 2009;20:566–570.
145. Block MS, Mercante DE, Lirette D, Mohamed W, Ryser M, Castellon P. Prospective evaluation of immediate and delayed provisional single tooth restorations. J Oral Maxillofac Surg 2009;67(11 suppl):89–107.
146. Al-Harbi SA, Edgin WA. Preservation of soft tissue contours with immediate screw-retained provisional implant crown. J Prosthet Dent 2007;98:329–332.
147. Tarnow DP, Cho SC, Wallace SS. The effect of inter-implant distance on the height of inter-implant bone crest. J Periodontol 2000;71:546–549.
148. Botticelli D, Persson LG, Lindhe J, Berglundh T. Bone tissue formation adjacent to implants placed in fresh extraction sockets: An experimental study in dogs. Clin Oral Implants Res 2006;17:351–358.
149. Araújo MG, Linder E, Lindhe J. Bio-Oss collagen in the buccal gap at immediate implants: A 6-month study in the dog. Clin Oral Implants Res 2011;22:1–8.
150. Tsuda H, Rungcharassaeng K, Kan JY, Roe P, Lozada JL, Zimmerman G. Peri-implant tissue response following connective tissue and bone grafting in conjunction with immediate single-tooth replacement in the esthetic zone: A case series. Int J Oral Maxillofac Implants 2011;26:427–436.
151. Barone A, Ricci M, Calvo-Guirado JL, Covani U. Bone remodelling after regenerative procedures around implants placed in fresh extraction sockets: An experimental study in Beagle dogs. Clin Oral Implants Res 2011;22:1131–1137.
152. Chen ST, Wilson TG Jr, Hämmerle CH. Immediate or early placement of implants following tooth extraction: Review of biologic basis, clinical procedures, and outcomes. Int J Oral Maxillofac Implants 2004;19 (suppl):12–25.
153. Schwartz-Arad D, Chaushu G. The ways and wherefores of immediate placement of implants into fresh extraction sites: A literature review. J Periodontol 1997;68:915–923.
154. Kan JY, Rungcharassaeng K, Lozada J. Immediate placement and provisionalization of maxillary anterior single implants: 1-year prospective study. Int J Oral Maxillofac Implants 2003;18:31–39.
155. Wilson TG Jr, Buser D. Timing of anterior implant placement postextraction: Immediate versus early placement. Clin Adv Periodontics 2011;1:61–76.
156. Huynh-Ba G, Pjetursson BE, Sanz M, et al. Analysis of the socket bone wall dimensions in the upper maxilla in relation to immediate implant placement. Clin Oral Implants Res 2010;21:37–42.

157. Januário AL, Duarte WR, Barriviera M, Mesti JC, Araújo MG, Lindhe J. Dimension of the facial bone wall in the anterior maxilla: A cone-beam computed tomography study. Clin Oral Implants Res 2011;22:1168–1171.
158. Cardaropoli G, Lekholm U, Wennström JL. Tissue alterations at implant-supported single-tooth replacements: A 1-year prospective clinical study. Clin Oral Implants Res 2006;17:165–171.
159. Becker W, Ochsenbein C, Tibbetts L, Becker BE. Alveolar bone anatomic profiles as measured from dry skulls. Clinical ramifications. J Clin Periodontol 1997;24:727–731.
160. Fickl S, Zuhr O, Wachtel H, Bolz W, Hürzeler M. Tissue alterations after tooth extraction with and without surgical trauma: A volumetric study in the beagle dog. J Clin Periodontol 2008;35:356–363.
161. Lekovic V, Kenney EB, Weinlaender M, et al. A bone regenerative approach to alveolar ridge maintenance following tooth extraction. Report of 10 cases. J Periodontol 1997;68:563–570.
162. Fickl S, Zuhr O, Wachtel H, Stappert CF, Stein JM, Hürzeler MB. Dimensional changes of the alveolar ridge contour after different socket preservation techniques. J Clin Periodontol 2008;35:906–913.
163. Vittorini Orgeas G, Clementini M, De Risi V, de Sanctis M. Surgical techniques for alveolar socket preservation: A systematic review. Int J Oral Maxillofac Implants 2013;28:1049–1061.
164. Vignoletti F, Matesanz P, Rodrigo D, Figuero E, Martin C, Sanz M. Surgical protocols for ridge preservation after tooth extraction. A systematic review. Clin Oral Implants Res 2012;23(suppl 5):22–38.
165. Barone A, Todisco M, Ludovichetti M, et al. A prospective, randomized, controlled, multicenter evaluation of extraction socket preservation comparing two bovine xenografts: Clinical and histologic outcomes. Int J Periodontics Restorative Dent 2013;33:795–802.
166. Lekovic V, Camargo PM, Klokkevold PR, et al. Preservation of alveolar bone in extraction sockets using bioabsorbable membranes. J Periodontol 1998;69:1044–1049.
167. Iasella JM, Greenwell H, Miller RL, et al. Ridge preservation with freeze-dried bone allograft and a collagen membrane compared to extraction alone for implant site development: A clinical and histologic study in humans. J Periodontol 2003;74:990–999.
168. Fu JH, Lee A, Wang HL. Influence of tissue biotype on implant esthetics. Int J Oral Maxillofac Implants 2011;26:499–508.
169. Araújo MG, Lindhe J. Dimensional ridge alterations following tooth extraction. An experimental study in the dog. J Clin Periodontol 2005;32:212–218.
170. Cook DR, Mealey BL, Verrett RG, et al. Relationship between clinical periodontal biotype and labial plate thickness: An in vivo study. Int J Periodontics Restorative Dent 2011;31:345–354.
171. Belser U, Bernard JP, Buser D. Implants in the esthetic zone. In: Lindhe J, Lang NP, Karring T (eds). Clinical Periodontology and Implant Dentistry, ed 5. Hoboken, NJ: Wiley Blackwell, 2008:1146–1174.
172. Spray JR, Black CG, Morris HF, Ochi S. The influence of bone thickness on facial marginal bone response: Stage 1 placement through stage 2 uncovering. Ann Periodontol 2000;5:119–128.
173. Teughels W, Merheb J, Quirynen M. Critical horizontal dimensions of interproximal and buccal bone around implants for optimal aesthetic outcomes: A systematic review. Clin Oral Implants Res 2009;20(suppl 4):134–145.
174. Abrahamsson I, Berglundh T, Wennström J, Lindhe J. The peri-implant hard and soft tissues at different implant systems. A comparative study in the dog. Clin Oral Implants Res 1996;7:212–219.
175. Linkevicius T, Apse P, Grybauskas S, Puisys A. Influence of thin mucosal tissues on crestal bone stability around implants with platform switching: A 1-year pilot study. J Oral Maxillofac Surg 2010;68:2272–2277.
176. Happe A, Korner G. Biologic interfaces in esthetic dentistry. Part II: The peri-implant/restorative interface. Eur J Esthet Dent 2011; 6:226–251.
177. Bouri A Jr, Bissada N, AL-Zahrani MS, Faddoul F, Nouneh I. Width of keratinized gingiva and the health status of the supporting tissues around dental implants. Int J Oral Maxillofac Implants 2008; 23:323–326.
178. Adibrad M, Shahabuei M, Sahabi M. Significance of the width of keratinized mucosa on the health status of the supporting tissue around implants supporting overdentures. J Oral Implantol 2009;35:232–237.
179. Schrott AR, Jimenez M, Hwang JW, Fiorellini J, Weber HP. Five-year evaluation of the influence of keratinized mucosa on peri-implant soft-tissue health and stability around implants supporting full-arch mandibular fixed prostheses. Clin Oral Implants Res 2009; 20:1170–1177.
180. Van der Velden U. Regeneration of the interdental soft tissues following denudation procedures. J Clin Periodontol 1982;9:455–459.
181. Romeo E, Lops D, Rossi A, Storelli S, Rozza R, Chiapasco M. Surgical and prosthetic management of interproximal region with single-implant restorations: 1-year prospective study. J Periodontol 2008;79:1048–1055.
182. Degidi M, Novaes AB Jr, Nardi D, Piattelli A. Outcome analysis of immediately placed, immediately restored implants in the esthetic area: The clinical relevance of different interimplant distances. J Periodontol 2008;79:1056–1061.
183. Gastaldo JF, Cury PR, Sendyk WR. Effect of the vertical and horizontal distances between adjacent implants and between a tooth and an implant on the incidence of interproximal papilla. J Periodontol 2004;75:1242–1246.
184. Kan JY, Rungcharassaeng K, Umezu K, Kois JC. Dimensions of peri-implant mucosa: An evaluation of maxillary anterior single implants in humans. J Periodontol 2003;74:557–562.
185. Choquet V, Hermans M, Adriaenssens P, Daelemans P, Tarnow DP, Malevez C. Clinical and radiographic evaluation of the papilla level adjacent to single-tooth dental implants. A retrospective study in the maxillary anterior region. J Periodontol 2001;72:1364–1371.
186. Jemt T. Regeneration of gingival papillae after single implant treatment. Int J Periodontics Restorative Dent 1997;17:326–333.
187. Chang M, Wennström JL, Odman P, Andersson B. Implant supported single-tooth replacements compared to contralateral natural teeth. Crown and soft tissue dimensions. Clin Oral Implants Res 1999;10:185–194.
188. Jemt T. Restoring the gingival contour by means of provisional resin crowns after single-implant treatment. Int J Periodontics Restorative Dent 1999;19:20–29.
189. Tarnow DP, Elian N, Fletcher P, et al. Vertical distance from the crest of bone to the height of the interproximal papilla between adjacent implants. J Periodontol 2003;74:1785–1788.
190. Grunder U. The inlay-graft technique to create papillae between implants. J Esthet Dent 1997;9:165–168.
191. Albrektsson T, Zarb G, Worthington P, Eriksson AR. The long-term efficacy of currently used dental implants: A review and proposed criteria of success. Int J Oral Maxillofac Implants 1986;1:11–25.
192. Novaes AB Jr, Papalexiou V, Muglia VA, Taba M Jr. Influence of interimplant distance on gingival papilla formation and bone resorption: Clinical-radiographic study in dogs. Int J Oral Maxillofac Implants 2006;21:45–51.
193. London RM. The esthetic effects of implant platform selection. Compend Contin Educ Dent 2001;22:675–682.
194. Raes F, Cosyn J, Crommelinck E, Coessens P, De Bruyn H. Immediate and conventional single implant treatment in the anterior maxilla: 1-year results of a case series on hard and soft tissue response and aesthetics. J Clin Periodontol 2011;38:385–394.
195. Adell R, Lekholm U, Rockler B, et al. Marginal tissue reactions at osseointegrated titanium fixtures (I). A 3-year longitudinal prospective study. Int J Oral Maxillofac Surg 1986;15:39–52.
196. Oates TW, West J, Jones J, Kaiser D, Cochran DL. Long-term changes in soft tissue height on the facial surface of dental implants. Implant Dent 2002;11:272–279.

197. Quiryen M, Bolen CM. The influence of surface roughness and surface-free energy on supra- and subgingival plaque formation in man. A review of the literature. J Clin Periodontol 1995;22:1–14.
198. Bollen CM, Papaioanno W, Van Eldere J, Schepers E, Quirynen M, Van Steenberghe D. The influence of abutment surface roughness on plaque accumulation and peri-implant mucositis. Clin Oral Implants Res 1996;7:201–211.
199. Elter C, Heuer W, Demling A, et al. Supra- and subgingival biofilm formation on implant abutments with different surface characteristics. Int J Oral Maxillofac Implants 2008;23:327–334.
200. Wataha JC. Biocompatibility of dental casting alloys: A review. J Prosthet Dent 2000;83:223–234.
201. Sjögren G, Sletten G, Dahl JE. Cytotoxicity of dental alloys, metals, and ceramics assessed by millipore filter, agar overlay, and MTT tests. J Prosthet Dent 2000;84:229–236.
202. Messer RL, Lockwood PE, Wataha JC, Lewis JB, Norris S, Bouillaguet S. In vitro cytotoxicity of traditional versus contemporary dental ceramics. J Prosthet Dent 2003;90:452–458.
203. Hao SQ, Lemons JE. Histology of dog dental tissues with Cu-based crowns [abstract 1125]. J Dent Res 1989;68SI:322.
204. Rechmann P. LAMMS and ICP-MS detection of dental metallic compounds in not-discolored human gingiva [abstract 672]. J Dent Res 1992;71SI:599.
205. Piccolomini R. Clinical and microbiological effects of different restorative materials on the periodontal tissues adjacent to subgingival class V restorations. 1-year results. J Clin Periodontol 2004;31:200–207.
206. Linkevicius T, Apse P. Influence of abutment material on stability of peri-implant tissues: A systematic review. Int J Oral Maxillofac Implants 2008;23:449–456.
207. Arvidson K, Fartash B, Moberg LE, Grafstrom R, Ericsson I. In vitro and in vivo experimental studies on single crystal sapphire dental implants. Clin Oral Implants Res 1991;2:47–55.
208. Kawahara H. Cellular responses to implant materials: Biological, physical and chemical factors. Int Dent J 1983;33:350–375.
209. Sailer I, Philipp A, Zembic A, Pjetursson BE, Hämmerle CH, Zwahlen M. A systematic review of the performance of ceramic and metal implant abutments supporting fixed implant reconstructions. Clin Oral Implants Res 2009;20(suppl 4):4–31.
210. Scarano A, Piattelli M, Vrespa G, Caputi S, Piattelli A. Bacterial adhesion on titanium nitride-coated and uncoated implants: An in vivo human study. J Oral Implantol 2003;29:80–85.
211. Kohal RJ, Weng D, Bachle M, Strub JR. Loaded custom-made zirconia and titanium implants show similar osseointegration: An animal experiment. J Periodontol 2004;75:1262–1268.
212. Gahlert M, Gudehus T, Eichhorn S, Steinhauser E, Kniha H, Erhardt W. Biomechanical and histomorphometric comparison between zirconia implants with varying surface textures and a titanium implant in the maxilla of miniature pigs. Clin Oral Implants Res 2007;18:662–668.
213. Jung RE, Sailer I, Hämmerle CH, Attin T, Schmidlin P. In vitro color changes of soft tissues caused by restorative materials. Int J Periodontics Restorative Dent 2007;27:251–257.
214. Park SE, Da Silva JD, Weber HP, Ishikawa-Nagai S. Optical phenomenon of peri-implant soft tissue. Part I. Spectrophotometric assessment of natural tooth gingiva and peri-implant mucosa. Clin Oral Implants Res 2007;18:569–574.
215. Rimondini L, Cerroni L, Carrassi A, Torricelli P. Bacterial colonization of zirconia ceramic surfaces: An in vitro and in vivo study. Int J Oral Maxillofac Implants 2002;17:793–798.
216. Scarano A, Piattelli M, Caputi S, Favero GA, Piattelli A. Bacterial adhesion on commercially pure titanium and zirconium oxide disks: An in vivo human study. J Periodontol 2004;75:292–296.
217. Degidi M, Artese L, Scarano A, Perrotti V, Gehrke P, Piattelli A. Inflammatory infiltrate, microvessel density, nitric oxide synthase expression, vascular endothelial growth factor expression, and proliferative activity in peri-implant soft tissues around titanium and zirconium oxide healing caps. J Periodontol 2006;77:73–80.
218. Zembic A, Sailer I, Jung RE, Hämmerle CH. Randomized-controlled clinical trial of customized zirconia and titanium implant abutments for single-tooth implants in canine and posterior regions: 3-year results. Clin Oral Implants Res 2009;20:802–808.
219. Loe H, Theilade E, Jensen SB. Experimental gingivitis in man. J Periodontol 1965;36:177–187.
220. Pontoriero R, Tonelli MP, Carnevale G, Mombelli A, Nyman SR, Lang NP. Experimentally induced peri-implant mucositis. A clinical study in humans. Clin Oral Implants Res 1994;5:254–259.
221. Heimdahl A, Kondell PA, Nord CE, Nordenram A. Effects of insertion of osseointegrated prosthesis on the oral microflora. Swed Dent J 1983;7:199–209.
222. Apse P, Ellen HP, Overall CM, Zarb GA. Microbiota and crevicular fluid collagenase activity in the osseointegrated dental implant sulcus: A comparison of sites in edentulous and partially edentulous patients. J Periodontol Res 1989;24:96–105.
223. Mombelli A, Buser D, Lang N. Colonization of osseointegrated titanium implants in edentulous patients. Early results. Oral Microbial Immunol 1988;3:113–120.
224. Loe H. Oral hygiene in the prevention of caries and periodontal disease. Int Dent J 2000;50:129–139.
225. Suomi J, Greene J, Vermillion J, Doyle J, Chang J, Leatherwood E. The effect of controlled oral hygiene procedures on the progression of periodontal disease in adults: Results after third and final year. J Periodontol 1971;42:152–160.
226. Van der Weijden F, Slot DE. Oral hygiene in the prevention of periodontal diseases: The evidence. Periodontol 2000 2011;55:104–123.
227. Sicilia A, Arregui I, Gallego M, Cabezas B, Cuesta S. Home oral hygiene revisited. Options and evidence. Oral Health Prev Dent 2003;1(suppl 1):407–422.
228. Husseini A, Slot DE, Van der Weijden GA. The efficacy of oral irrigation in addition to a toothbrush on plaque and the clinical parameters of periodontal inflammation: A systematic review. Int J Dent Hyg 2008;6:304–314.
229. Cancro LP, Fischman SL. The expected effect on oral health of dental plaque control through mechanical removal. Periodontol 2000 1995;8:60–74.
230. Deery C, Heanue M, Deacon S, et al. The effectiveness of manual versus powered toothbrushes for dental health: A systematic review. J Dent 2004;32:197–211.
231. Featherstone JD, Singh S, Curtis DA. Caries risk assessment and management for the prosthodontic patient. J Prosthodont 2011; 20:2–9.
232. Walker CB. Microbiological effects of mouthrinses containing antimicrobials. J Clin Periodontol 1988;15:499–505.
233. Veskler AE, Kayrouz GA, Newman MG. Reduction of salivary bacteria by pre-procedural rinses with chlorhexidine 0.12%. J Periodontol 1991;62:649–651.
234. Fardal O, Turnbull RS. A review of the literature on use of chlorhexidine in dentistry. J Am Dent Assoc 1986;112:863–869.
235. Esposito M, Worthington HV, Thomsen P, Coulthard P. Interventions for replacing missing teeth: Maintaining health around dental implants. Cochrane Database Syst Rev 2008;(1):CD003069.
236. Vandekerckhove B, Quirynen M, Warren PR, Strate J, Van Steenberghe D. The safety and efficacy of a powered toothbrush on soft tissues in patients with implant-supported fixed prostheses. Clin Oral Investig 2004;8:206–210.
237. Rasperini G, Pellegrini G, Cortella A, Rocchietta I, Consonni D, Simion M. The safety and acceptability of an electric toothbrush on peri-implant mucosa in patients with oral implants in aesthetic areas: A prospective cohort study. Eur J Oral Implantol 2008;1:221–228.
238. Slot DE, Wiggelinkhuizen L, Rosema NA, Van der Weijden GA. The efficacy of manual toothbrushes following a brushing exercise: A systematic review. Int J Dent Hyg 2012;10:187–197.
239. Ramfjord S, Morrison F, Burgett R, et al. Oral hygiene and maintenance of periodontal support. J Periodontol 1982;53:26–30.

240. Morrison E, Ramfjord S, Burgett F, Nissle R, Shick R. The significance of gingivitis during the maintenance phase of periodontal treatment. J Periodontol 1982;53:31–34.
241. Schallhorn R, Snider L. Periodontal maintenance therapy. J Am Dent Assoc 1981;103:227–231.
242. Shick R. Maintenance phase of periodontal therapy. J Periodontol 1981;52:576–583.
243. Orton GS, Steele DL, Wolinsky LE. The dental professional's role in monitoring and maintenance of tissue-integrated prosthesis. Int J Oral Maxillofac Implants 1989;4:305–310.
244. Fox SC, Moriarty ID, Kusy RP. The effects of scaling a titanium implant surface with metal and plastic instruments: An in vitro study. J Periodontol 1990;61:485–490.
245. Dmytryk JJ, Fox SC, Moriarty JD. The effects of scaling titanium implant surfaces with metal and plastic instruments on cell attachment. J Periodontol 1990;60:491–496.
246. Homiak AW, Cook PA, DeBoer J. Effect of hygiene instrumentation on titanium abutments: A scanning electron microscopy study. J Prosthet Dent 1992;67:364–369.
247. Speelman JA, Collaert B, Klinge B. Evaluation of different methods to clean titanium abutments. A scanning electron microscopic study. Clin Oral Implants Res 1992;3:120–127.
248. Rapley JW, Swan RH, Hallmon WW, Mills MO. The surface characteristics produced by various oral hygiene instruments and materials on titanium implant abutments. Int J Oral Maxillofac Implants 1990;5:47–52.

Preparation Design: Minimizing Soft Tissue Trauma

2

Ariel J. Raigrodski | Takafumi Otani

Tooth preparation design and procedures have an effect on soft tissue health and soft tissue esthetics, especially when the finish line of the tooth preparation is placed at or below the free gingival margins.[1–8] To provide patients with diagnostically driven tooth preparations, several guiding principles must be applied. Dental technicians may request more space for the restorative materials, while dental clinicians will follow the concept of tooth structure preservation as much as possible so as not to compromise tooth vitality or biomechanical durability.[9,10] The ultimate clinical goal is twofold: *(1)* to prepare teeth conservatively, from both biomechanical and periodontal perspectives, in terms of preserving a healthy dentogingival complex, and *(2)* to promote a durable and vital (when possible) tooth preparation while allowing the creation of a durable and functional restoration that fulfills the desired esthetic requirements.

Within the context of this chapter, the objective is to preserve the health of the dentogingival complex during the tooth preparation procedure while ensuring an adequate finish line placement customized to each clinical scenario. In general, the diagnostic wax-up, which serves as a treatment guide and provides clinicians and patients with a vision for the definitive treatment outcome, is used with an intraoral mock-up for enhancing a diagnostically driven tooth preparation for both anterior esthetic treatment (Fig 2-1) and complex, comprehensive patient care (Fig 2-2). Techniques and procedures for managing the soft tissue during tooth preparation procedures while maintaining its health and esthetics are discussed and demonstrated in this chapter in the context of ceramic veneers as well as conventional crowns and fixed dental prostheses (FDPs), particularly in areas where esthetics is of critical importance.

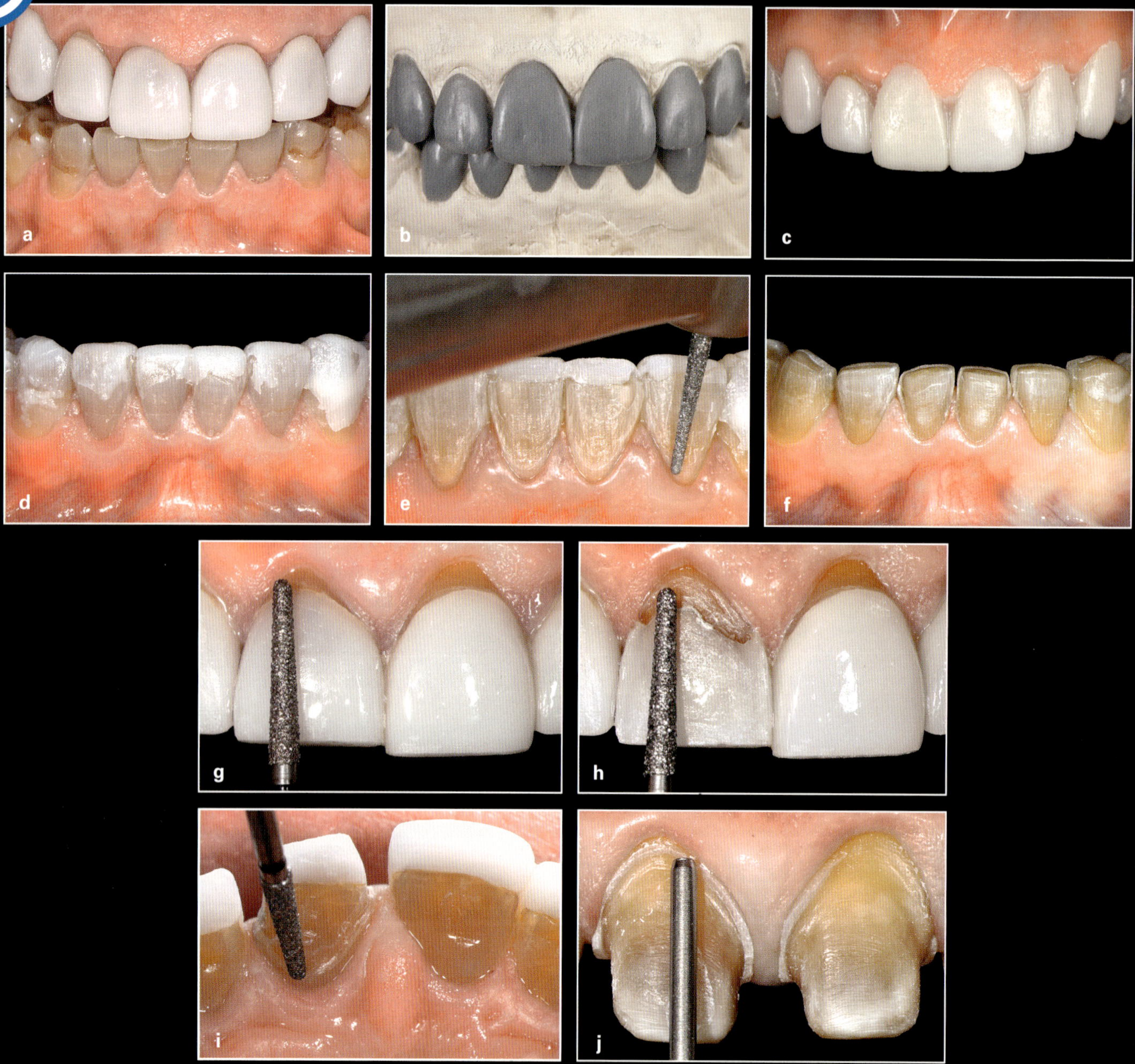

Fig 2-1 *(a)* Preoperative facial view in protrusive movement of a patient with ceramic veneers that are failing esthetically and because of secondary caries. Note the thick hyperplastic tissue in the maxillary anterior segment, the less than ideal maxillary gingival levels, and the inflamed interdental papillae. Also note the discolored mandibular anterior teeth and the enamel dysplasia on the mandibular canines and premolars. The mandibular anterior teeth are planned to be treated with ceramic veneers. The decision as to the type of restorations in the maxillary arch (veneers or crowns) will be made during the preparation visit depending on the clinical findings after the removal of the failing ceramic veneers. *(b and c)* An intraoral composite resin mock-up was fabricated following an initial diagnostic wax-up. It was tested intraorally and approved by the patient. An impression of the mock-up was made, and the cast was used for the fabrication of a guide for osseous crown lengthening surgery as well as a reference and guide for the subsequent restorative procedures. *(d)* Six months after osseous crown lengthening on the mandibular lateral incisors, an intraoral composite resin mock-up was made following a diagnostic wax-up. It was used as an aesthetic pre-evaluative temporary during the mandibular tooth preparation procedure for ceramic veneers. *(e)* An LVS4 high-speed diamond bur (Brasseler USA) was used to define and refine the finish lines of the preparations. *(f)* Facial view of the definitive tooth preparations for ceramic labial veneers with a well-defined, shallow chamfer finish line demonstrating healthy tissue. *(g)* Facial view of tooth preparation through the failing ceramic veneer. *(h)* Dental caries was detected beneath the failing maxillary ceramic veneers. It was decided to restore the teeth with ceramic zirconia-based crowns. *(i)* The palatal finish line was maintained coronal to the free gingival margins. *(j)* The finish line at the facial and interproximal aspects is dropped 0.5 to 1.0 mm below the free gingival margins with a tissue-protecting end-cutting bur.

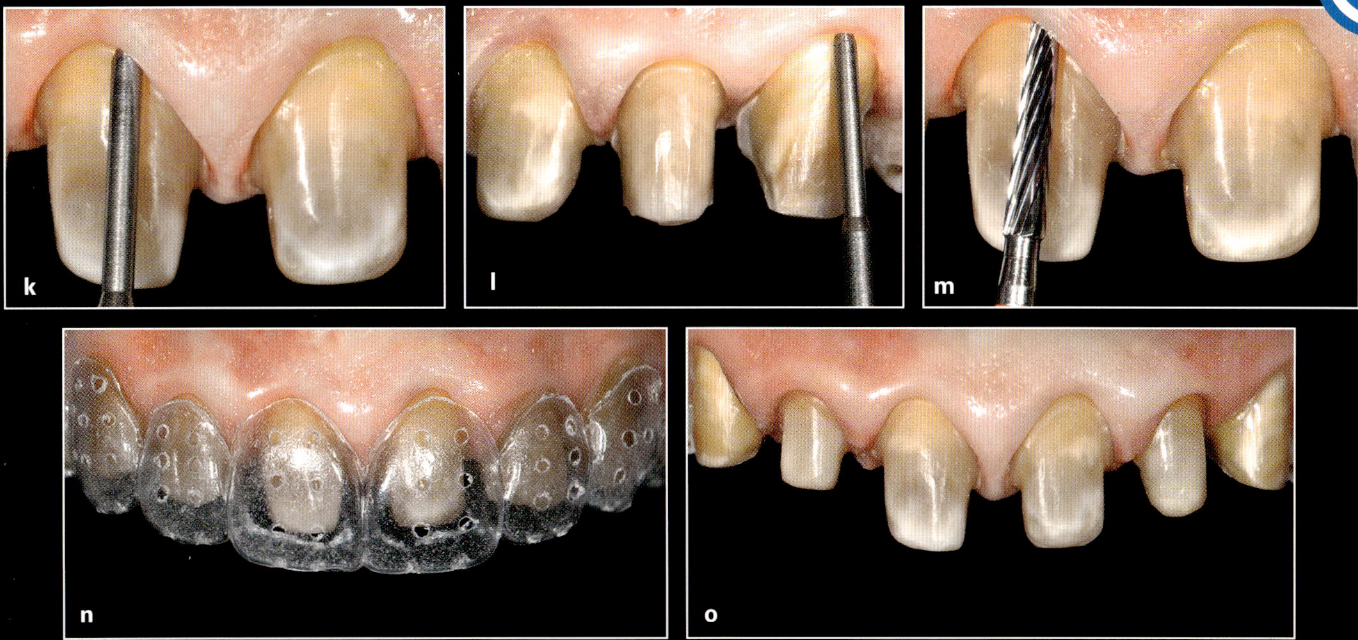

Fig 2-1 *(cont)* *(k)* Minimal trauma is caused to the soft tissue by the tissue-protecting beveled end-cutting bur. *(l)* At the facial and lingual aspects, the handpiece and the bur are kept on the finish line at a slight angle just away from the axial walls. *(m)* The finish line and the rest of the tooth preparation are polished with a 12-fluted carbide bur with minimal trauma to the tissue. *(n)* The tooth preparations and the amount of space created for the restorative materials were evaluated with a thermoplastic template made following the diagnostic mock-up. *(o)* Facial view of the completed definitive tooth preparations for the ceramic crowns.

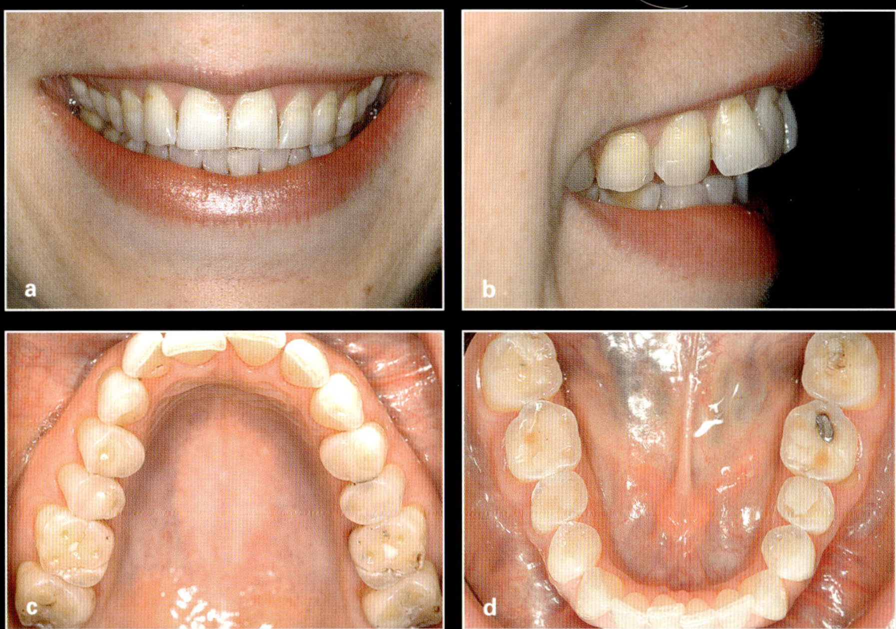

Fig 2-2 *(a)* Preoperative frontal smile view of a patient seeking therapy to improve function and esthetics in terms of tooth shade, form, and alignment. Note the short, square maxillary central incisors and the gingival display. *(b)* Preoperative lateral smile view. Note the extensive overjet and gingival display. *(c and d)* Maxillary and mandibular occlusal views of the patient's dentition, demonstrating signs of extensive wear related to erosion and parafunctional habits. In addition, note the failing restorations and the anterior crowding.

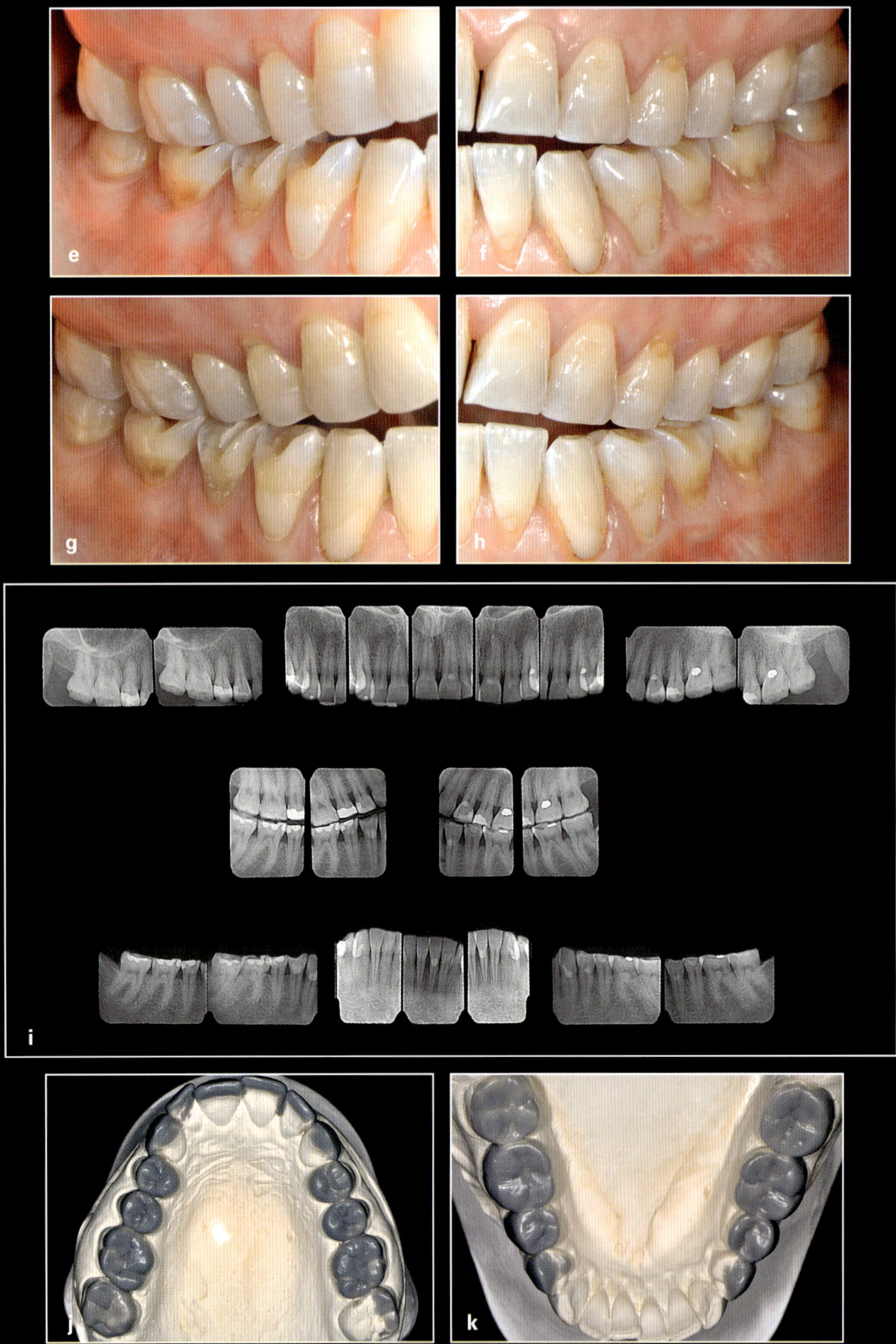

Fig 2-2 *(cont) (e and f)* Right and left lateral views of the patient in maximal intercuspal position. Note the history of recession and cervical restorations as well as the anterior open bite. *(g and h)* Right and left lateral views of the patient in working movements, demonstrating contact on the molars exclusively. In addition, protrusive movement demonstrated lack of anterior guidance. *(i)* A complete-mouth radiographic series demonstrating adequate bone levels and additional evidence of occlusal wear. The patient accepted the comprehensive treatment plan, which included orthodontic therapy and a complete-mouth restorative rehabilitation. *(j and k)* Maxillary and mandibular occlusal views of the diagnostic wax-up, which simulated the dentition restored to ideal dimensions. It was used to provide the patient with a functional bonded mock-up and then as a guide to facilitate the orthodontic therapy.

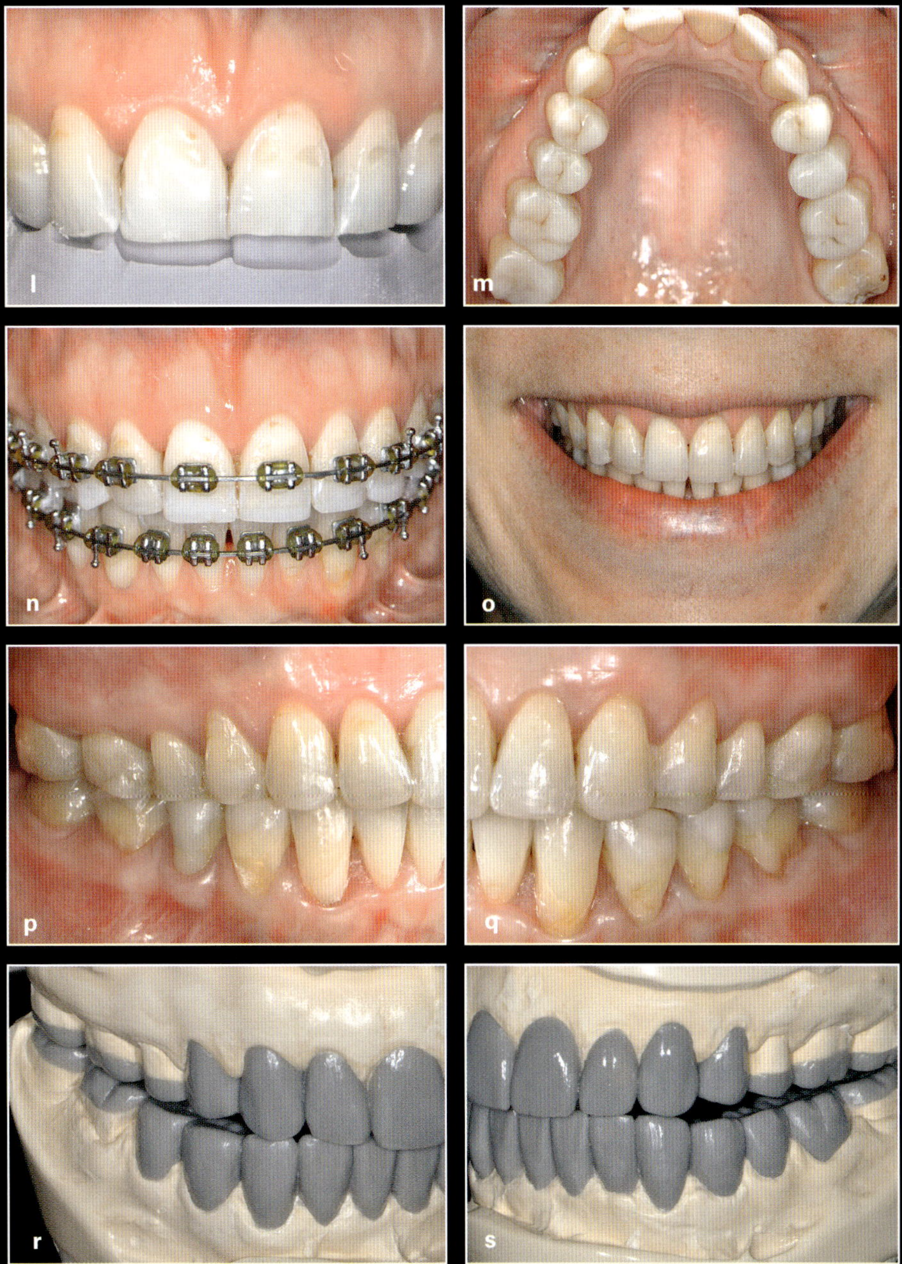

Fig 2-2 *(cont)* *(l)* Facial view of a silicone index used to restore the patient with a direct composite resin anterior functional mock-up. *(m)* Occlusal view of the maxillary arch with the bonded posterior indirect and anterior direct composite resin functional mock-up in place. *(n)* Facial view of the patient at the completion of orthodontic therapy. *(o)* The patient's smile demonstrated ideal alignment, occlusal plane, and incisal plane as well as the desired gingival levels. *(p and q)* Right and left lateral views in maximal intercuspal position, demonstrating adequate tooth position that will facilitate the desired occlusal scheme (mutually protected occlusion). *(r and s)* A new diagnostic wax-up demonstrated the creation of canine guidance in right and left lateral excursions.

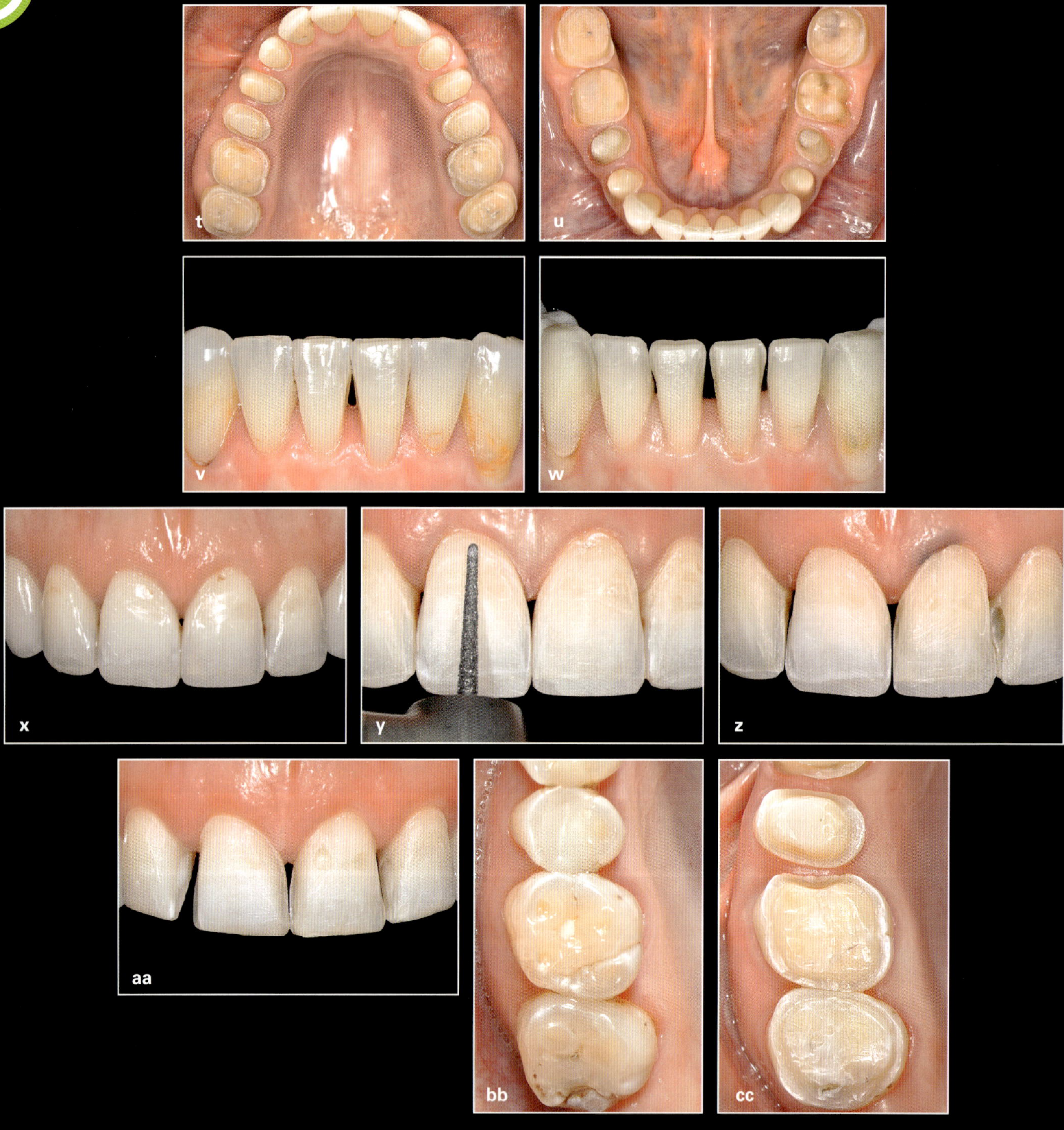

Fig 2-2 *(cont) (t and u)* Maxillary and mandibular occlusal views demonstrating the definitive posterior tooth preparations for both ceramic occlusal veneers and ceramic crowns. *(v)* Facial view of the anterior mandibular dentition with a mock-up for the fabrication of definitive ceramic veneers. Note that direct composite resin on the facial incisal aspect of the canines was used to facilitate the formation of canine guidance in lateral excursions. *(w)* Facial view of the definitive preparations for the mandibular ceramic labial veneers. Note that all of the direct composite resin restorations at the cervical aspect were replaced to eliminate any concerns of secondary caries. *(x)* Facial view of the anterior maxillary composite resin functional mock-up after the completion of orthodontic treatment. *(y)* Tooth preparations for ceramic labial veneers were performed on the four maxillary incisors, with supragingival finish line placement using the LVS3 high-speed bur (Brasseler USA). *(z)* Part of the cervical facial finish line at the left central maxillary incisor was placed subgingivally due to dental caries. Note the interproximal Class III cavity preparations after caries removal. *(aa)* Definitive tooth preparations demonstrating interproximal extension, due to the direct composite resin restorations, and slightly subgingival finish line placement to facilitate the closure of the diastemata and black triangles. *(bb)* Occlusal view of the right maxillary molars and second premolar. Note the wear as a result of parafunction and erosion. *(cc)* After the completion of orthodontic therapy, the teeth were prepared for occlusal veneers. The finish line was placed mostly coronal to the free gingival margins in enamel, except for the mesial proximal finish line of the first molar, which was placed equigingivally due to dental caries removal.

Finish Line Preparation for Ceramic Veneers

Enamel thickness

In the treatment planning and preparation design for ceramic veneers, a critical component is added to the guiding concepts previously discussed: enamel thickness.[11–14] The clinical success and survival of ceramic veneers is directly related to having sufficient enamel as a substrate for their adhesive cementation. Several clinical studies have demonstrated that when these restorations are bonded to enamel (with at least 50% of the bonding surface in enamel) and the finish line is placed supragingivally on enamel, these restorations are extremely successful with a high survival rate.[15–22] In addition, increased failure rates were associated with bruxism and nonvital teeth, and marginal discoloration was demonstrated to be more frequent in smokers.[23] Thus, to facilitate the long-term success and survival of ceramic veneers, clinicians should know the approximate mean enamel thickness at different areas of different teeth in the dental arches.[24,25] Enamel thickness may be reduced with advancing age[26,27] and may also vary based on ethnicity.[25] In general, the mean enamel thickness at the midfacial aspect of a maxillary central incisor is 0.9 mm. However, at the cervical aspect of that tooth, the mean enamel thickness is reduced to about 0.3 mm and sometimes even less. Consequently, the cervical part of the tooth is more challenging to prepare because of the need to create a shallow chamfer finish line that is still maintained in enamel. Therefore, it has been recommended to incorporate the diagnostic wax-up in the form of a composite resin mock-up, also known as an *aesthetic pre-evaluative temporary (APT)*, to facilitate the creation of adequate restorative space with minimal tooth reduction.[13,14]

Incisal edge preparation design

There is no consensus in the literature regarding the incisal edge preparation design. Some studies demonstrated that no incisal preparation or incisal preparation with a butt joint led to a better prognosis than incisal preparation with a lingual chamfer. In addition, incisal preparation with a lingual chamfer extended to the lingual concavity of the tooth may enhance the risk for porcelain fracture because of the concentration of tensile forces on the restoration at that area.[28,29] Nonetheless, some studies demonstrated that incisal preparation with a palatal chamfer is more beneficial in terms of fracture toughness.[30,31] However, an incisal preparation with a butt joint design results in a more conservative complete veneer preparation than such a design with a lingual chamfer, preserving more tooth structure. With a butt joint design, the preparation is going to be convex occlusogingivally, and the path of draw of the veneer is going to be from the facial to the lingual, which may further preserve the amount of enamel available for adhesive cementation of ceramic veneers. Labial veneer preparations with a lingual chamfer or conventional complete-coverage tooth preparations, on the other hand, have an occlusogingival path of draw. A labial veneer preparation design with such a path of draw may minimize the amount of enamel available for adhesive cementation.

Supragingival finish line placement

In an ideal clinical scenario, the finish line of the veneer preparation should be placed supragingivally so that the contact lens effect can be achieved. The *contact lens effect* is a concept related to the effect of a clear contact lens blending with the iris of the eye. The same principle can be applied to blending of ceramic labial veneers with natural tooth structure at the finish line. When ceramic labial veneers are cemented to the tooth structure, they blend optically with the substrate, becoming difficult to detect.[32] To achieve this goal, the tooth must not be discolored at the cervical area so that translucent light-polymerized composite resin cement can be used to bond the translucent ceramics at the cervical aspect of the veneer to the translucent enamel (Fig 2-3). As a result, the three bonded components will blend, mainly because of the design of the finish line, which is a very shallow chamfer. Consequently, the interface between the finish line of the tooth preparation and the margins of the ceramic veneer will become invisible, even when the patient presents with a high smile line. In addition, such finish line placement will *(1)* facilitate the fabrication of a provisional restoration with minimal impact on the soft tissues, *(2)* enhance impression procedures with minimal trauma, and *(3)* improve the prospective adhesive cementation of the veneers because gingival health and isolation can be achieved in a simple and straightforward manner.

To prepare and manage the finish line with minimal trauma to the soft tissue, a supragingival finish line is prepared with double-grit high-speed burs (LVS3 and LVS4, Brasseler USA) as described by Chiche (personal communication, 2005). The course-grit part *(green stripe)* is used for preparing the facial area of the tooth, whereas the fine-grit tip *(red stripe)* is used to define and refine a very shallow chamfer finish line (0.3 mm in width) (Fig 2-4). The use of an electric handpiece substantially improves the clinician's control in creating a continuous and smooth finish line that follows the scalloping of the free gingival margins[33,34] because the speed can be accurately reduced to 30,000 rpm. In addition, turning off the water spray and having the assistant spray air and occasionally water to clear the resulting dust also enables the creation of a crisp and refined finish line. No pressure should be applied with the bur, and the operator must continually follow the scalloping of the soft tissue as if drawing a very fine line with a very fine paintbrush.

Subgingival finish line placement

In many clinical scenarios, the finish line has to be placed slightly subgingivally. In such scenarios, a similar approach

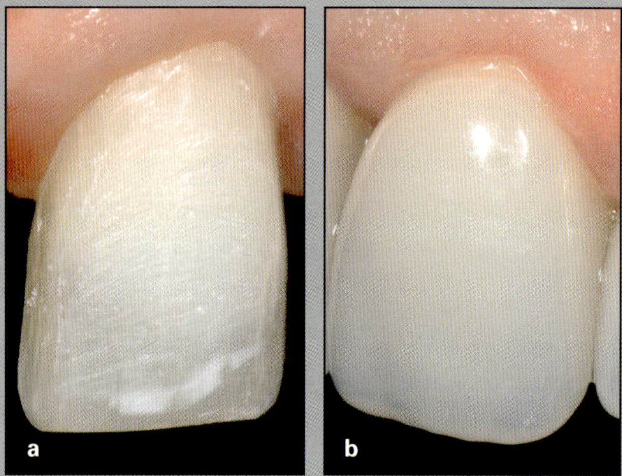

Fig 2-3 *(a)* Ceramic labial veneer preparation with supragingival finish line placement. *(b)* The interfaces between the finish line of the preparation, the translucent composite resin cement, and the margins of the ceramic veneer are well blended, leading to the contact lens effect.

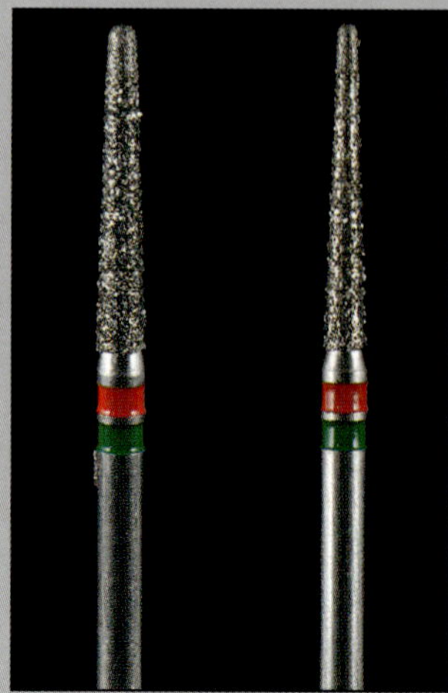

Fig 2-4 LVS3 and LVS4 high-speed burs. Note the coarse cutting area for the facial reduction and the fine tip for the creation of a shallow chamfer finish line.

with the same burs is used with the goal of reducing trauma to the soft tissue. The finish line is placed subgingivally as needed in the following clinical scenarios:

- When there is a need to close a diastema or a black triangle
- When a cervical direct composite resin restoration was previously placed with or without secondary caries (which requires restoration replacement)
- When cervical dental caries is present
- When the tooth is discolored in the cervical area

In such situations, a narrow-diameter cord (Ultrapak #000, Ultradent) can be placed below the free gingival margin to facilitate an atraumatic preparation. If the discoloration is limited to a specific area at the cervical aspect of a tooth, the finish line may be selectively placed below the free gingival margin at that area and gradually transitioned coronally in other areas to remain above the free gingival margin[11–13] (Fig 2-5). To close a diastema or a black triangle, the finish line must be placed slightly subgingivally exclusively at the interproximal areas to allow the ceramist to develop a gradual emergence profile for the ceramic veneers while reducing the likelihood of their overcontouring (see Figs 2-2x to 2-2aa).

Posterior occlusal veneers

Recently, posterior occlusal veneers have gained popularity as an alternative conservative treatment modality to posterior crowns, especially for young individuals affected by dental erosion. Although clinical evidence is still in its early stages, improved adhesive techniques in conjunction with improved tooth-colored restorative materials and technologies have contributed to the increasing use of lithium disilicate glass-ceramics and computer-aided design/computer-assisted manufacturing (CAD/CAM)–fabricated high-density polymers for such indications.[35–41] In general, the tooth preparation for such posterior occlusal veneers is minimal; in some clinical scenarios, no tooth preparation is required at all.

Placing a finish line for such restorations is still controversial, but even if a finish line is placed, it should be placed within enamel to facilitate long-term clinical success. Because the finish line for such posterior occlusal veneers is placed supragingivally in most clinical scenarios, preparation design, impression procedures, provisional restorations, or delivery of definitive restorations and their interface with the tooth structure rarely affect the health of gingival tissues. It is the authors' preference to place a finish line for such restorations to facilitate definitive and accurate seating of the restorations during the adhesive cementation procedures. In addition, subgingival finish line placement may be required in some clinical scenarios, such as when preexisting restorative materials or dental caries extend subgingivally. In such cases, the finish line must be selectively dropped subgingivally in the required area but gradually transitioned in other areas to be supragingival and placed in enamel. Two techniques are available for managing such a finish line while maintaining soft tissue health during the tooth preparation procedures: *(1)* the technique previously described for subgingival finish line placement for anterior ceramic veneers, and *(2)* a technique discussed in the fol-

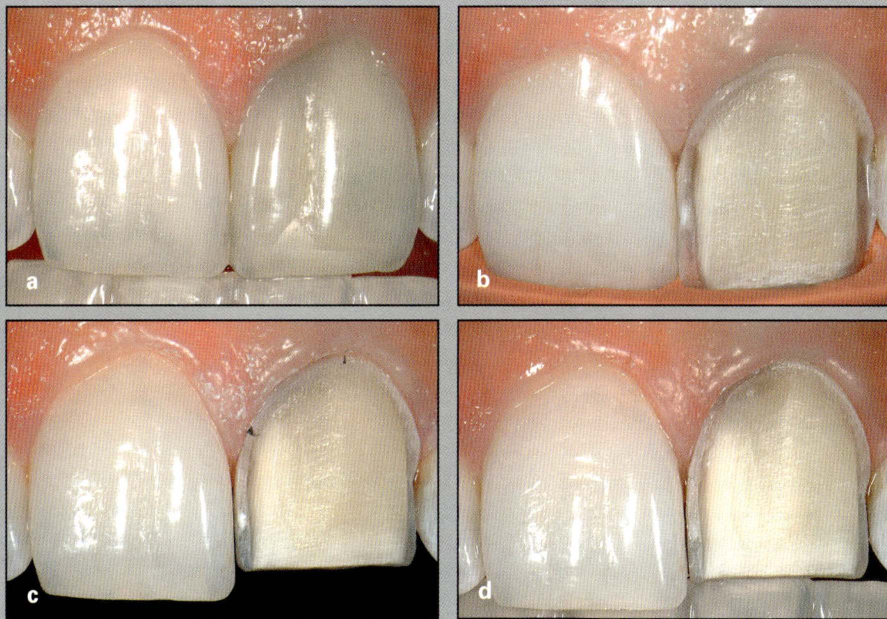

Fig 2-5 *(a)* Preoperative view of the patient's maxillary central incisors. The left central incisor is planned to be restored with a ceramic labial veneer. Note the discoloration on the mesial aspect of the facial cervical area. *(b)* Tooth preparation was performed with supragingival finish line placement. *(c)* The mesiodistal borders of the cervical discoloration area were marked with a pencil. *(d)* The finish line was selectively dropped below the free gingival margins at the area of discoloration, while the rest of the finish line remained coronal to the free gingival margins. (Treated with Dr Yen-Wei Chen.)

lowing section describing subgingival finish line placement for crowns and FDPs. The volume of the preexisting restoration or the extent of dental caries in the subgingival area will determine the more appropriate technique of the two (see Figs 2-2bb and 2-2cc).

Finish Line Preparation for Crowns and FDPs

In the treatment planning and preparation design for conventional crowns and FDPs in esthetically demanding areas in patients with a high smile line, material selection and finish line placement are critical in terms of achieving the desired esthetic outcome. Ceramic crowns are more predisposed to achieving a natural appearance at the soft tissue–restorative interface because of their translucency,[42,43] and they further enhance gingival tissue health because of their biocompatibility.[44,45] When a metal-ceramic crown is selected as a definitive restoration, however, the design of the metal framework at the margins is key to an esthetic result. Metal-ceramic crowns with porcelain butt margins are the design of choice to avoid the gray metal shadow seen through the gingival tissue.[46,47] For both ceramic and metal-ceramic restorative systems, subgingival finish line placement should be considered only in a healthy gingival crevice. If the marginal gingiva is not healthy, such finish line placement should be delayed until the desired gingival health is achieved.[1] When the cervical aspect of the tooth is not discolored, the finish line may be placed 0.5 mm below the free gingival margins to enhance a healthy gingival sulcus, thus minimizing the risk of violating the biologic width.[3,4,6,48] When the cervical aspect of the tooth is discolored, more apical placement of the finish line (up to 1.0 mm below the free gingival margin) will prevent biologic width violation while helping to conceal the cervical discoloration at the soft tissue–restorative interface. On the lingual aspect, the finish line should be placed supragingivally whenever possible depending on considerations such as resistance and retention form and the presence of preexisting restorations or caries lesions. Such a clinical approach enhances gingival health; facilitates impression procedures; facilitates adhesive cementation when needed; enhances residual excess cement removal during delivery procedures; and promotes health, esthetics, and longevity.

Subgingival finish line placement

The challenge clinicians confront with crown and FDP tooth preparations is placing the finish line subgingivally without causing irreversible trauma to the soft tissue. Many techniques have been suggested for performing this procedure predictably, such as cord placement to deflect the tissue with or without hemostatic agents,[49–51] surgical techniques using rotary instruments such as diamond burs in a high-speed turbine handpiece for gingival curettage,[52] electrosurgery,[53] laser surgery,[54] the use of extra-fine burs, and the use of special retractors.[55]

Placing a narrow-diameter cord in the gingival sulcus is a well-accepted technique. However, even with mild pressure, this cord may be pushed excessively into the gingival sulcus and may damage the epithelial and connective tissue attachments.[56] Moreover, placing such a cord for a long duration of time without the intent of immediately making master impressions may cause additional trauma to the gingival tissue,[56,57] especially in patients with the thin gingival phenotype; thin gingival tissue may react differently than thick gingival tissue and be more susceptible to gingival recession.[58,59] Such a procedure may also cause clinicians using the free gingival margin as a reference for finish line placement to lose that reference. This may result in an increased risk of placing the finish line too far apically and thereby violating the biologic width, which may translate to chronic gingival inflammation or gingival recession.[5]

Another technique advocated by Chiche is the use of a tissue-protecting beveled end-cutting bur.[60] This end-cutting bur with a smooth bevel at its tip is used to protect the tissue as the bur goes below the free gingival margins. Tissue-protecting beveled end-cutting burs are available from several manufacturers (Brasseler USA, Komet, Axis, Premier) in different diameters as needed for different clinical scenarios.

The rest of the tooth preparation, excluding the area requiring subgingival finish line placement, is accomplished with other burs while maintaining the finish line coronal to the free gingival margins (see Figs 2-1g to 2-1i). Subsequently, the finish line will be dropped with the tissue-protecting beveled end-cutting burs, creating a finish line that has a configuration of a rounded shoulder or a chamfer (see Figs 2-1j and 2-1k). This type of finish line design corresponds adequately with ceramic crowns and FDPs made of either zirconia or lithium disilicate with or without porcelain butt margins or with metal-ceramic restorations with porcelain butt margins.

Advantages of the beveled end-cutting bur

The advantages of the tissue-protecting beveled end-cutting bur are as follows:

- It causes minimal trauma to the gingival tissue.
- It will eliminate any trough also known as *J lipping* (acute cavosurface) that may have been created by previously used burs.
- It will not create a sharp line angle between the axial walls and the finish line.

As previously mentioned, this bur is available in different diameters that should be selected based on the desired width of the finish line, which relates to the restorative material preferred, its desired thickness, as well as the intended restoration design (eg, monolithic, hybrid, bilayered).[61] The recommended width of the finish line may change based on the type of restorative material used. However, a width of no more than 0.8 mm is usually recommended for the facial aspect of the finish line, and about 0.5 mm of finish line width is recommended on the lingual/palatal aspect. Interproximally, the finish line width will gradually transition from the facial to the lingual aspect.[62–64]

Guidelines for creating a smooth finish line

From a procedural perspective, there are a few guidelines that are recommended in order to facilitate the creation of an adequate, smooth, and well-defined finish line without causing trauma to the tissue:

- Examine the tip of the beveled end-cutting bur prior to using it; if needed, polish the tip of the bur with a diamond dresser to ensure a smooth line angle between the cutting aspect of the bur and the bevel (Fig 2-6).
- The use of an electric handpiece allows clinicians to reduce the speed of the handpiece dramatically in a controlled manner. Use an electric handpiece and reduce the speed from 200,000 to 30,000 rpm with ongoing air-water spray cooling.
- At the facial and lingual aspects of the preparation, keep the handpiece and the bur at a slight angle just away from the axial walls (see Fig 2-1l) and follow the scalloping of the soft tissues. At the interproximal areas, take special care to create a smooth, continuous transition from the facial to the lingual aspect adjacent to the papillae. This may be challenging, especially when prepping triangular teeth with increased scalloping of the soft tissue.
- Ensure constant back and forth movement with the bur as the finish line is dropped apically. Do not apply any pressure on the bur. Drop the finish line subgingivally while holding the handpiece as if drawing a very fine line with an ultrafine paintbrush using a light, feather touch. Do not pause with the bur at any point, because this may result in the creation of a ledge or step at the finish line. To remove such a step, more tooth structure must be lost that would be unnecessary otherwise.
- It is the authors' preference to polish the finish line with a 12-fluted carbide bur (H375R-012 or -014, Brasseler USA), which helps to create a smooth finish line without causing trauma to the tissue even when placed subgingivally with reduced speed of 30,000 rpm with ongoing air-water spray cooling (see Figs 2-1m to 2-1o).

Managing trauma

If, during the subgingival finish line placement procedure, any soft tissue trauma occurs, a hemostatic agent such as aluminum chloride (ViscoStat Clear, Ultradent; Hemodent, Premier Dental) should be applied at the exact point of soft

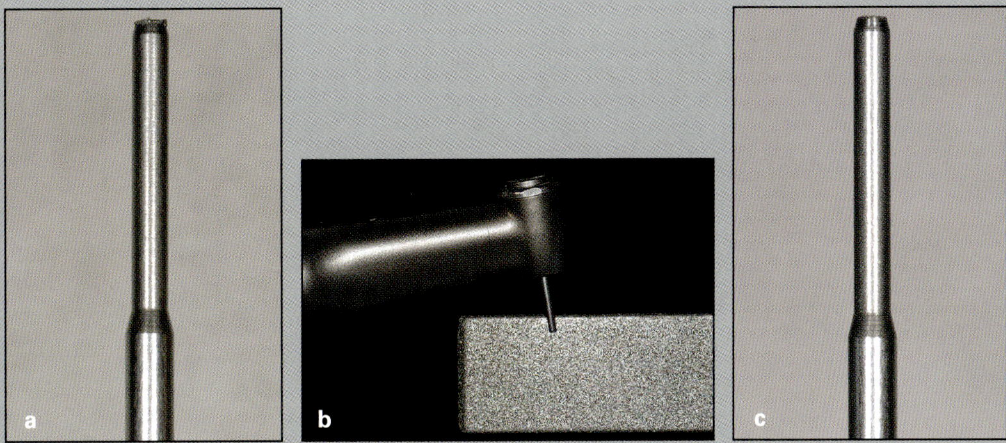

Fig 2-6 *(a)* View of a tissue-protecting beveled end-cutting bur. Excess diamond particles beyond the diameter of the tip of the bur may traumatize gingival tissue during finish line preparation. *(b)* The tip of the bur is polished by running the bur in the high-speed handpiece on a diamond dresser (grinding metal block coated with diamond particles) to ensure that no excess diamond particles are left beyond the diameter of the working tip of the bur. *(c)* After the tip of the bur has been polished, it presents with no excess particles and is ready for use.

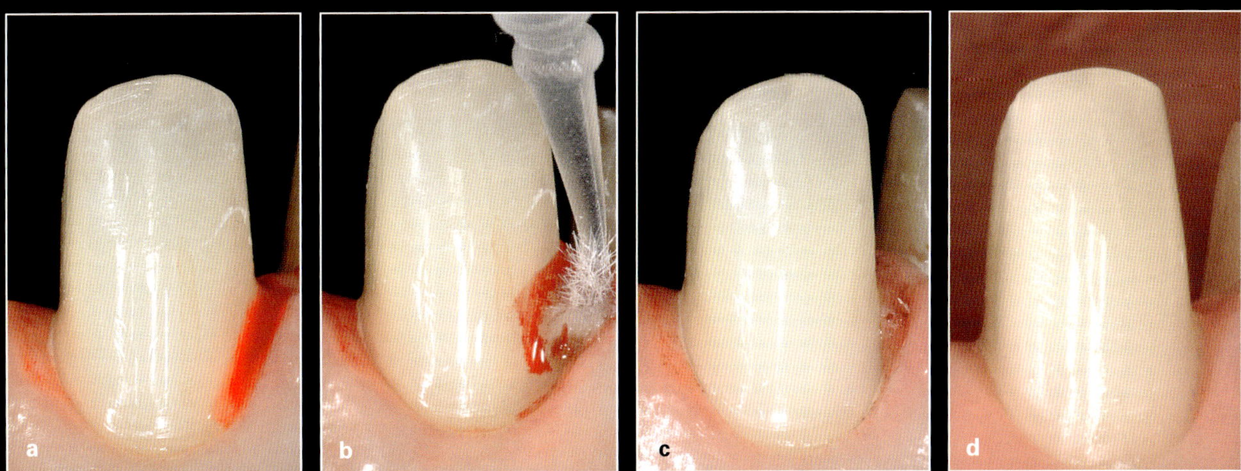

Continued from page 34

Fig 2-7 *(a)* During subgingival finish line placement, while preparing the tooth for a ceramic crown, heme is detected at the gingival tissue. *(b)* A hemostatic agent (aluminum chloride) was applied with a microbrush to the area where the tissue trauma occurred. *(c)* The tooth was rinsed, and coagulation was achieved. *(d)* View of the tooth several weeks after the tooth preparation procedure, demonstrating complete healing and gingival health.

tissue injury. It can be applied with either a cotton pellet or a microbrush to blot the traumatized area and stop the heme (Fig 2-7). Thus, only one area of the tissue is addressed rather than circumferential cord placement.

Insufficient or aggressive tooth preparation

If the amount of tooth preparation at the finish line is less than sufficient, one of the following compromised outcomes may result due to lack of space in terms of cervical width for definitive restoration (Fig 2-8):

- In an attempt to achieve an esthetic appearance for the ceramic material, the definitive restoration may be overcontoured. Gingival inflammation might be induced in this circumstance because of an inappropriate emergence profile.[65–71]
- If adequate cervical contours are maintained, the appearance of the definitive restoration might be compromised, demonstrating unnaturally high opacity or low value (depending on the color of the tooth) because of the lack of restorative material thickness.

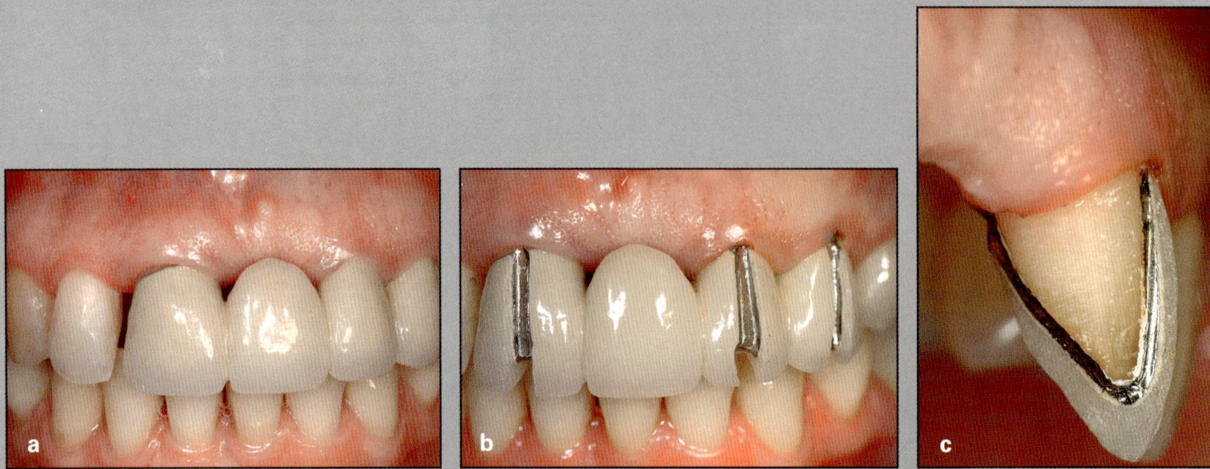

Fig 2-8 *(a)* Facial view of the failing metal-ceramic restoration, demonstrating adequate facial cervical contours on the right maxillary central incisor. However, the metal and the ceramic opaque layer are reflecting through the margins of the restoration. It seems that the teeth were not adequately prepared at the finish line, which led to compromised esthetics. *(b and c)* As the restoration is cut in the process of removal, it becomes evident that the width of the finish line, which looks like a feather-edge design, was less than adequate in this clinical scenario and caused an esthetic liability.

In the case of too aggressive tooth reduction at the finish line, postoperative hypersensitivity might be induced because of thin residual dentin over the pulp. Mechanical stimulation to the pulp tissue during the tooth preparation or chemical stimulation from the definitive cement may cause adverse effects; in extreme clinical scenarios, the abutment tooth may require endodontic therapy. Moreover, such aggressive tooth reduction may predispose the tooth to a higher risk of biomechanical complications such as tooth fracture after delivery of the definitive restoration.[72]

Summary

To minimize trauma and promote the health of the soft tissue during tooth preparation while seeking an esthetic clinical outcome and predictable long-term success, the following factors need to be well considered.

Tooth preparation for ceramic veneers

- The finish line should remain supragingival whenever possible. Thus, the gingival health can be well maintained and an esthetic outcome may be facilitated with the contact lens effect.
- When subgingival finish line placement is considered for selected areas in certain clinical scenarios, a narrow-diameter cord should be gently placed in these areas.
- Use of the recommended burs and the electric handpiece as discussed in this chapter may reduce the risk of soft tissue trauma while preparing a clear and well-defined finish line.

Tooth preparation for crowns and FDPs

- Subgingival finish line placement should be delayed until gingival health is achieved.
- A subgingival finish line should be placed conservatively in a healthy gingival crevice while avoiding biologic width violation.
- The use of beveled end-cutting burs without retraction cord is recommended to ensure that the finish line is ideally placed apicocoronally as relates to the free gingival margins with minimal soft tissue trauma.
- An adequate amount of tooth structure must be removed at the finish line to minimize the likelihood of esthetic and biologic complications such as gingival inflammation, caused by overcontoured restorations, or unnatural and opaque ceramic appearance, caused by inadequate space for the restorative materials (especially with discolored abutment teeth).
- Rotary cutting instruments should be well controlled by using an electric handpiece to achieve a smooth, clear, and well-defined finish line and to minimize trauma to the gingival tissues.

References

1. Wilson RD, Maynard G. Intracrevicular restorative dentistry. Int J Periodontics Restorative Dent 1981;1(4):34–49.
2. Nevins M, Skurow HM. The intracrevicular restorative margin, the biologic width, and the maintenance of the gingival margin. Int J Periodontics Restorative Dent 1984;4(3):30–49.
3. Newcomb GM. The relationship between the location of subgingival crown margins and gingival inflammation. J Periodontol 1974; 45:151–154.
4. Dragoo MR, Williams GB. Periodontal tissue reactions to restorative procedures. Int J Periodontics Restorative Dent 1981;1(1):8–23.
5. Tarnow D, Stahl SS, Magner A, Zamzok J. Human gingival attachment responses to subgingival crown placement. Marginal remodelling. J Clin Periodontol 1986;13:563–569.
6. Günay H, Seeger A, Tschernitschek H, Geurtsen W. Placement of the preparation line and periodontal health—A prospective 2-year clinical study. Int J Periodontics Restorative Dent 2000;20:171–181.
7. Kancyper SG, Koka S. The influence of intracrevicular crown margins on gingival health: Preliminary findings. J Prosthet Dent 2001;85:461–465.
8. Knoernschild KL, Campbell SD. Periodontal tissue responses after insertion of artificial crowns and fixed partial dentures. J Prosthet Dent 2000;84:492–498.
9. Edelhoff D, Sorensen JA. Tooth structure removal associated with various preparation designs for anterior teeth. J Prosthet Dent 2002;87:503–509.
10. Edelhoff D, Sorensen JA. Tooth structure removal associated with various preparation designs for posterior teeth. Int J Periodontics Restorative Dent 2002;22:241–249.
11. Roulet JF, Blunck U, Janda R. Adhesion. In: Gürel G (ed). The Science and Art of Porcelain Laminate Veneers. Chicago: Quintessence, 2003:113–134.
12. Magne P, Belser U. Bonded Porcelain Restorations in the Anterior Dentition: A Biomimetic Approach. Chicago: Quintessence, 2002.
13. Gürel G. Improving the esthetics of healthy teeth with porcelain laminate veneers. In: Cohen M (ed). Interdisciplinary Treatment Planning: Principles, Design, Implementation. Chicago: Quintessence, 2008:461–502.
14. Gürel G. Predictable, precise, and repeatable tooth preparation for porcelain laminate veneers. Pract Proced Aesthet Dent 2003; 15:17–24.
15. Friedman MJ. A 15-year review of porcelain veneer failure—A clinician's observations. Compend Contin Educ Dent 1998;19:625–636.
16. Fradeani M. Six-year follow-up with Empress veneers. Int J Periodontics Restorative Dent 1998;18:216–225.
17. Fradeani M, Redemagni M, Corrado M. Porcelain laminate veneers: 6- to 12-year clinical evaluation—A retrospective study. Int J Periodontics Restorative Dent 2005;25:9–17.
18. Burke FJT. Survival rates for porcelain laminate veneers with special reference to the effect of preparation in dentin: A literature review. J Esthet Restor Dent 2012;24:257–265.
19. Layton DM, Walton TR. The up to 21-year clinical outcome and survival of feldspathic porcelain veneers: Accounting for clustering. Int J Prosthodont 2012;25:604–612.
20. Gürel G, Sesma N, Calamita MA, Coachman C, Morimoto S. Influence of enamel preservation on failures rates of porcelain laminate veneers. Int J Periodontics Restorative Dent 2013;33:31–39.
21. Layton DM, Clarke M. A systematic review and meta-analysis of the survival of non-feldspathic porcelain veneers over 5 and 10 years. Int J Prosthodont 2013;26:111–124.
22. Layton DM, Clarke M, Walton TR. A systematic review and meta-analysis of the survival of feldspathic porcelain veneers over 5 and 10 years. Int J Prosthodont 2012;25:590–603.
23. Beier US, Kapferer I, Burtscher D, Dumfahrt H. Clinical performance of porcelain laminate veneers for up to 20 years. Int J Prosthodont 2012;25:79–85.
24. Ferrari M, Patroni S, Balleri P. Measurement of enamel thickness in relation to reduction for etched laminate veneers. Int J Periodontics Restorative Dent 1992;12:407–413.
25. Hall NE, Lindauer SJ, Tüfekçi E, Shroff B. Predictors of variation in mandibular incisor enamel thickness. J Am Dent Assoc 2007;138:809–815.
26. Atsu SS, Aka PS, Kucukesmen HC, Kilicarslan MA, Atakan C. Age-related changes in tooth enamel as measured by electron microscopy: Implications for porcelain laminate veneers. J Prosthet Dent 2005;94:336–341.
27. Ellis DM, Bogacki RE. The effects of aging on enamel thickness for maxillary incisors and its impact on porcelain laminate preparations [abstract 2591]. Presented at the 80th General Session of the International Association for Dental Research, San Diego, March 2002.
28. Castelnuovo J, Tjan AH, Phillips K, Nicholls JI, Kois JC. Fracture load and mode of failure of ceramic veneers with different preparations. J Prosthet Dent 2000;83:171–180.
29. Stappert CFJ, Ozden U, Gerds T, Strub JR. Longevity and failure load of ceramic veneers with different preparation designs after exposure to masticatory simulation. J Prosthet Dent 2005;94:132–139.
30. Schmidt KK, Chiayabutr Y, Phillips KM, Kois JC. Influence of preparation design and existing condition of tooth structure on load to failure of ceramic laminate veneers. J Prosthet Dent 2011;105:374–382.
31. Li Z, Yang Z, Zuo L, Meng Y. A three-dimensional finite element study on anterior laminate veneers with different incisal preparations. J Prosthet Dent 2014;6:1–9.
32. Materdomini D, Friedman MJ. The contact lens effect: Enhancing porcelain veneer esthetics. J Esthet Dent 1995;7:99–103.
33. Kenyon BJ, Van Zyl I, Louie KG. Comparison of cavity preparation quality using an electric motor handpiece and an air turbine dental handpiece. J Am Dent Assoc 2005;136:1101–1105.
34. Ercoli C, Rotella M, Funkenbusch PD, Russell S, Feng C. In vitro comparison of the cutting efficiency and temperature production of ten different rotary cutting instruments. Part II: Electric handpiece and comparison with turbine. J Prosthet Dent 2009;101:319–331.
35. Johnson AC, Tantbirojn D, Ahuja S. Fracture strength of CAD/CAM composite and composite-ceramic occlusal veneers. J Prosthodont Res 2014;58:107–114.
36. Edelhoff D, Beuer F, Schweiger J, Brix O, Stimmelmayr M, Güth JF. CAD/CAM-generated high-density polymer restorations for the pretreatment of complex cases: A case report. Quintessence Int 2012;43:457–467.
37. Güth JF, Edelhoff D, Ihloff H, Mast G. Complete mouth rehabilitation after transposition osteotomy based on intraoral scanning: An experimental approach. J Prosthet Dent 2014;11:1–5.
38. Güth JF, Almeida E Silva JS, Ramberger M, Beuer F, Edelhoff D. Treatment concept with CAD/CAM-fabricated high-density polymer temporary restorations. J Esthet Restor Dent 2011;24:310–318.
39. Magne P, Schlichting LH, Maia HP, Baratieri LN. In vitro fatigue resistance of CAD/CAM composite resin and ceramic posterior occlusal veneers. J Prosthet Dent 2010;104:149–157.
40. Schlichting LH, Maia HP, Baratieri LN, Magne P. Novel-design ultra-thin CAD/CAM composite resin and ceramic occlusal veneers for the treatment of severe dental erosion. J Prosthet Dent 2011;105:217–226.
41. Fabbri G, Zarone F, Dellificorelli G, et al. Clinical evaluation of 860 anterior and posterior lithium disilicate restorations: Retrospective study with a mean follow-up of 3 years and a maximum observational period of 6 years. Int J Periodontics Restorative Dent 2014;34:165–177.
42. Meyenberg KH. Dental esthetics: A European perspective. J Esthet Dent 1994;6:274–281.
43. Touati B, Miara P. Light transmission in bonded ceramic restorations. J Esthet Dent 1993;5:11–18.

44. Wataha JC. Biocompatibility of dental casting alloys: A review. J Prosthet Dent 2000;83:223–234.
45. Sadowsky SJ. An overview of treatment considerations for esthetic restorations: A review of the literature. J Prosthet Dent 2006; 96:433–442.
46. Swain VL, Pesun IJ, Hodges JS. The effect of metal ceramic restoration framework design on tooth color. J Prosthet Dent 2008; 99:468–476.
47. Paniz G, Kim Y, Abualsaud H, Hirayama H. Influence of framework design on the cervical color of metal ceramic crowns. J Prosthet Dent 2011;106:310–318.
48. Block PL. Restorative margins and periodontal health: A new look at an old perspective. J Prosthet Dent 1987;57:683–689.
49. Donovan TE, Gandara BK, Nemetz H. Review and survey of medicaments used with gingival retraction cords. J Prosthet Dent 1985;53:525–531.
50. Benson BW, Bomberg TJ, Hatch RA, Hoffman W. Tissue displacement methods in fixed prosthodontics. J Prosthet Dent 1986; 55:175–181.
51. Donovan TE, Chee WWL. Current concepts in gingival displacement. Dent Clin North Am 2004;48:433–444.
52. Azzi R, Tsao TF, Carranza FA, Kenney EB. Comparative study of gingival retraction methods. J Prosthet Dent 1983;50:561–565.
53. Ruel J, Schuessler PJ, Malament K, Mori D. Effect of retraction procedures on the periodontium in humans. J Prosthet Dent 1980;44:508–515.
54. Scott A. Use of an erbium laser in lieu of retraction cord: A modern technique. Gen Dent 2005;53:116–119.
55. Tebrock OC. Tissue retraction for esthetic ceramometal crowns. J Prosthet Dent 1986;55:21–23.
56. Loe H, Silness J. Tissue reactions to string packs used in fixed restorations. J Prosthet Dent 1963;13:318–323.
57. Harrison JD. Effect of retraction materials on the gingival sulcus epithelium. J Prosthet Dent 1961;11:514–521.
58. Cook DR, Mealey BL, Verrett RG, et al. Relationship between clinical periodontal biotype and labial plate thickness: An in vivo study. Int J Periodontics Restorative Dent 2011;31:345–354.
59. Kao RT, Pasquinelli K. Thick vs. thin gingival tissue: A key determinant in tissue response to disease and restorative treatment. J Calif Dent Assoc 2002;30:521–526.
60. Harrison JD, Chiche G, Pinault A. Tissue managment for the maxillary anteior region. In: Chiche GJ, Pinault A (eds). Esthetics of Anterior Fixed Prosthodontics.Chicago: Quintessence, 1994:143–160.
61. Raigrodski AJ. Managing prosthetic challenges with a CAD/CAM zirconia from bilayered to monolithic. J Cosmet Dent 2014;30:34–46.
62. Goodacre CJ, Campagni WV, Aquilino SA. Tooth preparations for complete crowns: An art form based on scientific principles. J Prosthet Dent 2001;85:363–376.
63. Goodacre CJ. Designing tooth preparations for optimal success. Dent Clin North Am 2004;48:359–385.
64. Kunzelmann KH, Kern M, Pospiech P, et al. All-Ceramics at a Glance: Introduction to Indications, Material Selection, Preparation and Insertion of All-Ceramic Restorations. Ettlingen, Germany: AG Keramik, 2007.
65. Wagman SS. The role of coronal contour in gingival health. J Prosthet Dent 1977;37:280–287.
66. Yuodelis RA, Weaver JD, Sapkos S. Facial and lingual contours of artificial complete crown restorations and their effects on the periodontium. J Prosthet Dent 1973;29:61–66.
67. Weisgold AS. Contours of the full crown restoration. Alpha Omegan 1977;70:77–89.
68. Perel ML. Axial crown contours. J Prosthet Dent 1971;25:642–649.
69. Becker CM, Kaldahl WB. Current theories of crown contour, margin placement, and pontic design. J Prosthet Dent 1981;45:268–277.
70. Perel ML. Periodontal considerations of crown contours. J Prosthet Dent 1971;26:627–630.
71. Ehrlich J, Hochman N. Alterations on crown contour—Effect on gingival health in man. J Prosthet Dent 1980;44:523–525.
72. Goodacre CJ, Bernal G, Rungcharassaeng K, Kan JY. Clinical complications in fixed prosthodontics. J Prosthet Dent 2003;90:31–41.

Therapeutic Provisional Restorations

3

Ariel J. Raigrodski

The *Glossary of Prosthodontic Terms* defines a *provisional* or an *interim prosthesis* as "a fixed or removable dental or maxillofacial prosthesis designed to enhance aesthetics, stabilization and/or function for a limited period of time, after which it is to be replaced by a definitive dental or maxillofacial prosthesis. Often such prostheses are used to assist in determination of the therapeutic effectiveness of a specific treatment plan, or the form and function of the planned definitive prosthesis."[1] The role of the provisional restoration has broadened with the increased demand for a highly advanced level of restorative dentistry in terms of esthetics, function, and oral health.[2,3] A clear understanding of the patient's expectations and the limitations of restorative therapy must be confirmed prior to providing the patient with the definitive restoration. To enhance such an understanding, the designed provisional restoration allows both the restorative dentist and the patient to see a common vision for the definitive restoration. Once tested, evaluated, and adjusted as needed, the provisional restoration will serve as a blueprint or template for the design and fabrication of the definitive restoration from both functional and esthetic perspectives.[4,5]

Provisional restorations can also be regarded as therapy prostheses, especially in the context of managing the soft tissue around crowns and fixed dental prostheses (FDPs), ovate pontics, and implant-supported restorations.[6–12] With such provisional restorations that provide the patient with the desired function and hard and soft tissue esthetics, clinicians have an opportunity to "test-drive" and evaluate new occlusal schemes, esthetic enhancements, and functional modifications prior to committing to the ultimate design of the definitive restoration.[13]

One of the main objectives of the provisional phase of therapy is to use the provisional restoration as a restorative tool for developing the prospective prosthetic recipient site. An additional major role of the provisional restoration is to assist in creating a harmonious soft tissue–restorative interface where the abutments (prepared teeth or implant abutments), restorations, and surrounding tissues all come together in a manner that will promote soft tissue esthetics and health.[7–9]

A well-contoured provisional restoration should facilitate the tissue's ability to heal to the desired cervical contours with an emergence profile that will subsequently be transferred to the definitive prosthesis.[14,15] As a general concept, all biologic, functional, and esthetic objectives must be met in the provisional phase prior to moving forward with the next steps of the restorative sequence toward the fabrication and placement of the definitive restoration.[4]

Rationale

Reduce sensitivity and protect the pulp

A properly constructed provisional restoration will protect the pulp from thermal changes in the mouth. Marginal adaptation is critical in maintaining a seal around the finish line from bacterial invasion.[16] Marginal leakage of a provisional restoration could be the consequence of an inadequate fabrication process and improper occlusal scheme leading to micromovement of the provisional restoration, resulting in open margins and cement wash. It may cause several types of biologic complications, including irreversible pulpal irritation and secondary caries.[16,17]

Protect teeth from fracture

A provisional restoration must satisfy the requirement of maintaining the structural integrity of the tooth throughout the restorative therapy sequence until the definitive restoration is delivered.[18,19] A provisional restoration must be strong and durable enough to sustain occlusal functional forces during mastication as well as to withstand parafunctional forces.[20–22]

Prevent tooth movement

A provisional restoration has to maintain the prepared teeth in a stable position in relation to the adjacent and opposing dentition.[23] It should prevent the mesiodistal and buccolingual migration of the abutment teeth and prevent their supraeruption.

Provide interim esthetics

An optimal interim restoration must be provided immediately after the tooth preparation to enhance the patient's psychosocial comfort.[24] In esthetically demanding areas, the provisional restoration may be designed based on a mock-up followed by a diagnostic wax-up, which allows patients to perceive a significant improvement in their smile on the day the provisional restoration is placed.

Serve as a diagnostic guide for function and esthetics

Provisional restorations serve as a diagnostic adjunct and guide in oral rehabilitation, particularly when extensive esthetic and functional changes are expected.[5,7,8,25] The relative ease of modifying the provisional restoration provides clinicians with the unique opportunity to address patients' individual esthetic requests while addressing and meeting functional needs. Data collection from the patient based on the clinician's experience with the provisional restoration provides a valuable tool for the clinician in the continuous evaluation and refinement of the treatment plan, which translates to further refinement of the cervical, occlusal, facial, and incisal contours of the definitive restoration.[4,13]

Shape and enhance the soft tissue health and contours

The health of the surrounding periodontal structure is maintained by creating a provisional restoration that has proper and relatively flat contours, adequate gingival adaptation, and optimal gingival embrasure spaces.[14,15,26,27] A well-made provisional complete-coverage restoration should provide a preview of the future prosthesis while enhancing the health of the abutment teeth or the implant-abutment complex and the soft tissue. In areas where esthetics is critical, provisional restorations aid in the development of appropriate soft tissue contours in order to achieve an acceptable emergence profile and appropriate tissue topography, thus facilitating the pink esthetic component of the patient's smile.[28–31]

This is particularly important in the context of ovate pontics and implant-supported restorations where critical, active soft tissue shaping occurs in the process of creating the desired emergence profile of the previously lost tooth. The ovate pontic site may be modified in order to shape the soft tissue selectively with the provisional restoration as needed. The same approach is used for implant-supported restorations: The emergence profile is created from the level of the implant platform to the level of the free gingival margin. This procedure may vary in different clinical situations, such as delayed and immediate implant placement and delayed and immediate implant provisionalization.[11,12,30] Once the ideal soft tissue contours have been achieved for implant-supported restorations and for ovate pontics, it is recommended that clinicians wait at least 3 months for tissue stabilization before proceeding with the master impression and fabrication of the definitive restoration.

Furthermore, properly contoured and fit provisional restorations can positively impact the overall gingival health of the patient, thereby facilitating prospective restorative procedures such as impression-making and the delivery of the definitive restorations.[7,8,32] In particular, scenarios requiring predictable bonding procedures to enhance the longevity of tooth-colored restorations rely on successful soft tissue management.[33,34]

Principles

Biologic, biomechanical, esthetic, and communication principles must be followed for good patient care, particularly in areas where the appearance of the restoration and soft tissue esthetics are critical.

Biologic

Clinicians must ensure that no harm is done to the dental pulp or the supporting tissues.[35] The provisional restorations must have an excellent seal to prevent marginal leakage from occurring. High polish[36] and adequate contours as well as perfect margins are essential to minimize soft tissue irritation.[4,7,32]

Biomechanical

The provisional restoration has to be durable enough to withstand occlusal functional forces and parafunctional forces, all the while avoiding fracture or dislodgment.[22] Inter- and intra-arch stability must be maintained with optimal proximal and occlusal contacts both in centric occlusion and in lateral and protrusive movements. Additionally, an uneventful removal of the provisional restoration should occur in an easy and atraumatic manner with respect to the supporting dentition and surrounding tissues.

As previously mentioned, the provisional restoration is used as a tool to modify the soft tissue contours at the level of the free gingival margins at the cervical and interproximal areas. The emergence profile of the provisional restoration is modified mainly for ovate pontics and implant-supported restorations but also for crowns and FDP retainers.[9,37] Concurrently, an evaluation of the occlusal scheme, new vertical dimension of occlusion, and guidance in protrusive and lateral movements can be carried out with the provisional restoration.[5] If any of the proposed changes does not coincide with the patient's adaptability and the envelope of parafunction, complications may occur and must be addressed in the provisional phase. Such complications may be manifested in the repeated fracture of the provisional restoration, loss of retention, or movement of the provisional restoration, which may result in marginal leakage, cement wash, and secondary caries.

Esthetic

A provisional restoration must provide the patient with psychosocial comfort in terms of esthetics and appearance, even when long-term provisionals are required due to reasons such as healing after surgery, orthodontics, testing of new occlusal schemes, or esthetics, among others. The provisional phase of treatment is often where the significant transformation occurs for the patient from an esthetic standpoint. Instead of comparing the preoperative situation to the postoperative definitive situation, a comparison can be made between the preoperative situation and the refined and agreed-upon provisional restoration. Subsequently, the transition from the provisional restoration to the definitive one should be uneventful, facilitating patient acceptance of the definitive restoration.[24,38,39]

Conceptually, fixed provisional restorations have a similar function in terms of assessing and determining the desired esthetics as wax trial dentures for complete denture patients. Tooth shape, length, position and angulation, shade (to a certain extent), incisal edge position, and display as well as lip support, incisal plane, and occlusal plane are all evaluated and finalized in the provisional phase.

Communication

As a communication tool, the provisional restoration helps in facilitating the mutual understanding between clinicians and patients with regard to treatment outcomes in terms of realistic treatment expectations and limitations. The provisional restoration is an excellent communication tool not only with the patient but also between the restorative dentist and the other members of the treating team (ie, other specialists and the dental technician). Communication with the oral surgeon and the periodontist may be facilitated by duplicating the provisional restoration and modifying it to serve as a radiographic and surgical guide in different procedures such as osseous crown lengthening, ridge augmentation, and implant placement. With the orthodontist, a provisional restoration with an ideal contour and size provides a visual aid for moving the teeth to the correct position while also facilitating space appropriation and orthodontic anchorage.[40,41]

A replica cast of the provisional restoration serves as a blueprint for the definitive restoration. It transfers both the function and esthetics generated in the patient's mouth to the dental laboratory. Ultimately, once the functional contours of the provisional restoration—including the occlusal aspects of posterior teeth, palatal and incisal aspects of maxillary anterior teeth, and facial and incisal aspects of the mandibular anterior teeth—are confirmed as needed and the desired esthetics are evaluated and agreed upon, an impression of the provisional restoration is made. Subsequently, the resulting casts are mounted on the articulator to serve as a guide for the dental technician in fabricating the definitive restoration.[5] Consequently, the individual character of the patient's smile and the customized cervical and functional contours will be copied from the cast of the provisional restoration and accurately reproduced by the dental technician in the definitive restoration. The fundamental difference between the provisional and definitive restorations should be the material used and the characterization level and surface texture, which can be achieved at a much higher level by the dental ceramist.[4,24]

Box 3-1 Desired properties and attributes of materials for provisional restorations

- High strength to minimize the likelihood of fracture during function and parafunction (with no inherent defects or voids when CAD/CAM technology is used)
- Adequate modulus of elasticity to reduce the likelihood of fracture mainly of FDP connectors
- Low brittleness to reduce the likelihood of fracture mainly of FDP connectors
- Wear resistance to maintain the newly proposed occlusal scheme and a newly proposed vertical dimension of occlusion for long-term function as needed
- Biocompatibility so as not to compromise the dental pulp and the soft tissues
- Low exothermic reaction to reduce the likelihood of trauma to the pulp and surrounding tissues
- Ease of predictable repairability to allow for repeated relines at the margins and other repairs as needed
- Low to no polymerization shrinkage to facilitate reline and repair procedures
- Color stability for enhanced long-term esthetics as needed
- Esthetic, with several shades, different levels of translucency, and ease of characterization
- Able to achieve excellent marginal integrity with different types of techniques
- High polishability to enhance soft tissue response and patient comfort
- Adequately retained and easily removed
- Cost-effective

Materials

Materials for provisional restorations have evolved from traditional acrylic resins (eg, polymethyl methacrylate [PMMA] and polyethyl methacrylate [PEMA]) to newer composite resin materials (eg, bis-acryl, bisphenol glycidyl methacrylate [bis-GMA], urethane dimethacrylate [UDMA], and triethylene glycol dimethacrylate [TEGDMA]).[42] In addition, the use of computer-aided design/computer-assisted manufacturing (CAD/CAM) technology and new three-dimensional (3D) printing technologies has facilitated the fabrication of provisional restorations for several treatment modalities while enhancing the quality of these provisional restorations.[42] From a clinician's perspective, an ideal material for provisional restorations possesses several properties and attributes that enhance the ability of such restorations to completely fulfill their clinical role in numerous clinical scenarios for different treatment modalities (Box 3-1).

Unfortunately, no single class of material meets all of these desired properties and attributes, and it is important that clinicians select the proper material for the proper clinical indication. Thus, clinicians must understand various materials' properties and, more importantly from a clinical perspective, master various materials' handling properties. The most common materials currently used for provisional restorations are categorized in the following sections.

Autopolymerized acrylic resins

PMMAs and PEMAs have been used for many years for the fabrication of provisional restorations. With a long track record and proven cost-effectiveness, PMMAs have been the standard for the fabrication of complete-coverage fixed provisional restorations.[7,15] PMMAs offer a cost-effective, adequate option for meeting the criteria of a proper material for provisional restorations in terms of physical properties providing adequate strength[43,44] with acceptable color stability, depending on the brand used.[45–48] Depending on the technique and the brand used, excellent marginal integrity can be achieved with such materials.[16,17] However, its relatively high polymerization shrinkage, limited wear resistance,[18] high exothermic reaction,[49,50] concerns of hypersensitivity, and strong apparent odor release restrict its popularity in the dental clinic.[51–53] Nonetheless, it is still considered the material of choice in particular for multiple-unit long-span provisional restorations, sometimes with the use of additional metal castings or fiber reinforcement.[5,54–56] For more complex treatments, especially for multiunit, multipontic clinical situations that require long-term durability, the ability to effectively reline the provisional restorations' margins and repair fractures in a relatively simple manner is extremely advantageous. Thus, PMMA provisional materials are generally considered the material of choice for such complex clinical scenarios. Excellent marginal integrity with PMMA provisional restorations is critical not only for reducing the risk of pulpal irritation and secondary caries but also for facilitating favorable gingival reaction when the finish line is placed slightly below the free gingival margins.[57] Recently, these materials have been introduced for processing via CAD/CAM technology, which addresses the concerns of lack of consistency within the material.[42,58,59]

Composite resin provisional materials

Composite resin materials were developed for provisional restorations to address some of the drawbacks and concerns expressed with regard to PMMAs.[60] These materials retain improved physical properties, particularly in terms of strength and wear resistance. With these materials, the fabrication of provisional single crowns is less technique sen-

Box 3-2 Conceptual sequence of steps for using provisional restorations as a comprehensive diagnostic tool

1. Perform an esthetic and functional analysis with the use of a mock-up to assess and determine prospective gingival levels, incisal edge position, occlusal plane, and occlusal scheme.
2. Make diagnostic impressions and mount the diagnostic casts on the articulator.
3. Fabricate a diagnostic wax-up on duplicates of the mounted diagnostic casts. These will be used later in various manners during the fabrication process of the definitive restorations.
4. Deliver the provisional restorations.
5. Clinically assess the provisional restorations for various durations of time depending on the type of therapy prescribed.
6. Make alterations to the provisional restorations as needed to meet the patient's esthetic and functional requirements.
7. Make impressions of the provisional restorations, which are then mounted on the articulator to serve as the blueprint for the fabrication of the definitive restorations. The mounted casts of the provisional restorations also serve as a guide for the fabrication of a custom incisal guide table for transferring the functional contours of the anterior dentition from the patient's mouth to the articulator. These casts are cross-mounted with the definitive casts using interocclusal records.

sitive and more predictable.[61] However, they are not without limitations. Composite resins for chairside fabrication of provisional restorations are based on either bis-acryl or bis-GMA, whereas laboratory-based materials are based on UDMA and TEGDMA as well.

Newer composite resin materials for provisional restorations have been introduced to eliminate the challenges associated with traditional PMMAs. They can be autopolymerized, dual-polymerized, or light-polymerized. These materials, mainly bis-acryl materials, have gained rapid acceptance due to their relative ease of use, low exothermic reaction,[62] low polymerization shrinkage, improved surface microhardness, good marginal adaptation, improved color stability,[48] improved polishability, and improved wear resistance.[18,61,63] In terms of soft tissue response, a recent study demonstrated no difference between PMMAs and bis-acryl materials in terms of inducing gingival inflammation.[64]

Despite their multiple superior properties, the main disadvantage of these materials is related to their brittle nature, particularly in areas of increased stress such as the connectors of provisional FDPs.[65] However, it was demonstrated that after aging, the newer bis-acryl materials demonstrated higher fracture resistance compared with their predecessors and PMMAs.[66] Though debatable, repairability and reline procedures may be challenging with these materials as compared with PMMAs.[65] In general, these materials are ideal for single-unit restorations and should be limited to short-span multiple-unit provisional restorations.[67] Caution should be applied with these materials in the presence of severe undercuts beneath the prepared tooth abutments so as not to lock the provisional restoration in the patient's mouth or create a fracture of the restoration. The overall clinical situation in terms of the patient's functional considerations and occlusion will determine whether these materials are the best choice for any given clinical scenario.

Light-polymerized direct composite resins

Light-polymerized direct composite resins are also available for use as a material of choice for provisional restorations. These materials combine the advantages of composite resin–based materials for provisional restorations with the benefits of flexible manipulation and extended working time, which are a direct derivative of their polymerization procedure. It is the author's preference to use these materials, which have a wide array of shades, for provisional veneers. In addition, because of their excellent polishability and ease of use, these materials can be used at the subgingival emergence area between the free gingival margins and the implant platform for implant-supported provisional restorations.

Techniques

Whether PMMAs or composite resin–based materials are selected to fabricate fixed provisional restorations, the main goals of such restorations remain the same: the construction of properly contoured, well-fitting, well-polished, and functional and esthetic provisional restorations that maintain their integrity throughout a reasonable period from tooth preparation to the completion and delivery of the definitive restorations. Several techniques may be employed for the fabrication of provisional restorations, and they may be categorized as direct, indirect, or indirect-direct.[23,24,68] Regardless of the technique used, similar conceptual steps are used during the provisional treatment sequence depending on the complexity of the treatment plan, starting with a dentofacial analysis and the use of some type of a mock-up in the patient's mouth to provide an initial reference for function and esthetics[69–71] (Box 3-2).

Direct technique

The direct technique is a convenient chairside method of constructing provisional restorations.[4,6] However, it has significant disadvantages such as potential pulp and soft tissue trauma with the use of PMMAs. Therefore, prefabricated polycarbonate (Polycarbonate Crowns, 3M ESPE) or malleable composite resin crowns (Protemp Crown Temporization Material, 3M ESPE) may be used with this technique, thus reducing the likelihood of trauma to the pulp and tissue and reducing the need for extensive occlusal adjustment. This technique can be used with or without silicone matrices/templates.[4,6,72]

The direct technique mainly applies for fabricating posterior single provisional crowns in areas where esthetics is of limited importance or for fabricating up to two anterior provisional veneers with direct light-polymerized composite resin material where esthetics can be achieved via composite resin layering procedures. However, the direct technique is not the focus of this chapter and therefore is not described further. For multiple-unit provisional veneers, which are discussed later in this chapter, a different direct approach is described with the use of a special rigid, clear matrix derived from a diagnostic wax-up.

Indirect technique

The indirect technique involves complete fabrication of the provisional restoration in the dental laboratory. This technique has several advantages over the direct technique. When a PMMA is selected for use, there is no contact of free monomer with the prepared teeth or with the gingival tissues, thereby resulting in less pulpal trauma or soft tissue irritation than the direct technique. In addition, the axial contours of the provisional restoration and the occlusal contacts can be managed and controlled much more readily. Moreover, the indirect technique produces provisional restorations with excellent fit and marginal integrity.[73] Although repairs at the margins may sometimes be required during the delivery of such provisional restorations made using traditional indirect techniques, the use of CAD/CAM technology for fabricating such restorations has facilitated a superior marginal fit.

However, this technique is not without shortcomings, mainly in the context of provisional restorations for natural dentition. Unless the clinician retains a chairside CAD/CAM unit or employs an in-house dental laboratory technician, a total of at least two sets of provisional restorations are required for managing the patient. The first one is delivered on the day of teeth preparation and impression-making (for making the indirect provisional restoration), and the second one is delivered at the next appointment. Such an approach increases chair time with the patient and may further increase irritation to the tissue due to delivery and removal of two sets of provisional restorations. In addition, the cost of the provisional restorations made in the dental laboratory must be factored into the financial equation.[4,68,74]

Within the context of implant-supported restorations, the indirect technique is advantageous. With these restorations, control of all axial contours and subgingival emergence areas often requires further reshaping and is especially challenging with multiple-unit provisional implant-supported restorations. Impressions are made for fabricating such indirect provisional restorations (whether screw- or cement-retained), and these restorations can be fabricated in the dental laboratory to address all esthetic, occlusal, and functional requirements. Subsequently, these restorations are delivered in the patient's mouth with minimal to no occlusal adjustment and with excellent fit.[75] To date, indirect provisional restorations may be predictably fabricated via CAD/CAM technology, leading to a more durable provisional restoration for both tooth-borne and implant-supported provisional restorations.[3,58] The indirect technique is not the focus of this chapter and therefore is not described further.

Indirect-direct combination technique with provisional restoration eggshell

The indirect-direct combination technique produces a custom-made preformed cameo (external) surface form, which is used as a provisional restoration eggshell (PRES). Subsequently, it is relined intraorally immediately after tooth preparation has been completed. The axial and cervical contours, embrasures, and occlusal surfaces are designed in the diagnostic wax-up and transferred to the PRES during its fabrication.

The indirect-direct procedure offers clinicians several advantages. Because the PRES is fabricated prior to the patient's appointment, chair time may be reduced depending on how extensive the provisional restoration is. Enhanced control over the provisional restoration's contours minimizes the time required for chairside adjustments, particularly with regard to occlusal adjustments, provided that the PRES is seated adequately in the patient's mouth during the reline procedure. Less of the provisional material will polymerize while in contact with the prepared abutment teeth, leading to decreased heat generation, less chemical irritation, and reduced polymerization shrinkage compared with the direct technique if PMMA is used. In addition, because the contact between the monomer and the soft tissues is reduced, the risk of soft tissue trauma is minimized as well.[68] Moreover, because there is no need to use a matrix (as is used sometimes with the direct technique and which may prevent access to excess provisional material removal if PMMA is the material used), the majority of excess provisional material used during the reline procedure may be removed prior to its complete polymerization. This reduces the risk of excess material being locked in tissue undercuts and more importantly reduces pulpal and soft tissue trauma, polymerization shrinkage, and the time required for excess material trimming with a bur after the material polymerization is completed.

The disadvantage of this technique is the relatively limited dental laboratory phase prior to tooth preparation.[4] If the PRES is not prepared adequately and thinned to a thickness of 0.5 mm or less, adjustments may be required to seat it completely and adequately on the prepared teeth prior to the intraoral reline procedure. Adequate seating of the PRES is critical for ease of reline while maintaining adequate incisal edge position, gingival levels, and the occlusal plane. In addition, in complex cases in which the occlusal scheme and the vertical dimension of occlusion are modified, references and indexes should be carefully used for adequate seating of the PRES prior to and during the reline procedure.[5,15]

The choice of material for the PRES and the reline procedure could be either PMMA or bis-acryl composite resins. It is recommended to use a bis-acryl composite resin system to fabricate the PRES, taking into consideration its strength, color stability, wear resistance, polishability, and esthetics. PMMA is applied as the reline material in order to take advantage of its repairability, marginal integrity, flexibility, and lack of brittleness. In addition, it should be emphasized that the use of the multiple reline technique, as advocated by Amsterdam and Fox,[76] later by Yuodelis and Faucher,[15] and later described and slightly modified by Chiche,[77,78] may facilitate better marginal integrity. Moreover, the use of a disposable plastic syringe with a curved tip to inject the reline material around the tooth preparation finish line (in a similar manner to injecting a light-body impression material around the finish line while making a master impression) enhances the fabrication of a provisional restoration with excellent marginal integrity.[79]

Procedures for Provisional Veneers

Making provisional restorations for patients treated with ceramic veneers is a time-consuming and technique-sensitive procedure. The challenge is to provide patients with provisional restorations that not only are functional and durable but also provide adequate interim esthetics without compromising the soft tissue health.[33,34,80,81] As with crowns and FDPs, the role of the provisional restoration is to test-drive the proposed definitive treatment outcome both functionally and esthetically. Yet it is essential that such provisional restorations do not compromise the health of the gingiva. With provisional veneers, this is a critical concern because the prospective bonding procedure of the definitive restorations can be compromised by uncontrolled heme and crevicular fluid contamination.[82] Thus, the longevity of the definitive restorations may be completely compromised.

As previously described, for up to two anterior provisional veneers, light-polymerized composite resin materials may be the materials of choice when using the direct technique with the aid of silicone matrices that are based on the diagnostic wax-up. Furthermore, excellent esthetics can be achieved via composite resin layering procedures. However, with multiple-unit restorations, such a procedure can be extremely time-consuming and cost-prohibitive.

Many techniques have been described in the dental literature for multiple-unit provisional veneers.[33,34,80,81] The custom rigid clear matrix (CRCM) technique mentioned earlier uses a direct approach with direct composite resin light-polymerized restorative material.

Custom rigid clear matrix technique (A)

The procedure for the CRCM technique is as follows (Fig 3-1):

Prior to tooth preparation

1. Have the dental technician fabricate a diagnostic wax-up with ideal incisal edge position, occlusal plane, and tooth contours as needed. The diagnostic wax-up is based on a mock-up that was made in the patient's mouth as part of the esthetic and functional analysis during the diagnostic phase of therapy. Re-evaluate the diagnostic wax-up.
2. Once approved, duplicate the cast of the diagnostic wax-up in dental stone (see Fig 3-1a).
3. Mix polyvinyl siloxane (PVS) putty and apply it as a spacer on the duplicate cast. The putty is applied on the teeth to be prepared as well as the teeth distal to them (and on the anterior part of the hard palate adjacent to the palatal free gingival margins of the teeth when making a provisional restoration for the maxillary arch). It should have a thickness of approximately 3 mm. The putty acts in a similar manner to a wax spacer that is applied during the fabrication of a custom tray (see Fig 3-1b).
4. Take a clear light-polymerized tray material (Triad, Dentsply) and apply it on top of the putty spacer and slightly beyond for fabricating a custom tray. Polymerize it as per the manufacturer's instructions (see Fig 3-1c).
5. Once the tray is polymerized, remove it from the cast. Dispose of the putty and leave only the tray and the cast on the laboratory bench.
6. Seat the tray on the cast, mark the midline with a black marker, and mark the areas corresponding to the free gingival margins of the teeth on the cast. Using a low-speed acrylic bur, scallop the tray following the scalloping of the soft tissue.
7. Take a round acrylic bur and create perforations in the tray, which will enhance the retention of the material to be used in the next step (see Fig 3-1d).
8. Take a clear PVS material (TransBite, SciCan; Memosil, Heraeus Kulzer; Clear Bite, Discus Dental) and syringe it into the tray. Make an impression of the duplicate of the wax-up with the clear PVS material (see Fig 3-1e).

9. Once it has set, remove the tray from the cast. Trim the PVS material following the scalloping of the soft tissue using a Bard-Parker knife or a surgical blade. If needed, trim the tray further following the scalloping of the soft tissue to ensure open gingival embrasures and that the tray and the PVS clear material are short of the free gingival margins by at least 1 to 2 mm (see Fig 3-1f).

The CRCM that has been created will be used for the fabrication of the provisional veneers in the patient's mouth with light-polymerized direct composite resin material with a shade that was selected in advance.

After tooth preparation and master impressions

The following procedures are performed after the teeth to be veneered have been prepared for the ceramic veneers and a master impression and interocclusal records have been made (see Fig 3-1g):

1. As a seating index in the maxillary arch, use the palatal aspect of the matrix and the areas of the teeth distal to the teeth that were prepared. As a seating index in the mandibular arch, use the teeth distal to the teeth that were prepared. This will ensure adequate seating of the tray in the patient's mouth.
2. Evaluate the matrix in the patient's mouth. Ensure that the gingival embrasures of the matrix are open and that the tray is shy of the facial free gingival margin by at least 1 to 2 mm.
3. If areas of the dentin have been exposed and the immediate dentin sealing approach is used, apply and polymerize the bonding agent prior to making the master impression.[83] While preparing for the fabrication of the provisional restoration, apply a thin layer of petroleum jelly (Vaseline) on the area of exposed dentin.
4. Spot-etch the midfacial aspect of the tooth preparation (see Fig 3-1h), apply a bonding agent (Scotchbond Universal, 3M ESPE) on that specific spot (spot bond), and light-polymerize (see Fig 3-1i).
5. Use a composite resin warmer or a mixing bowl with boiling water to warm up cartridges of a light-polymerized direct restorative composite resin material (such as nanocomposite resin material [Filtek Supreme, 3M ESPE]). This will reduce the viscosity of the material and facilitate the flow of composite resin into the areas to be restored with the CRCM. Fill the tray with the composite resin material in the relevant areas (see Fig 3-1j).
6. Immediately seat the CRCM in the patient's mouth and observe the excess composite resin flowing out of the CRCM through the gingival embrasures and at the facial areas (see Fig 3-1k).
7. While keeping the tray in the patient's mouth, remove as much excess composite resin material as possible from the facial-cervical and interproximal areas with a sickle-shaped explorer (see Fig 3-1l). Because a light-polymerized material is used for making the provisional restoration, there is no limit in terms of working time, and all excess material can be easily removed prior to polymerization, ensuring that no excess remains at the gingival embrasures and apical to the finish lines.
8. Once all of the excess composite resin material has been removed, light-polymerize the material through the tray for at least 40 seconds per tooth surface (see Fig 3-1m).
9. Remove the CRCM from the patient's mouth and assess the provisional restoration (see Fig 3-1n). Fill any voids within the provisional restorations with the same composite resin material (freehand).
10. Because the CRCM was short of the prospective finish line and the margins of the provisional restoration are incomplete, complete the cervical areas freehand with the same composite resin (see Fig 3-1o). Clinicians can choose to cut back the incisal and incisal-facial aspects of the provisional restoration and further characterize it incrementally.
11. Polish at the margins with sandpaper disks and composite resin silicone polishing points. Care should be taken so as not to compromise the finish lines of the tooth preparations, which have been already impressed (see Fig 3-1p).
12. Assess the occlusion and esthetics. Because the provisional restorations are all splinted, ensure that the patient can clean interproximally with floss and a threader.

Continued from chapter 2

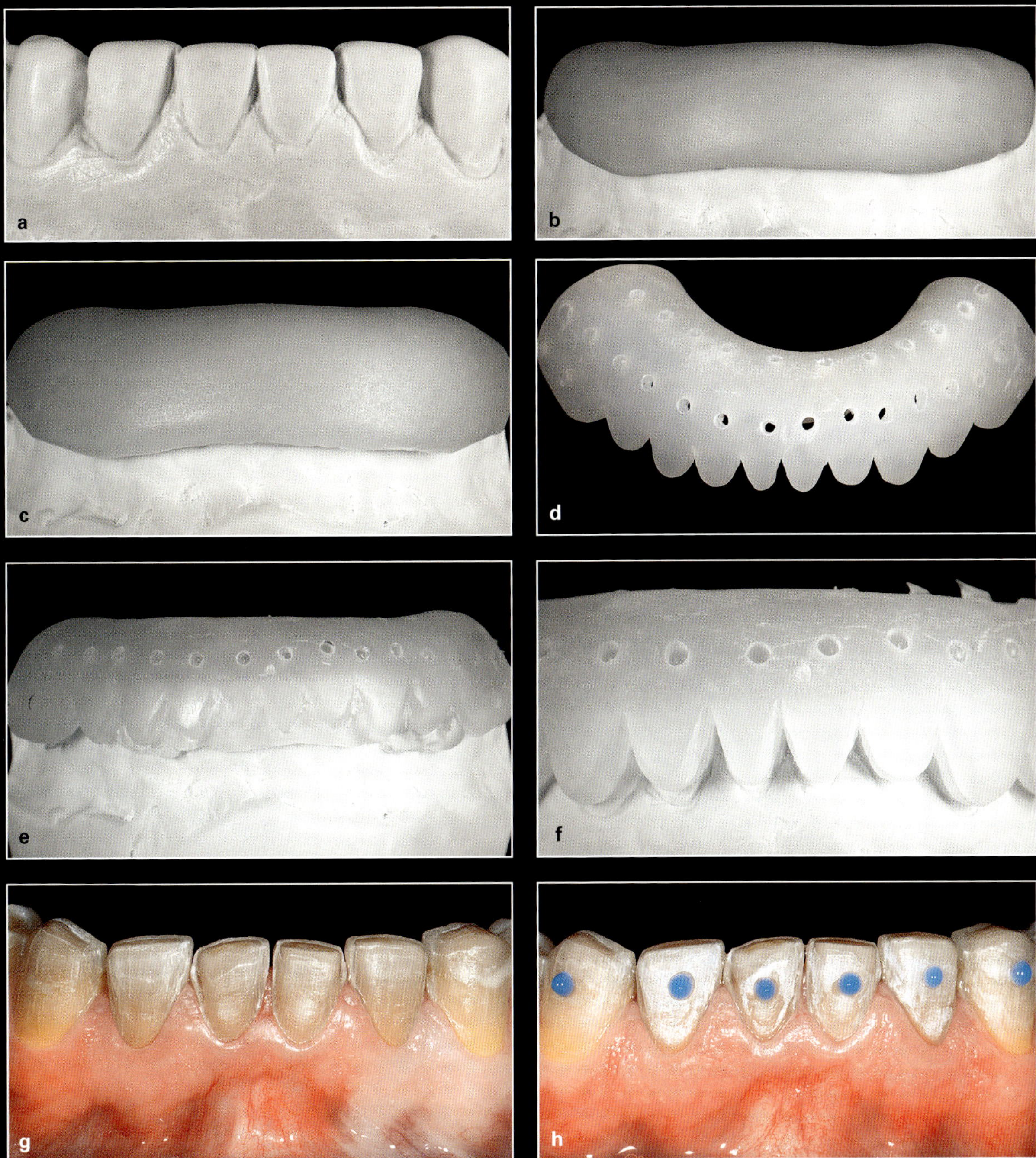

Fig 3-1 The CRCM technique. *(a)* A stone cast duplicate of a diagnostic wax-up for mandibular ceramic veneers. *(b)* Putty serving as a spacer is placed on the teeth to be prepared. *(c)* A light-polymerized clear tray material is placed on the putty spacer and then polymerized. *(d)* View of the complete CRCM with the scalloping following the free gingival margins on the stone casts and with retentive holes. *(e)* An impression of the teeth to be prepared is made on the stone cast with a clear PVS material. *(f)* The impression material is trimmed following the scalloping of the free gingival margins on the stone cast. Verification of adequate trimming is made on the cast. *(g)* Facial view of the definitive preparations for ceramic labial veneers. Note the severe discoloration. *(h)* The teeth are spot-etched.

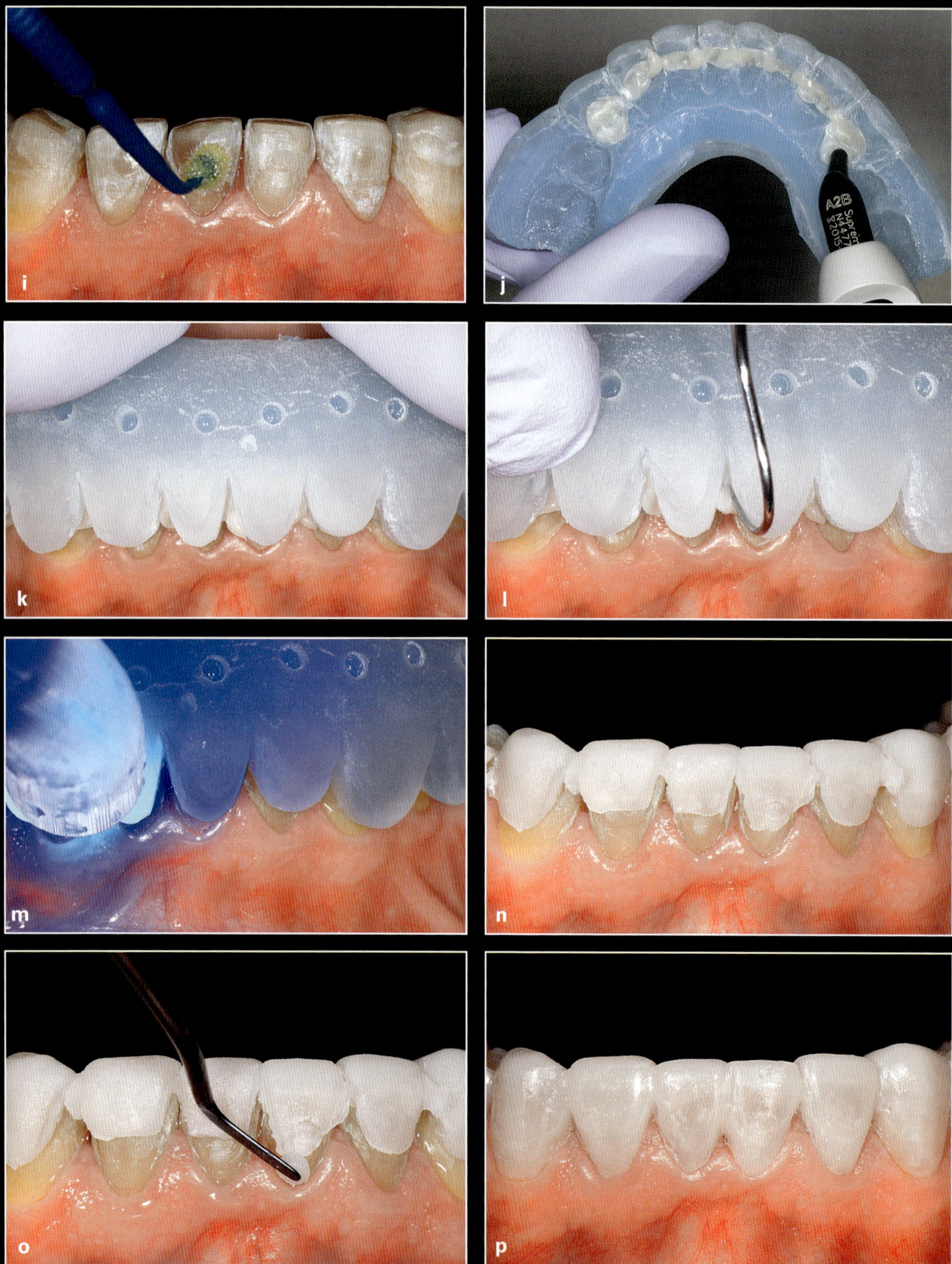

Fig 3-1 *(cont) (i)* A bonding agent is applied to the spot-etched areas and light-polymerized. *(j)* A warmed-up composite resin restorative material is injected into the impression. *(k)* Facial view of the CRCM filled with the composite resin material seated in the patient's mouth. Note the excess composite resin flowing out of the gingival embrasures. *(l)* Excess composite resin material is removed using an explorer. *(m)* The material is light-polymerized through the clear CRCM. *(n)* Facial view of the polymerized composite resin after removal of the CRCM. *(o)* Additional composite resin is added freehand to the interproximal and cervical areas and light-polymerized. *(p)* Facial view of the complete provisional restoration. Note the relatively healthy and untraumatized soft tissue.

Box 3-3 Advantages and limitations of the CRCM technique

Advantages:
- Relatively esthetic and functional
- Allows a relatively accurate transfer of the wax-up to the mouth (length, angulation, shape, and surface texture)
- Maintains the health of the soft tissue throughout the provisional phase, which is critical for predictable delivery of the definitive ceramic veneers
- May be used long-term
- May be removed with minimal trauma to the hard and soft tissues
- The matrix may be easily reused when needed

Limitations:
- Involves both laboratory and chairside procedures
- Has a learning curve
- Technique sensitive depending on the number of units involved

After fabrication of the definitive restoration

Once the definitive restoration has been fabricated and is ready for try-in, the following steps should be taken:

1. Break the provisional restoration gently with a curette and a curved hemostat.
2. Remove residual composite resin at the spot-etched area with a high-speed diamond bur. Any residual composite resin or bonding agent may compromise the seating of the restoration during the try-in phase, cause stresses and/or cracks within the veneer, or even cause a ceramic fracture.
3. Proceed with the try-in and adhesive cementation procedures of the definitive ceramic veneers.

Summary

Provisional veneers that enhance the health of the soft tissue are paramount for successful prospective delivery procedures and for enhancing the longevity of the definitive ceramic veneers. This technique is one of many that can be used and modified based on the presented clinical scenario for both anterior labial ceramic veneers and occlusal veneers in the posterior segments. Box 3-3 lists its advantages and limitations.[34]

Procedures for Provisional Crowns and FDPs

This section describes the indirect-direct combination technique—a simple technique for fabricating durable and esthetic provisional restorations in the office with limited to no in-house dental laboratory support (as compared with the indirect technique)—for crowns and FDPs. It is the author's experience that if adequately fabricated, provisional restorations made with this technique may be used long-term (ie, for many months) with minimal maintenance. This method does not require major investment in expensive equipment and laboratory space and can be used in the everyday restorative dental practice in a relatively simple manner; some of the preclinical procedures such as the fabrication of the PRES may be delegated to the dental auxiliary staff and performed prior to the patient's definitive tooth preparation visit.

PRES indirect-direct combination technique C D

The procedure for the indirect-direct combination technique for crowns and FDPs is as follows (Figs 3-2 and 3-3):

Prior to tooth preparation

1. Have the dental technician fabricate a diagnostic wax-up with an ideal incisal edge position, occlusal plane, and tooth contours. Such a design is based on a mock-up that was made in the patient's mouth as part of the esthetic and functional analysis during the diagnostic phase of therapy. Re-evaluate the diagnostic wax-up (see Figs 3-2a to 3-2d).
2. Once approved, duplicate the diagnostic wax-up in stone (see Figs 3-2e and 3-2f).
3. Add additional wax on the cervical third of the teeth on the duplicate cast of the diagnostic wax-up, thus widening the prospective provisional restoration shell to compensate for any minimal potential shrinkage of the material used for the fabrication of the PRES.[15]
4. The duplicate cast of the wax-up with the modified cervical contours is impressed in an impression tray with PVS reversible hydrocolloid (alginate) substitute impression material (Position PentQuick, 3M ESPE) or with alginate and is used as a template for the fabrication of the PRES. The advantage of the PVS alginate substitute is that the PVS template created can be easily maintained in the patient's records for future use if needed (see Fig 3-2g).

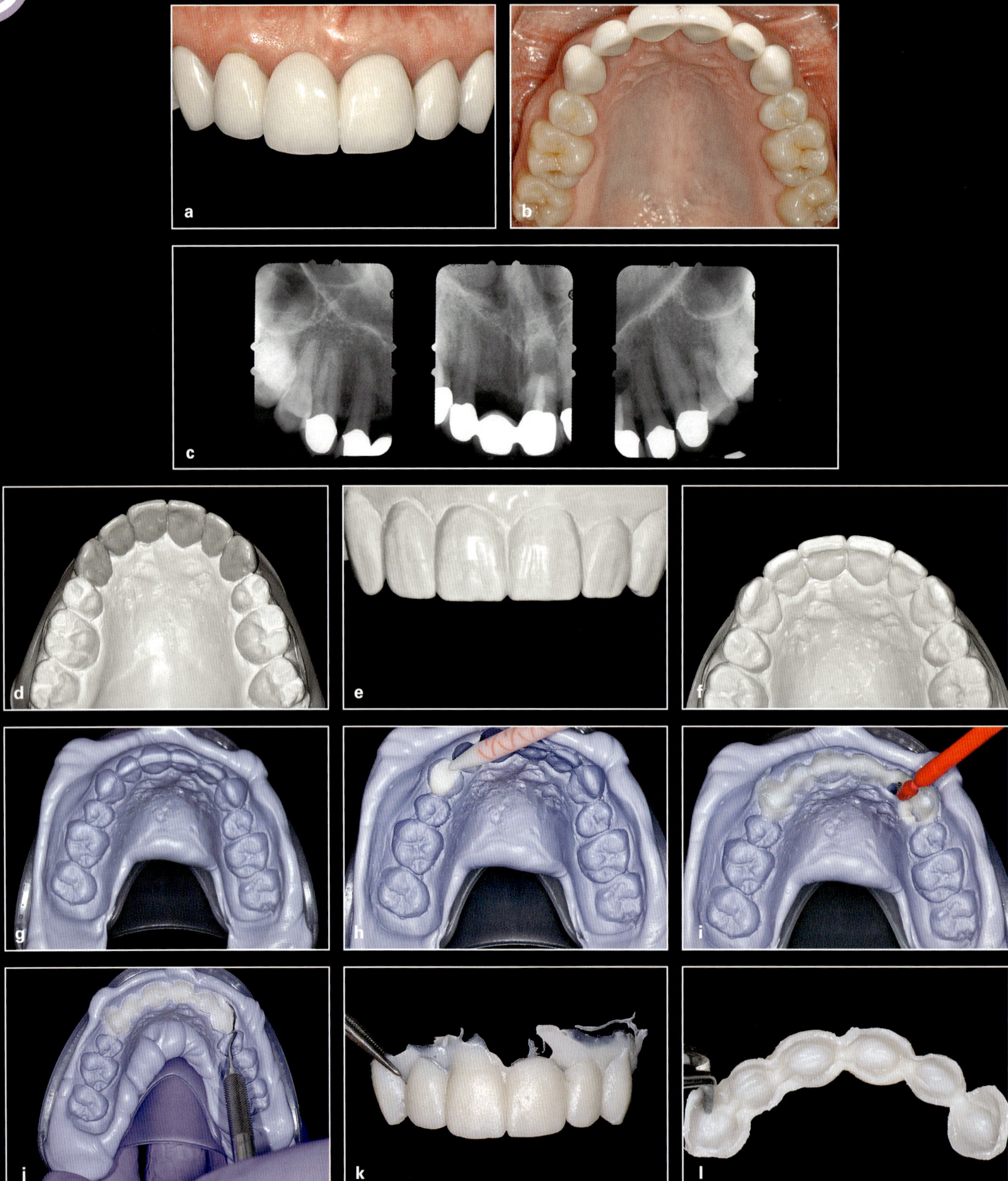

Fig 3-2 The PRES indirect-direct combination technique. *(a and b)* Preoperative facial and occlusal views of esthetically failing metal-ceramic restorations in the anterior maxillary segment. *(c)* Preoperative radiograph demonstrating a history of endodontic and surgical periapical therapy on the maxillary left central incisor. *(d)* Occlusal view of the diagnostic wax-up. *(e and f)* Facial and occlusal views of the duplicate cast of the diagnostic wax-up. *(g)* Complete-arch impression made with an alginate substitute in an impression tray. *(h and i)* The bis-acryl material of choice is injected and "painted" onto the intaglio surface of the relevant areas of the PVS impression to fabricate a PRES. *(j)* The PRES is gently retrieved from the impression with a hand instrument. *(k and l)* Excess material at the cervical aspects is trimmed with a high-speed diamond bur. The intaglio surface is trimmed to ensure that the PRES thickness does not exceed 0.5 mm. The intaglio interproximal areas are trimmed as well.

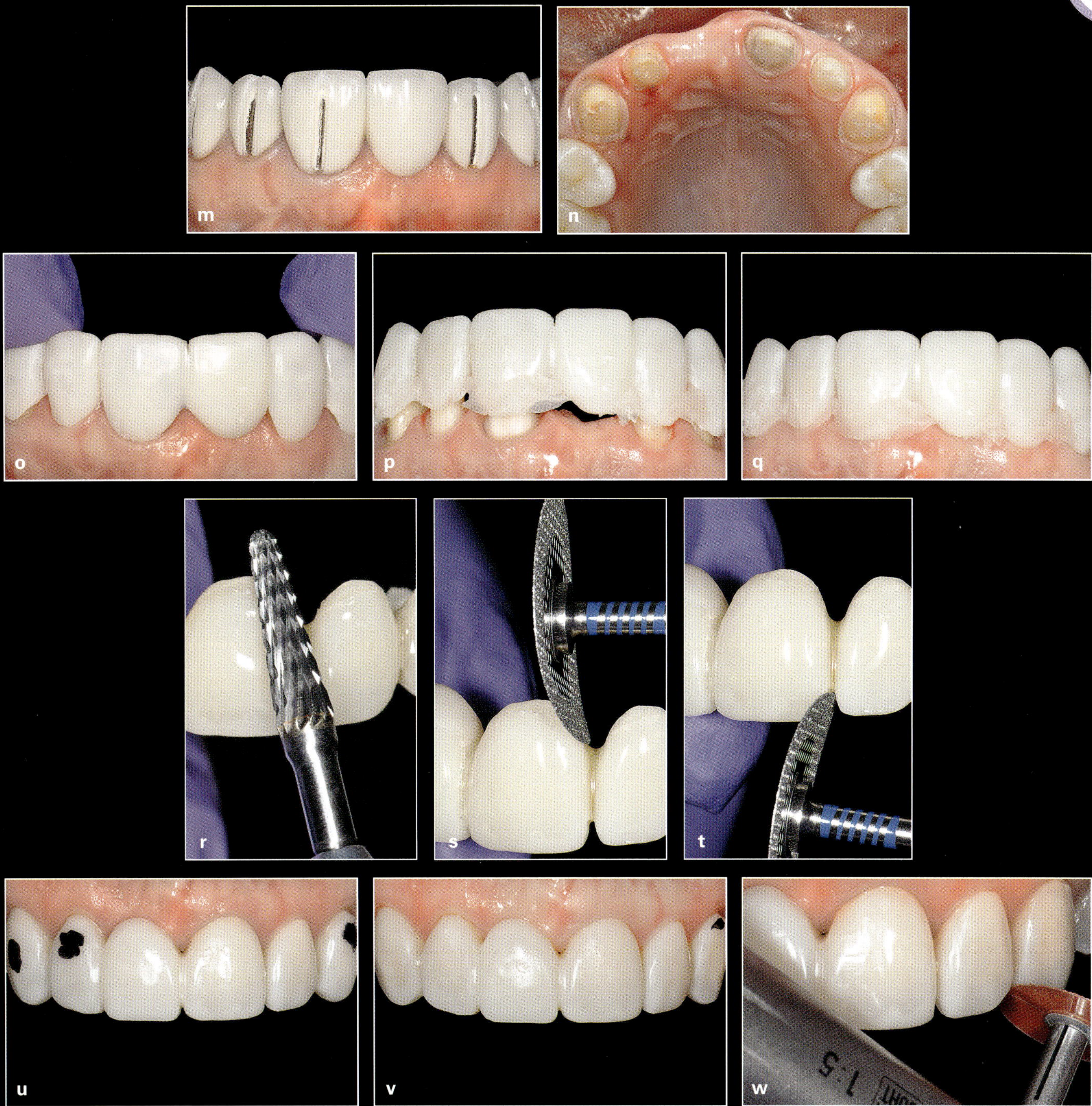

Fig 3-2 *(cont) (m and n)* The failing restorations are removed. Note the severity of the horizontal residual alveolar ridge deficiency at the pontic site. *(o)* The fit of the PRES is verified in the patient's mouth prior to commencing the reline procedure. *(p and q)* Once the reline PMMA material is applied, the provisional restoration is teased and removed (a couple of millimeters) from the finish line of the abutment teeth. The teeth are sprayed with water for lubrication and to offset the polymerization shrinkage and exothermic reaction. The fit, incisal plane, and occlusal contacts are verified. *(r)* Excess PMMA reline material at the cervical aspect is trimmed with an extra-fine carbide bur. *(s and t)* The gingival embrasures and cervical contours at the line angles as well as the incisal embrasures are trimmed with flexible, perforated diamond disks. *(u and v)* The contours and esthetics of the provisional restoration are evaluated in the patient's mouth when the patient is in an upright position. Overcontoured areas are marked with a marker and subsequently trimmed with a 12-fluted high-speed carbide bur intraorally. *(w)* Incisal edges and incisal embrasures may be adjusted with sandpaper disks.

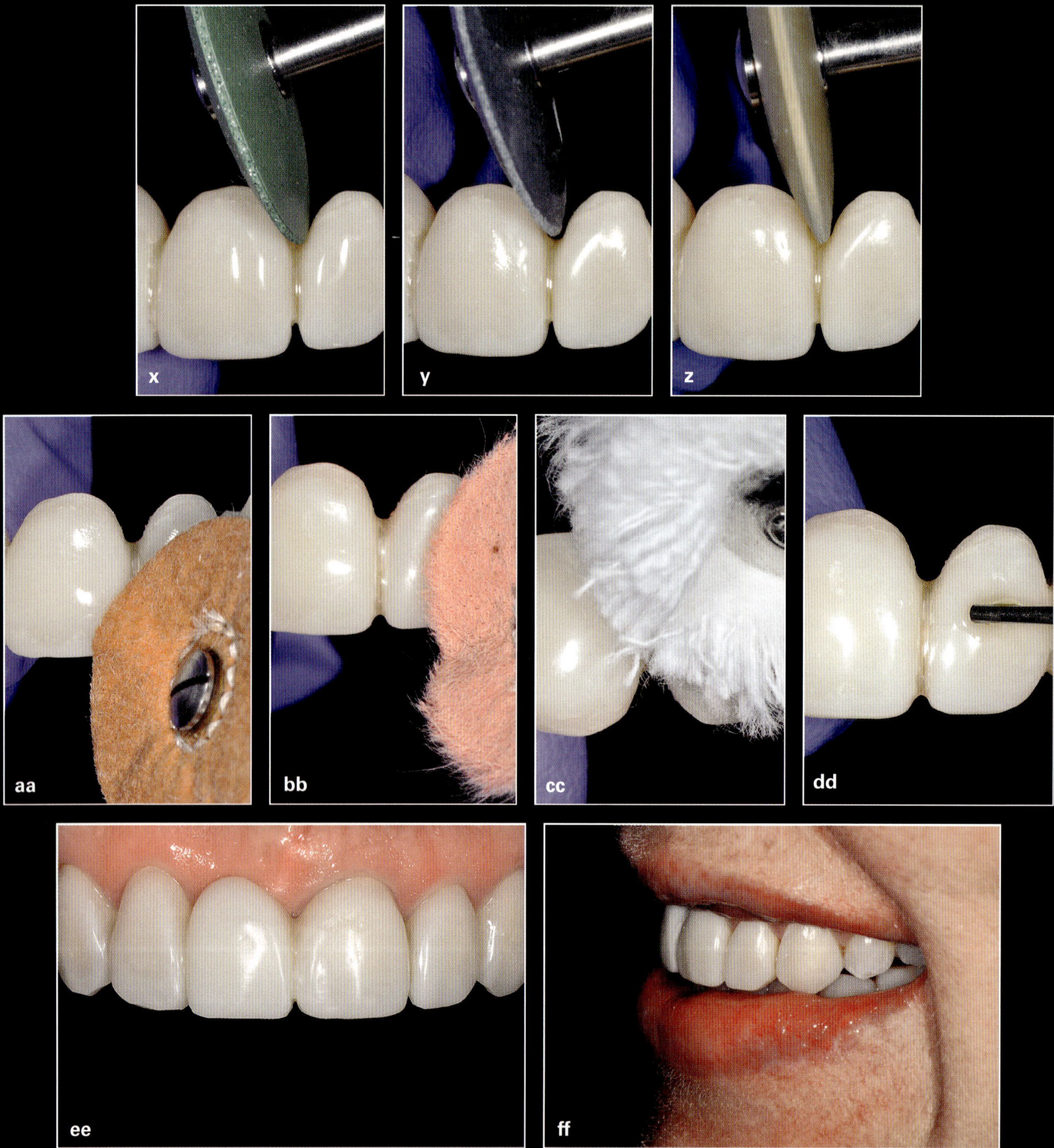

Fig 3-2 *(cont) (x to z)* Low-speed silicone polishing disks are used to polish the embrasures, whereas corresponding silicone points are used to polish all other surfaces. *(aa and bb)* Aluminum oxide–impregnated cotton buffs are used next. *(cc)* The final polished surface is achieved with a flannel or felt cloth buff impregnated with alumina-based buffing compound to provide high luster. *(dd)* Further luster is achieved with a thin coat of unfilled resin that is then light-polymerized. *(ee)* Facial view of the provisional restoration several weeks after delivery. *(ff)* Lateral view of the patient's smile demonstrating esthetic integration of the provisional restoration.

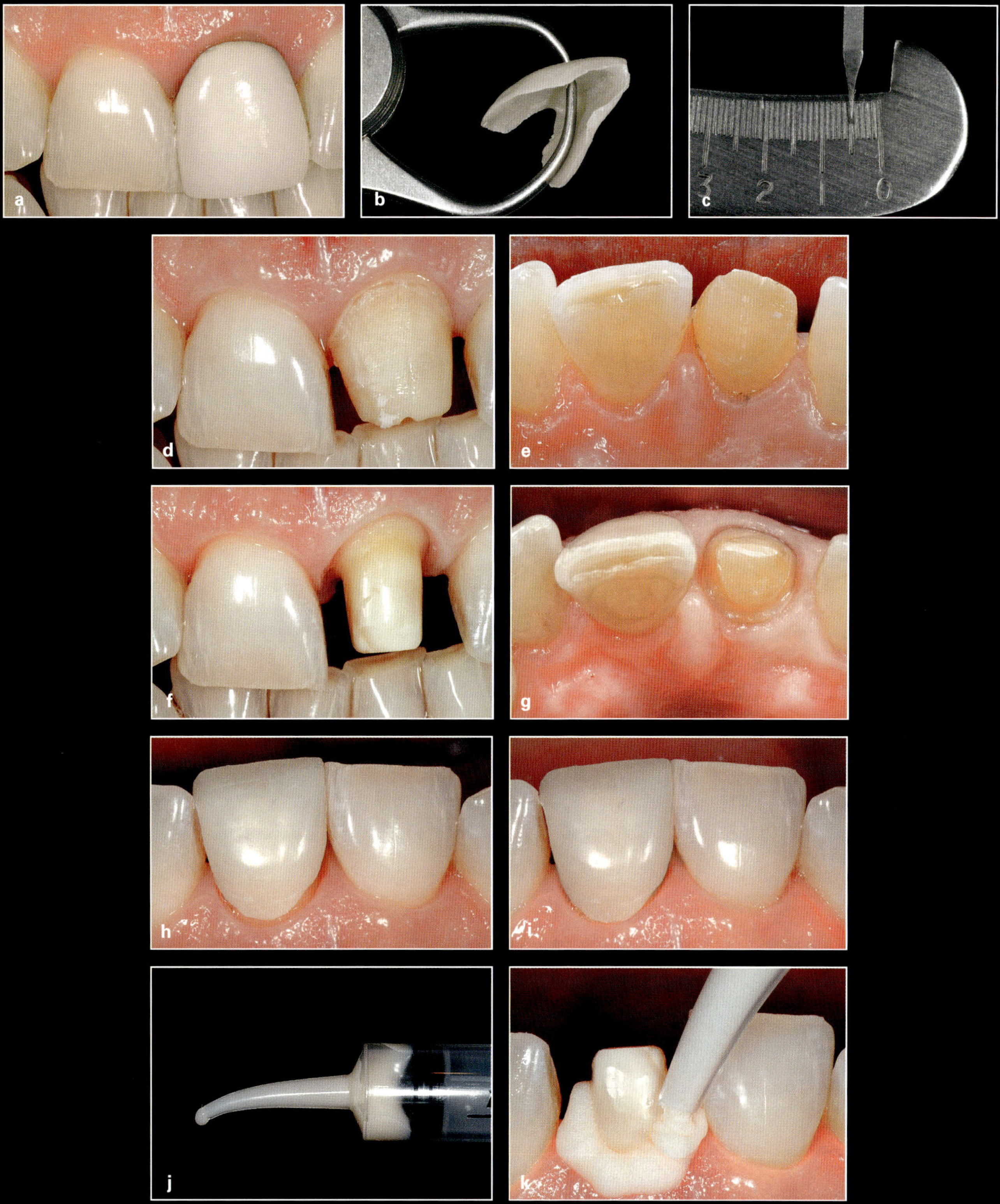

Fig 3-3 The PRES indirect-direct combination technique. *(a)* Facial view of a failing crown on the maxillary left central incisor. *(b and c)* An evaluation of the fabricated PRES demonstrates a thickness of 0.5 mm at the midfacial aspect. Also, note the open interproximal areas to facilitate adequate seating of the PRES during try-in and reline procedures. *(d and e)* Facial and occlusal views of the maxillary left central incisor after removal of the failing crown. *(f and g)* Facial and occlusal views of the maxillary left central incisor after refining the tooth preparation. *(h and i)* Views of the PRES tried in the patient's mouth. Once the interproximal contacts are slightly adjusted, the PRES is seated adequately and ready for the reline procedure. *(j and k)* The PMMA is mixed and inserted into the disposable syringe. It is injected onto the intaglio surface of the PRES. Once the luster of the mixed material is gone, the material is injected around the finish line of the tooth preparation as if a master impression of the prepared tooth is being made.

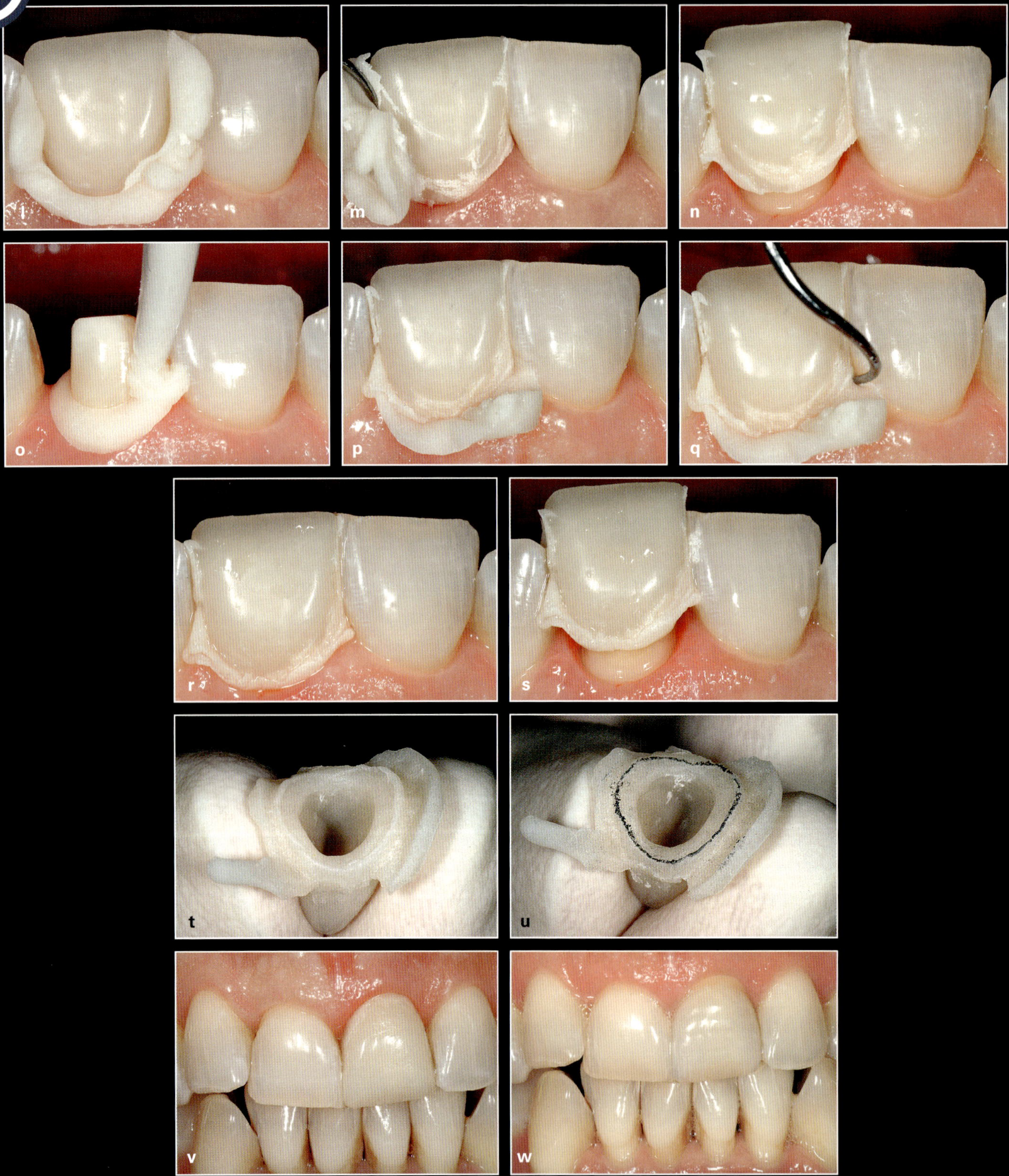

Fig 3-3 *(cont) (l to n)* Once the PRES is seated, the patient is instructed to gently close until posterior contacts are achieved. Excess PMMA is removed with an explorer. Subsequently, the provisional restoration is slightly removed from the tooth, and water is sprayed on the finish line. *(o to s)* Prior to complete setting of the first PMMA mix, a new second mix in a runny consistency is injected circumferentially on the finish line of the preparation, and the steps in parts *l* to *n* are repeated until complete polymerization of the PMMA is achieved. *(t and u)* View of the intaglio surface of the crown demonstrates the crisp and clear margin of the provisional restoration. It is marked with a sharp graphite pencil to ensure a clear reading of the margins during the excess trimming procedure. *(v)* Facial view of the provisional restoration at the completion of the procedure. Note that the mesial interproximal contours can be further adjusted and that the level of polish in the facial cervical area may be further improved. *(w)* Facial view of the definitive restoration at the 7-year follow-up. Note the gingival health.

5. Mix the bis-acryl (Protemp Plus, 3M ESPE), and lightly inject and "paint" it onto the intaglio surface of the relevant areas of the PVS impression to fabricate the cameo surface of the PRES (see Figs 3-2h and 3-2i). Bis-acryl sets much quicker and shrinks less than PMMA, hence its selection as the material of choice for the shell. When using bis-acryl as the PRES material, "paint" in no more than three to four units at a time. If more units are to be created, inject additional material into the areas of the additional units (only after the previously injected material is set), and connect the two segments at the interproximal area while relying on the presence of the oxygen-inhibited layer.
6. Gently retrieve the PRES from the PVS template, and carefully trim the intaglio surface with a super-coarse high-speed diamond bur to achieve even thickness of no more than 0.5 mm (see Fig 3-2j and Figs 3-3a to 3-3c). If the provisional restoration contains pontics for restoring missing teeth, ensure that the pontic and connector areas are hollowed as well (see Figs 3-2k and 3-2l). Consequently, once the reline procedure is complete, the connector areas are less susceptible to fracture because their bulk is made mostly of PMMA, which is less brittle. Fabricating the intaglio surface of the connectors out of PMMA will also facilitate any repairs of fractures that may occur. Ensure that the interproximal gingival areas of the PRES are open so that no internal binding in the interproximal areas prevents the placement of the PRES completely and adequately in the patient's mouth.[76]
7. If the provisional PRES is accidentally perforated, place it back into the PVS template, apply bonding agent, and light-polymerize. Then apply flowable composite resin with the corresponding shade and light-polymerize it. Afterward, remove the PRES from the PVS template.
8. Roughen the cervical third of the cameo surface of the PRES either with airborne-particle abrasion or with a coarse, high-speed diamond bur.

After tooth preparation

The following procedures are performed after the teeth to be restored have been prepared for complete-coverage restorations:

1. Prepare the abutment teeth with the aid of a clear vacuum-formed preparation guide as described in chapter 2 (see Figs 3-2m and 3-2n and Figs 3-3d to 3-3g).
2. Try in the PRES in the patient's mouth to confirm its complete seating and fit (see Fig 3-2o). Carefully assess—either tactilely or with a silicone disclosing agent (Fit Checker, GC America)—any areas of internal binding. Make adjustments to the intaglio surface of the PRES as needed (see Figs 3-3h and 3-3i). If the patient's occlusal scheme is maintained, have the patient gently occlude to ensure that other teeth are in contact with the PRES in place, thus facilitating control of the occlusion prior to starting the procedure.
3. Once adequate seating of the PRES is verified, use a microbrush to paint the abutment teeth with a thin layer of petroleum jelly (Vaseline).
4. Paint the intaglio surface and the cervical third of the cameo surface of the PRES with monomer to facilitate retention to the reline material.
5. Prepare a disposable plastic syringe with a curved tip. For extensive cases, use Monoject 412 curved-tip syringe (Tyco/Healthcare-Kendall). For limited cases, use the 1.2-mL syringe with black minitip (Ultradent). Cut off 4 to 5 mm of the tip of the nozzle of the Monoject syringe to ensure a larger diameter at the tip.
6. Have the dental assistant mix the PMMA powder and liquid. Load a runny mix of PMMA into the disposable syringe (see Fig 3-3j), and then inject the PMMA onto the intaglio surface of the PRES. Once the initial gloss of the PMMA disappears from the intaglio surface of the PRES, carefully inject the same PMMA mix onto the finish line of the abutment teeth in a similar manner to injecting a light-body impression material to capture the finish line while making a master impression[79] (see Fig 3-3k).
7. Position the PRES (loaded with the PMMA) in the patient's mouth at the level of the predetermined incisal and occlusal plane. Have the patient bite down to control the occlusion (if the occlusal scheme is to remain the same); otherwise, hold the PRES in place using an index based on the newly planned occlusal scheme (see Fig 3-3l).
8. Remove the PMMA excess with a sickle-shaped dental explorer. With this approach, excess material, esthetic orientation, and the occlusion can all be controlled during the same procedure (see Fig 3-3m).
9. Slightly tease and remove (by a couple of millimeters) the provisional restoration from the finish line of the abutment teeth, spray water on the finish line, and reposition the provisional restoration after a few seconds[77] (see Fig 3-3n). Perform this procedure several times to offset the polymerization shrinkage and for lubrication. Keep spraying the tooth and the provisional restoration at the cervical areas with water to eliminate the thermal effect on the pulp and the surrounding soft tissue.[84]
10. At the same time, have the dental assistant mix a second very runny PMMA mix and place it in a new disposable syringe. As the first reline material reaches the doughy stage on the tissue surface, remove the provisional restoration and dispense the second PMMA runny mix onto the finish line of the tooth preparations exclusively to capture the finish line in detail, with the purpose of generating a crisp margin in the provisional restoration (see Fig 3-3o). Remove excess material with a dental explorer and repeat step 9 (see Figs 3-3p to 3-3s). Have the patient continue closing until adequate occlusal contacts are achieved to minimize subsequent

occlusal adjustment, which could compromise the occlusal anatomy generated in the diagnostic wax-up used for the fabrication of the PRES (see Figs 3-2p and 3-2q).

11. Once definitive polymerization is achieved, retrieve the provisional restoration from the patient's mouth. Identify and mark the crisp definitive margin of the provisional restoration with graphite pencil (see Figs 3-3t and 3-3u).
12. Once a clear reading of the margins is achieved, trim the excess material with a carbide bur (H79EF, Brasseler USA) (see Fig 3-2r). Use flexible perforated diamond disks (Visionflex, Brasseler USA) to trim any excess interproximally. These disks facilitate control of the gingival embrasures and cervical contours at the line angles as well as the incisal embrasures (allowing for clear vision of the gingival embrasures while flexing and adjusting the disk to the desired contours) (see Figs 3-2s and 3-2t).
13. Reposition the provisional restoration on the prepared teeth, and reassess the marginal integrity, proper contours, and proper proximal and occlusal contacts.
14. If a small area of inadequate marginal integrity is detected, use a small-diameter sable brush to pick up PMMA monomer and powder, and add it to that specific area of the margin exclusively.[85] It is critical for the patient to bite down while the material polymerizes. Overcontour that area of the margin and continue applying monomer to address concerns of porosity. Remove the provisional restoration from the patient's mouth and trim it to ideal contours once polymerization is complete.
15. Face the patient and evaluate the esthetics when the patient is in an upright position. Manage the facial contours with a 12-fluted high-speed carbide bur (H375R-012 or -014, Brasseler USA) (see Figs 3-2u and 3-2v), and trim the incisal edges with sandpaper disks (Sof-Lex, 3M ESPE) as needed (see Fig 3-2w). Individualize the provisional restorations by accenting the line angles and interproximal facial areas and by opening incisal embrasures with a diamond disk using a straight, low-speed handpiece.
16. During the initial polishing procedures, the cameo surface of the provisional restoration should be polished sequentially by using low-speed polishing silicones and brushes (green [coarse], black [medium], and yellow [fine] AcrylPro disks/points; Soft Abbot-Robinson polishing brushes, Brasseler USA) (see Figs 3-2x to 3-2z).
17. Continue polishing with aluminum oxide–impregnated cotton buffs (orange and pink ProviPro Polishers, Brasseler USA) (see Figs 3-2aa and 3-2bb) and subsequently with a flannel or a felt cloth buff impregnated with alumina-based buffing compound (Fabulustre, Grobet USA) to provide high luster (Fig 3-2cc).
18. The provisional restoration may be further characterized using stains such as ceramic external stain powders mixed with unfilled resin (eg, PermaSeal, Ultradent; Palaseal, Heraeus Kulzer; Optiglaze, GC America). Any stain must be light-polymerized (see Figs 3-2dd to 3-2ff and Figs 3-3v and 3-3w).

Managing ovate pontic sites

In those clinical scenarios in which a patient must undergo soft tissue ridge augmentation for the management of an ovate pontic site, the following steps may be taken (Fig 3-4):

1. On the day of ridge augmentation, shorten the intaglio surface of the pontic of the provisional restoration to allow for a space between the augmented soft tissue and the pontic. This will prevent the creation of pressure from the pontic to the pontic site that may compromise the healing of the augmented pontic site (see Figs 3-4a to 3-4e).
2. After 3 months, once healing is complete, remove the provisional restoration from the patient's mouth (see Figs 3-4f and 3-4g).
3. Anesthetize the patient, and sound to the bone at the pontic site in a vertical direction to assess the distance between the pontic site and the underlying bone (see Figs 3-4h and 3-4i).
4. Subsequently, use a football-shaped, super-coarse, high-speed diamond bur and trim the tissue to an ovate pontic site shape. Manage any bleeding that occurs by blotting the site with a microbrush impregnated with 25% aluminum chloride hemostatic agent (ViscoStat Clear, Ultradent) (see Figs 3-4j and 3-4k). While trimming the soft tissue in an apicocoronal direction, stay slightly coronal of the ideal gingival level of the pontic site and trim the soft tissue 0.5 to 1.0 mm shy of the ideal gingival level (see Figs 3-4l and 3-4m).
5. Clean the provisional restoration of any residual temporary cement.
6. Roughen the intaglio surface of the pontic with a super-coarse, high-speed diamond bur (see Fig 3-4n). Then apply a bonding agent (Scotchbond Universal) and light-polymerize it (see Figs 3-4o and 3-4p).
7. Follow with the application of direct composite resin restorative material in increments as needed (Filtek Supreme). Mold the material to a convex contour with composite resin hand instruments as needed to the desired ovate pontic shape, and light-polymerize it (see Figs 3-4q to 3-4s).
8. Try in the provisional restoration in the patient's mouth and assess the seating for marginal integrity and soft tissue response and contours. Expect to experience blanching at the pontic site due to pressure created by the provisional restoration. If the margins are still open and the blanching does not disappear within 10 to 15 minutes, readjust the contours of the provisional ovate pontic until the desired marginal integrity is achieved and the soft tissue contours are close to adequate (see Figs 3-4t and 3-4u). No blanching indicates the likelihood that the tissue at the pontic site will adapt rather than creating a pressure point, which may cause tissue necrosis and/or a recession (see Figs 3-4v and 3-4w).

Continued from page 56

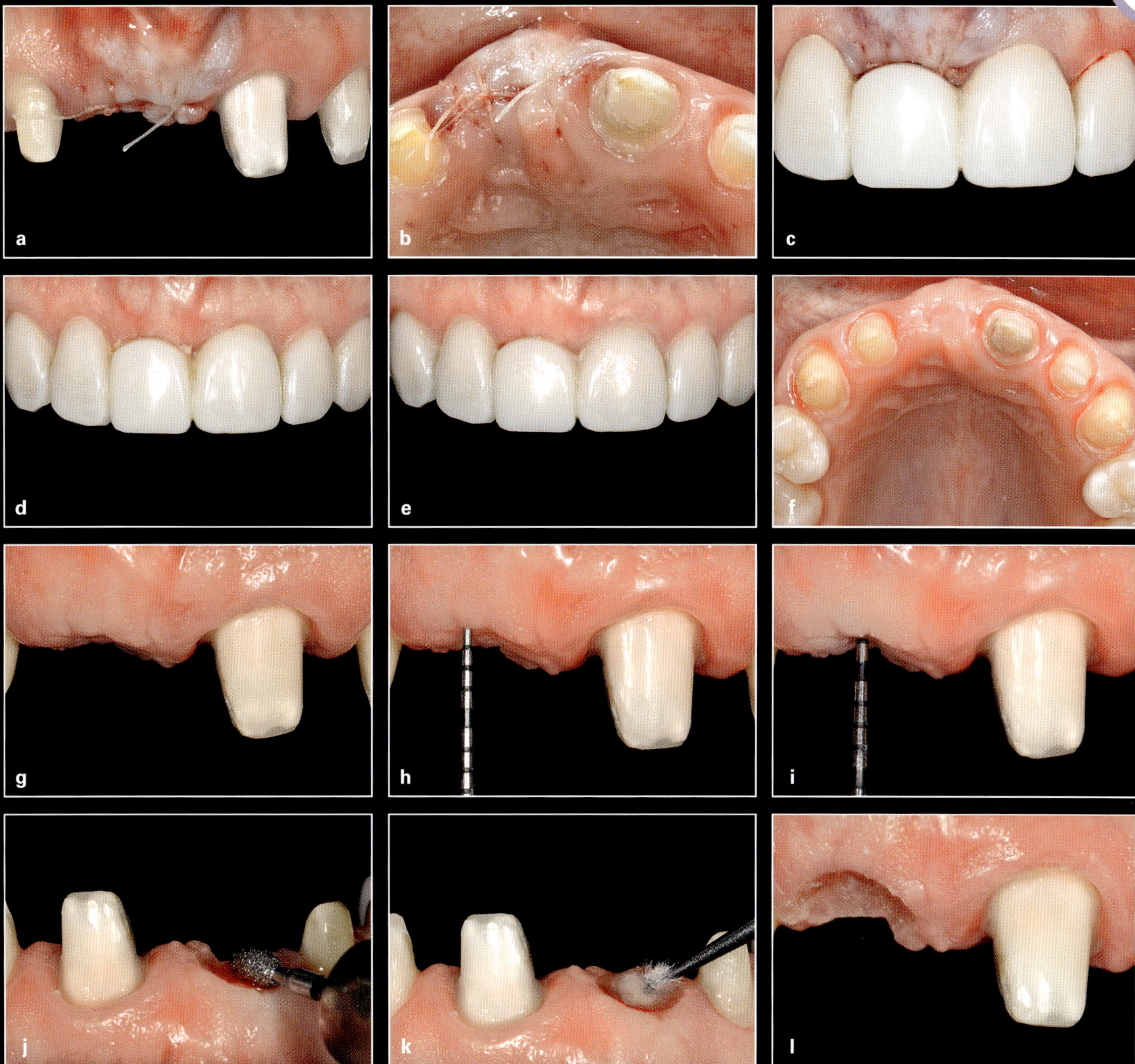

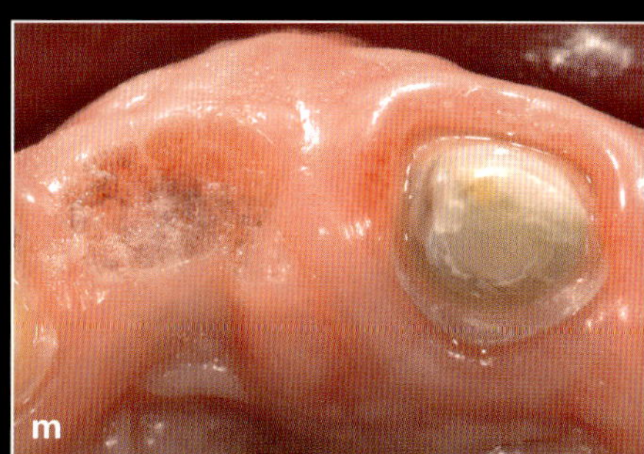

Fig 3-4 *(a and b)* Soft tissue augmentation of the residual alveolar ridge was performed using acellular dermal matrix to eliminate the horizontal ridge deficiency at the pontic site. *(c)* The pontic was shortened at the cervical aspect to eliminate pressure at the augmented site, and the provisional restoration was delivered. *(d and e)* Facial views of the provisional restoration 4 weeks and 4 months after surgery, respectively. *(f and g)* Occlusal and facial views of the pontic site once healed 4 months after surgery. *(h and i)* Vertical bone sounding is performed to assess the distance between the anesthetized pontic site and the underlying bone. *(j and k)* The ovate pontic site is trimmed with a football-shaped, super-coarse, high-speed diamond bur, and the heme is managed by blotting the site with a microbrush impregnated with a hemostatic agent . *(l and m)* Facial and occlusal views of the pontic site after control of the heme has been achieved.

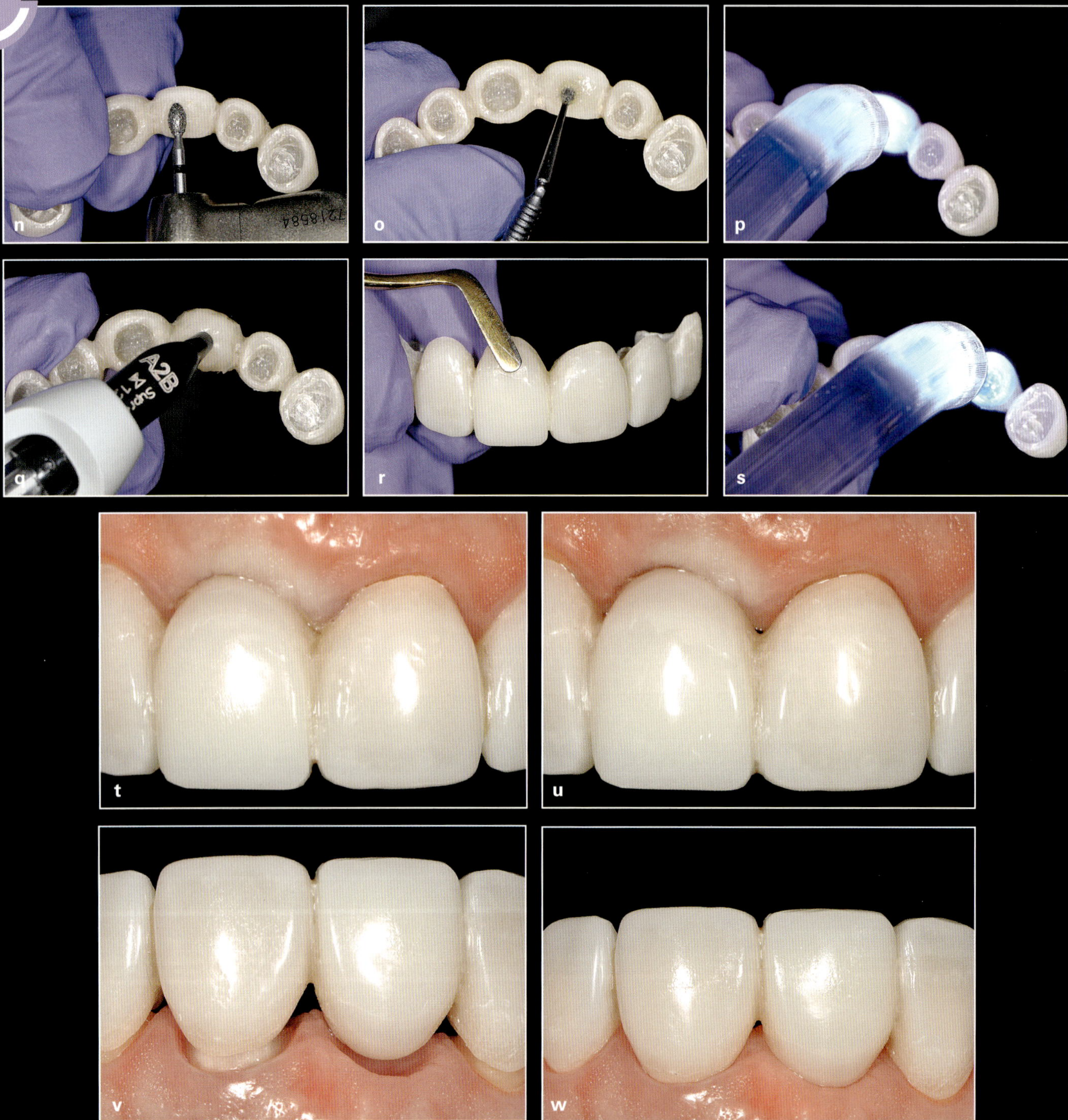

Fig 3-4 *(cont) (n)* The intaglio surface of the pontic is roughened with a super-coarse, high-speed diamond bur. *(o and p)* A bonding agent is applied to the intaglio surface of the pontic and light-polymerized. *(q to s)* Direct composite resin restorative material is applied in increments to the intaglio surface of the pontic and to the cervical facial aspect. It is then shaped to the convex desired contours with composite resin hand instruments and light-polymerized. *(t and u)* The modified provisional restoration with the augmented pontic is evaluated in the patient's mouth and assessed for marginal integrity and soft tissue response and contours. The transient blanching and the compromised seating of the provisional restoration prompt additional adjustment of the pontic. *(v and w)* Facial views of the pontic and pontic site 2 months after final adjustment of the pontic, demonstrating the complete adjustment and healing of the soft tissue and the complete seating of the restorations.

Box 3-4 Advantages and limitations of the PRES indirect-direct combination technique

Advantages:
- Incorporates advantages of both materials
  - Bis-acryl: strength, polishability, wear resistance, color stability, and esthetics
  - PMMAs: reline and repair capabilities, flexural strength and flexibility (allowing easy removal with a less than ideal path of draw), and lack of brittleness
- Relatively esthetic and functional
- Accurate transfer of wax-up to the mouth in terms of length, angulation, shape, surface texture, and occlusion
- Maintains and may serve to enhance the health of the soft tissue
- May be used long-term
- May be removed with minimal trauma to the hard and soft tissues
- The matrix may be easily reused when needed

Limitations:
- Technique sensitive depending on the complexity of the case and the experience of the operator
- Has a learning curve and is time-consuming
- More complex for long-span provisional restorations (for up to three units with a path of draw, reline with bis-GMA or bis-acryl material; for four or more units, reline with PMMA)

9. Next, polish the modified provisional restoration and recement it in place, ensuring complete excess cement removal.
10. Reassess the provisional restoration 2 to 3 weeks after cementation, and make further adjustments to the provisional restoration at the pontic site as needed.
11. Once the ideal convex pontic contours have been achieved and the patient has reported comfort and ability to maintain oral hygiene at the pontic site, leave the provisional restoration in place and allow the soft tissue to stabilize for 3 months[10,29,86] (as discussed in chapter 1).

Summary

Although it has a learning curve, the PRES indirect-direct combination technique incorporates the advantages of two materials—bis-acryl composite resin and PMMA—creating a synergistic effect (Box 3-4). From a clinical perspective, the polishability, wear resistance, color stability, and esthetics achieved with the bis-acryl materials, in conjunction with the ability to reline and achieve excellent marginal integrity while maintaining excellent repair capabilities of PMMAs, provide clinicians with an opportunity to offer their patients an esthetic and functional vision of the definitive outcome. Such restorations can be utilized long-term, if needed, while maintaining excellent soft tissue health. In addition, the procedure is relatively cost-effective compared with the indirect technique and can be managed and performed in the restorative dental practice with limited laboratory support.

In extensive patient care, the technique allows an accurate transfer of the restoration design (as proposed in the diagnostic wax-up) from the cast to the patient's mouth and enhances control of the occlusion from the initial steps of the procedure (Figs 3-5a to 3-5l). During the reline procedure, it is recommended to use indexes made out of PVS, thermoplastic templates, or resins to facilitate the maintenance of ideal incisal and occlusal planes, the desired vertical dimension of occlusion, and the desired occlusal scheme (Figs 3-5m to 3-5o). The exposed cervical contours of the PRES facilitate a relatively easy removal of excess reline material prior to the material's complete setting (Fig 3-5p). The controlled amount of the reline PMMA material reduces the thermal trauma to the pulp and the surrounding soft tissue. Following the finishing and polishing procedures, the interface between the PMMA and the bis-acryl blends very well (Figs 3-5q to 3-5u).

The main goal of such a procedure should be the construction of a properly contoured and well-fitting provisional restoration that maintains its integrity throughout a reasonable time frame from tooth preparation to completion of definitive treatment while maintaining and facilitating health of the soft tissue. It is the author's opinion that by controlling the cervical contours as designed in the diagnostic wax-up and by practically making an impression of the finish line with PMMA using the curved disposable syringe, excellent margins and contours may be achieved. This may reduce the likelihood of the patient developing secondary caries and may enhance the health of the supporting tissues.

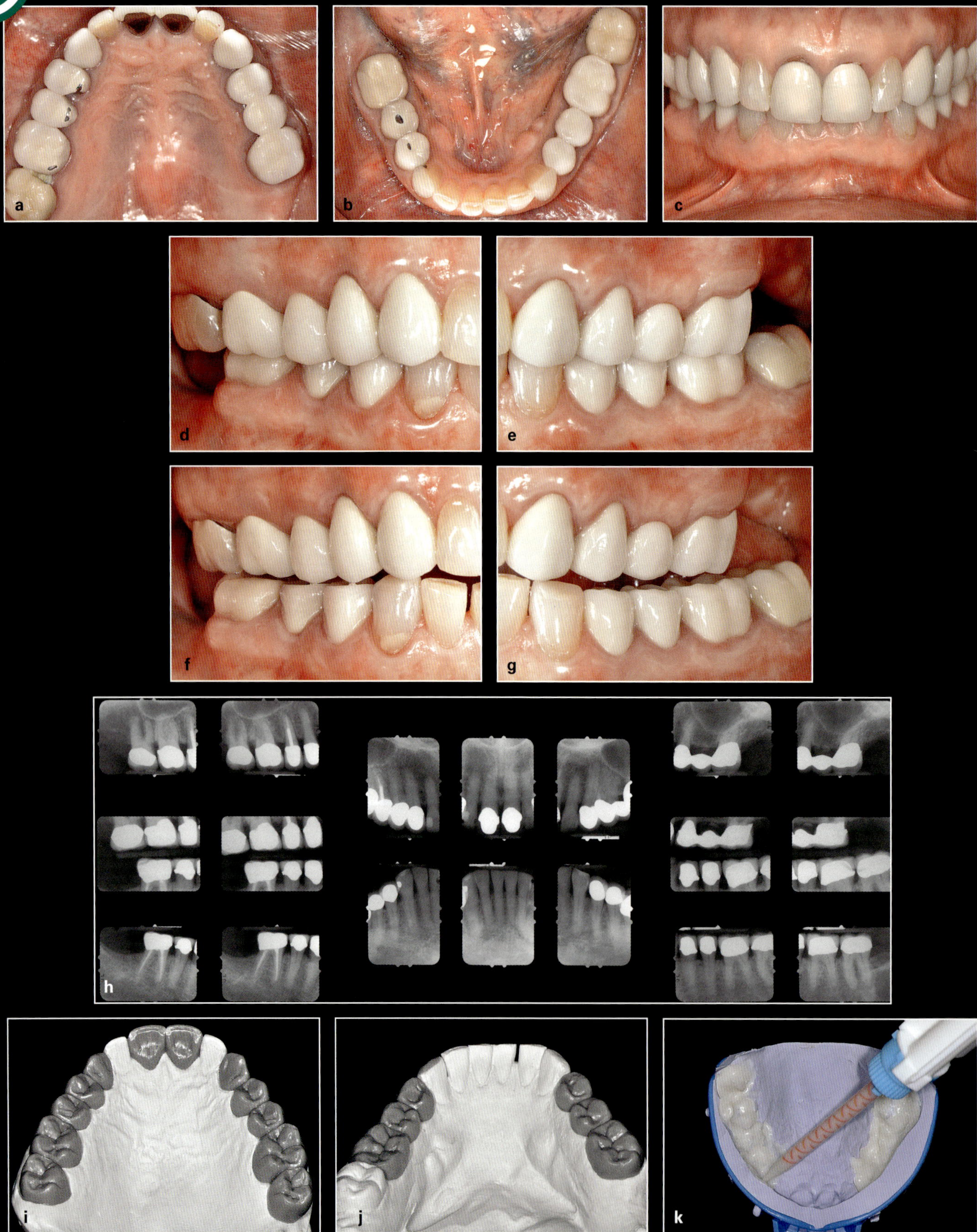

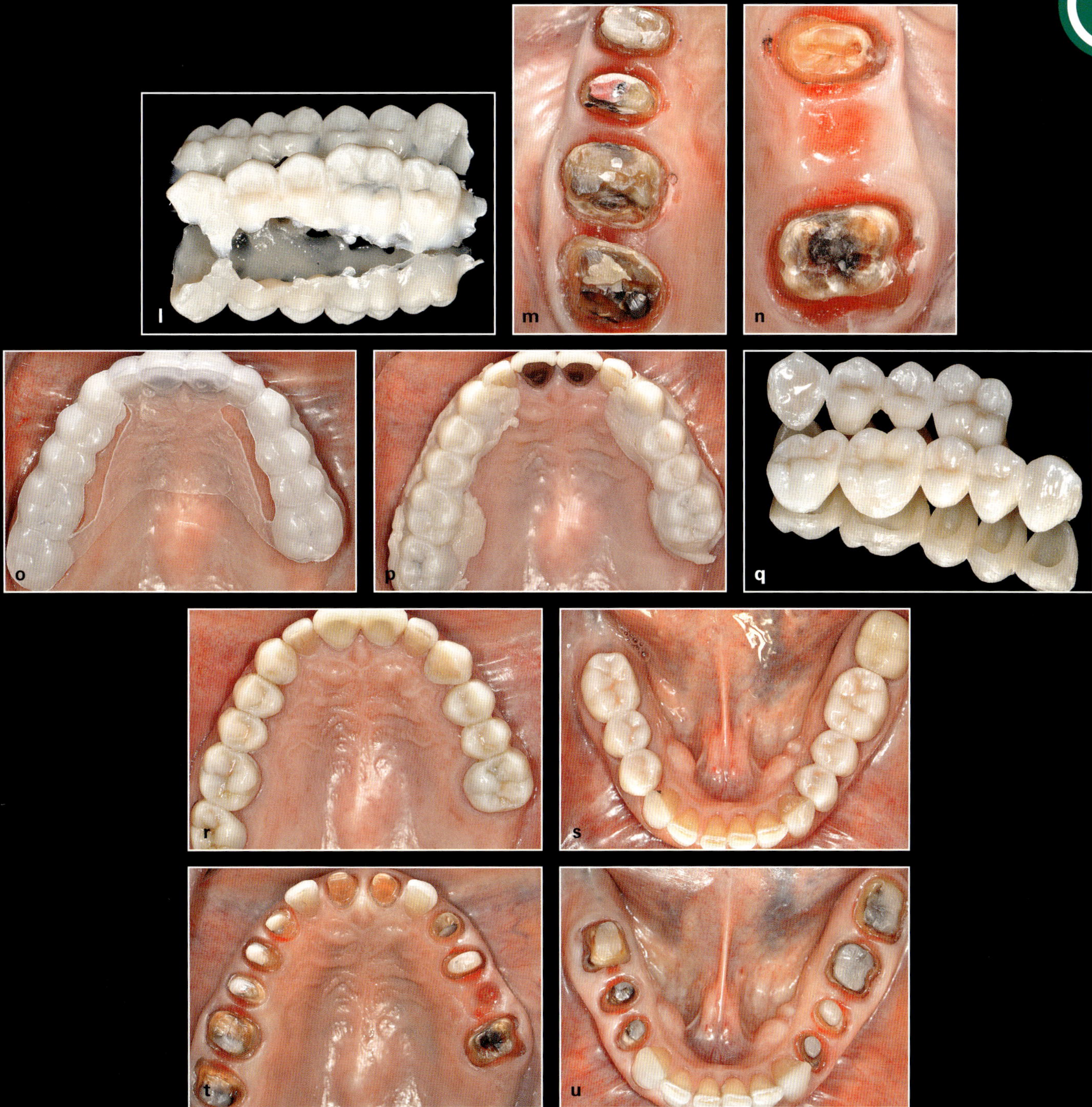

Fig 3-5 *(a and b)* Preoperative maxillary and mandibular occlusal views of a patient with a failing complete-mouth rehabilitation. Note the wear presented in the dentition and restorations and the porcelain fractures on the maxillary right posterior crowns. *(c)* Preoperative facial view of the patient in maximal intercuspal position. Note the color-match discrepancies of the restorations with the remaining dentition and the recession at the maxillary central incisors. *(d and e)* Right and left lateral views of the patient's dentition in maximal intercuspal position. *(f and g)* Right and left lateral views of the patient's dentition in lateral excursions. The patient presented with bilateral initial group function occlusion transitioning to canine guidance. *(h)* Complete-mouth periapical radiographs. *(i and j)* Occlusal views of the maxillary and mandibular wax-ups, which were later duplicated in dental stone. (Note that the mandibular left second molar was not restored.) Impressions of the duplicate casts were made with an alginate substitute. *(k)* View of the maxillary impression of the duplicate cast in the process of being injected with bisacryl material for the fabrication of the posterior PRES. *(l)* View of the maxillary posterior PRES immediately after removal from the impression. *(m and n)* Occlusal views of the maxillary posterior teeth after removal of the failing restorations. *(o)* A thermoplastic template made from the duplicate cast of the diagnostic wax-up is used as an index for seating the PRES during the reline procedure while maintaining an ideal occlusal plane at the desired vertical dimension of occlusion. Note the seating of the PRES in the template and the palatal windows in the template, which are used to facilitate the removal of excess reline material prior to its complete polymerization. *(p)* Occlusal view of the maxillary arch once complete polymerization of the reline PMMA material has been achieved. *(q)* The provisional restorations have been trimmed, polished, and stained. They were further characterized using ceramic external stain powders mixed with unfilled resin, which was then light-polymerized. *(r and s)* Occlusal views of the maxillary and mandibular provisional restorations. *(t and u)* Occlusal views of the finalized tooth preparations prior to making master impressions.

Cementation

Several types of temporary cements are available for cementing such provisional restorations. Some are resin based and are translucent (tooth-colored) to facilitate the esthetic outcome and reduce the likelihood of an extremely opaque provisional restoration. Other cements are white and opaque with zinc oxide as the main ingredient, with or without eugenol. It is the author's opinion that the temporary cement of choice should be easily used without compromising the integrity of the soft tissue or of the provisional restoration. Temporary cement must be clinically visible for ease of cleaning and excess cement removal, and it should be easily removed. In addition, it should contain no eugenol, because eugenol not only may compromise prospective bonding procedures but will also cause disintegration of PMMA, thus eliminating the ability to repair, add, or reline at areas of the provisional restoration made of PMMA and in contact with the cement.[87,88] Therefore, zinc oxide–based white and opaque temporary cements that can be easily cleaned and contain no eugenol are recommended for simplified clinical use. Removal of the provisional restoration cemented with such cements may be easily performed in an atraumatic manner for the abutment teeth, the soft tissue, and the provisional restoration with the use of a curved hemostat or with special pliers (KY Pliers, GC America).[5] Once the provisional restoration is removed, clinicians may assess the presence of cement wash (Figs 3-6a to 3-6c) as well as measure the thickness of the complete provisional restoration with the cement still attached to the intaglio surface to ensure adequate space for the definitive restorative materials (Figs 3-6d to 3-6f).

Recent studies evaluated some of the zinc-oxide eugenol-free temporary cements and demonstrated their antibacterial activity.[89] The antibacterial capability of zinc oxide–based temporary cements can be further enhanced by mixing them with fluoride (in particular with sodium fluoride [NaF]); this antibacterial activity may last for up to 6 months[90] without compromising the tensile strength of the cement (eg, RelyX Temp, 3M ESPE).[89] Such an approach may facilitate caries prevention during the provisional phase, especially in patients who are at high risk for dental caries[91] or who are in need of a longer-term provisional restoration due to surgical or functional considerations.

Continued from page 62

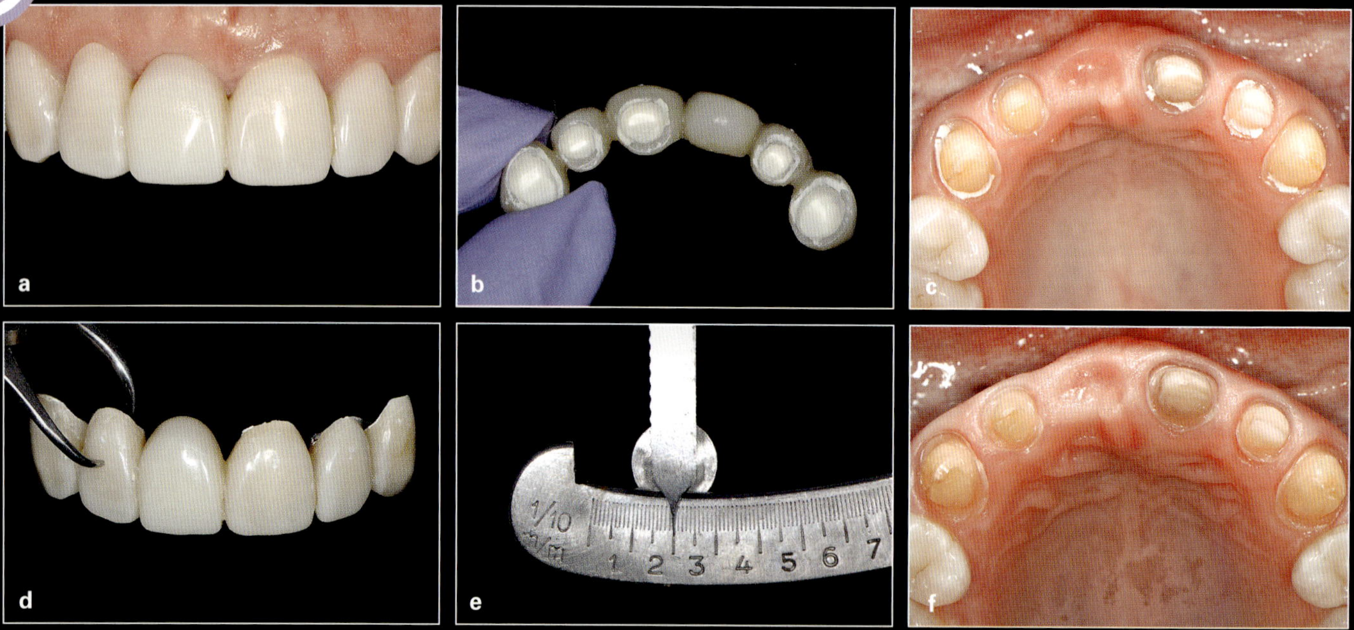

Fig 3-6 *(a)* Facial view of the provisional restoration 9 months after its initial delivery. Note the integration of the pontic with the pontic site. *(b and c)* Views of the intaglio surface of the provisional restoration and of the prepared teeth, demonstrating no cement wash. *(d and e)* The thickness of the complete provisional restoration is measured with a caliper while the temporary cement is still attached to its intaglio surface to ensure that adequate thickness may be achieved for the definitive restorative materials. *(f)* Occlusal view of the final tooth preparations and the matured and healed soft tissue prior to impression making.

Procedures for CAD/CAM Provisional Restorations

The application of CAD/CAM technology for the fabrication of definitive restorations has been growing rapidly with the increased demand for esthetics as well as efficiency. Currently, precision-milled, high-density acrylate polymer provisional restorations have become available. Traditional techniques for fabricating provisional restorations use either a powder and liquid system as with PMMA or a paste-paste system as with bis-acryl resin and other materials.[42] The polymerization of these materials under various uncontrolled conditions may cause porosity and lack of homogeneity, which may compromise durability and esthetics, causing discoloration, wear, and inferior cameo surface polish.[42]

CAD/CAM provisional restorations are milled from uniform, high-density resin blocks composed mainly of either PMMA or bis-GMA[42,58] (Table 3-1). The machinable resin blocks are fabricated under ideal industrial conditions to optimize their mechanical and physical properties.[92,93] Provisional restorations made out of the strengthened, highly cross-linked homogenous PMMA blocks can be used as long-term provisional restorations in extensive and complex rehabilitation cases while serving as a diagnostic tool for managing wear and occlusal conditions.[42] In addition, the milling process of a completely polymerized resin block eliminates the concerns of dimensional changes that accompany polymerization of similar materials used with traditional techniques. The CAM precision process enhances the physical properties, dimensional stability, and marginal integrity (if an indirect approach is used) of the provisional restorations while also allowing the fabrication of a CAD/CAM PRES with a thickness as thin as 0.3 mm, which can be used with the indirect-direct combination technique.[59] With their enhanced mechanical properties, such materials may be used as long-term provisional restorations, and because esthetics may be of importance in such clinical scenarios, the high range of translucency offered by different high-density polymers may provide an additional advantage.[94]

Chairside CAD/CAM systems provide an alternative convenient solution for designing and milling provisional restorations in a single clinical appointment for relatively small-scale, simple restorations.[3,95] However, to justify the initial high cost of such systems and the need for special training of the operators, the system must be used with high frequency for other definitive treatment modalities in the dental practice. For extensive and complex patient treatment, laboratory-based CAD/CAM systems provide a more efficient solution due to superior scanning and milling capabilities and better efficiency. One must remember, however, that the collaboration between clinicians and dental technicians across all phases of restoration design is a crucial step in achieving provisional restorations with optimal quality.

As with traditional techniques, a prerequisite for the fabrication of a CAD/CAM-based provisional restoration with the desired attributes is the fabrication of a diagnostic wax-up based on data collected during the diagnostic phase of therapy, with the goal of creating a blueprint for a durable, functional, and esthetic restoration. The diagnostic wax-up is scanned to provide the cameo, axial, and occlusal contours of the prospective restorations and the surrounding structures to the CAD unit.

With the indirect approach, laboratory-based CAD/CAM systems may enhance the fabrication of provisional restorations that fit the tooth preparations with minimal to no need for additional intraoral adjustments. Therefore, with this approach, a scan of the prepared teeth must be performed, or a master impression of the teeth preparations must be made, poured, and scanned (if traditional impressions are to be used) (Figs 3-7a and 3-7b). Subsequently, the digitized data of the definitive cast and the cast of a removable wax-up made on the definitive cast are to be superimposed for the fabrication of the complete provisional restoration (Figs 3-7c and 3-7d). As with any other indirect technique, such restorations exhibit excellent fit and marginal integrity (Fig 3-7e) as well as axial and occlusal cameo contours that, once delivered, easily follow the desired incisal and occlusal planes. Such an approach also eliminates the need for major modifications in terms of axial contours and occlusal surfaces and contacts as well as subsequent reline procedures. In addition, multiple individual units may be fabricated without compromising the incisal edge position and occlusal plane while allowing the patient to floss easily (Figs 3-7f to 3-7i). As previously described, the limitation of this technique is that these provisional restorations are usually delivered at the following appointment after tooth preparation and are used as a second set unless the clinician owns an in-house dental laboratory or the practice is located in close proximity to one. Another limitation is the additional cost for the fabrication of these restorations and the added chair time. A

CAD/CAM systems also allow the fabrication of a PRES that can be milled down to a minimal thickness of 0.3 mm prior to the patient's tooth preparation visit. Such CAM capability reduces the likelihood of binding to the teeth and to other oral structures while seating the PRES during the try-in and reline procedures. Following this approach, the diagnostic wax-up is duplicated, and the duplicate cast is scanned and digitized on the CAD unit to provide the cameo axial and occlusal contours of the prospective provisional restorations and the surrounding structures. Subsequently, the teeth to be treated are prepared on the same duplicate cast of the diagnostic wax-up by the dental technician and scanned. The digitized data of both scans are then superimposed for the design and fabrication of a PRES (Figs 3-8a to 3-8h). Such a PRES can be subsequently milled down to a thickness of 0.3 mm for multiple types of provisional restorations (Figs 3-8i to 3-8n). Once tried in, the PRES is relined in the patient's mouth and delivered at the day of tooth preparation as previously described with the PRES indirect-direct combination technique (Fig 3-8o). Thus, as with the traditional PRES indirect-direct combination technique, a B

Table 3-1 Overview of high-density polymers for CAD/CAM manufacturing

Trade name (manufacturer)	Indication(s)	Description	CAD/CAM system
Ambarino High-class (Creamed Creative Medizintechnik)	Definitive single-tooth restorations and FDPs, telescopic prostheses, tertiary structures, fully/partially anatomically milled restorations, milled emergence profiles, implant superstructures, and abutments	Highly cross-linked polymer blends (bis-GMA, urethane methacrylate, butanediol dimethacrylate, 70.1 wt% ceramic-type anorganic silicate glass fillers)	Micron 400 (Micron), M7 Dental (Datron); all systems with circular blank automaton holder and corresponding templates
artBloc Temp (Merz Dental)	Long-term provisionalization of crowns, partial crowns, and FDPs; immediate implant restorations	Ingot made of highly cross-linked, interpenetrated PMMA (or OMP networks)	Cerec (Sirona)
Artegral imCrown (Merz Dental)	Long-term provisionalization of single crowns in the anterior region	Semifinished blanks made of unfilled PMMA material with highly cross-linked macromolecular structure (or IPNs)	Cerec (Sirona)
CAD-Temp (Vita Zahnfabrik)	Single- and multiunit, fully and partially long-term provisional restorations with up to two pontics	High-molecular cross-linked acrylic polymer containing 14 wt% microfillers (or MRP)	
cara PMMA prov (Heraeus Kulzer)	Tooth-colored PMMA for the CAD/CAM manufacturing of provisional crowns and fixed partial dentures	PMMA and cross-linked copolymers of methacrylic acid	cara (Heraeus Kulzer)
Cercon base PMMA (Degudent)	Provisional crowns and multiunit FDPs with up to 16 units (with one pontic between the abutment teeth) for a period of clinical service of up to 6 months	PMMA and cross-linked copolymers of methacrylic acid	Cercon System (Degudent)
Everest C-Temp (KaVo)	Frameworks for provisional FDPs with veneering and with a span up to 60 mm	Glass fiber–reinforced high-density polymer as framework material	Everest (KaVo)
New Outline CAT (anaxdent)	Provisional single and FDP frameworks up to two pontics, for a period of clinical service of 3 to 12 months, relinable	PMMA and copolymers of methacrylate, n-alkyl methacrylate, and pigments	Organical (Rübeling & Klar), Open Zeno (Wieland)
Organic Composit (R+D CAD/CAM Technologie)	Approved for definitive restorations of up to three units	1.4 butanediol dimethacrylate UDMA bis-GMA	Organical (Rübeling & Klar)
Paradigm MZ 100 (3M ESPE)	Final inlays, onlays, veneers, and single crowns	Polymer consisting of bis-GMA and TEG-DMA matrix with 85 wt% zirconia microfillers	Cerec 3 (Sirona), E4D (DVD)
polycon ae (Straumann CAD/CAM)	Long-term provisional restorations, crowns, and FDPs with one pontic in the anterior and posterior region	PMMA-based acrylate resin with IPN	Straumann CAD/CAM
Telio CAD (Ivoclar Vivadent)	Long-term provisional restorations, from single-tooth restorations up to four-unit FDPs including restorations on implants	99.5% PMMA polymer	Procera (Nobel Biocare), Cerec (Sirona)
Zenotec Pro Fix (Wieland Dental)	Long-term provisional restorations, fully anatomical crowns, and FDPs up to two pontics in the anterior and posterior region	Fiber-free, homogenous, methacrylate-based acrylomer	All Zenotec (Wieland)

OMP, organic modified polymer; IPN, interpenetrated network polymer; MRP, microfiller-reinforced polyacrylic. (Reprinted from Edelhoff et al[42] with permission.)

Continued from page 52

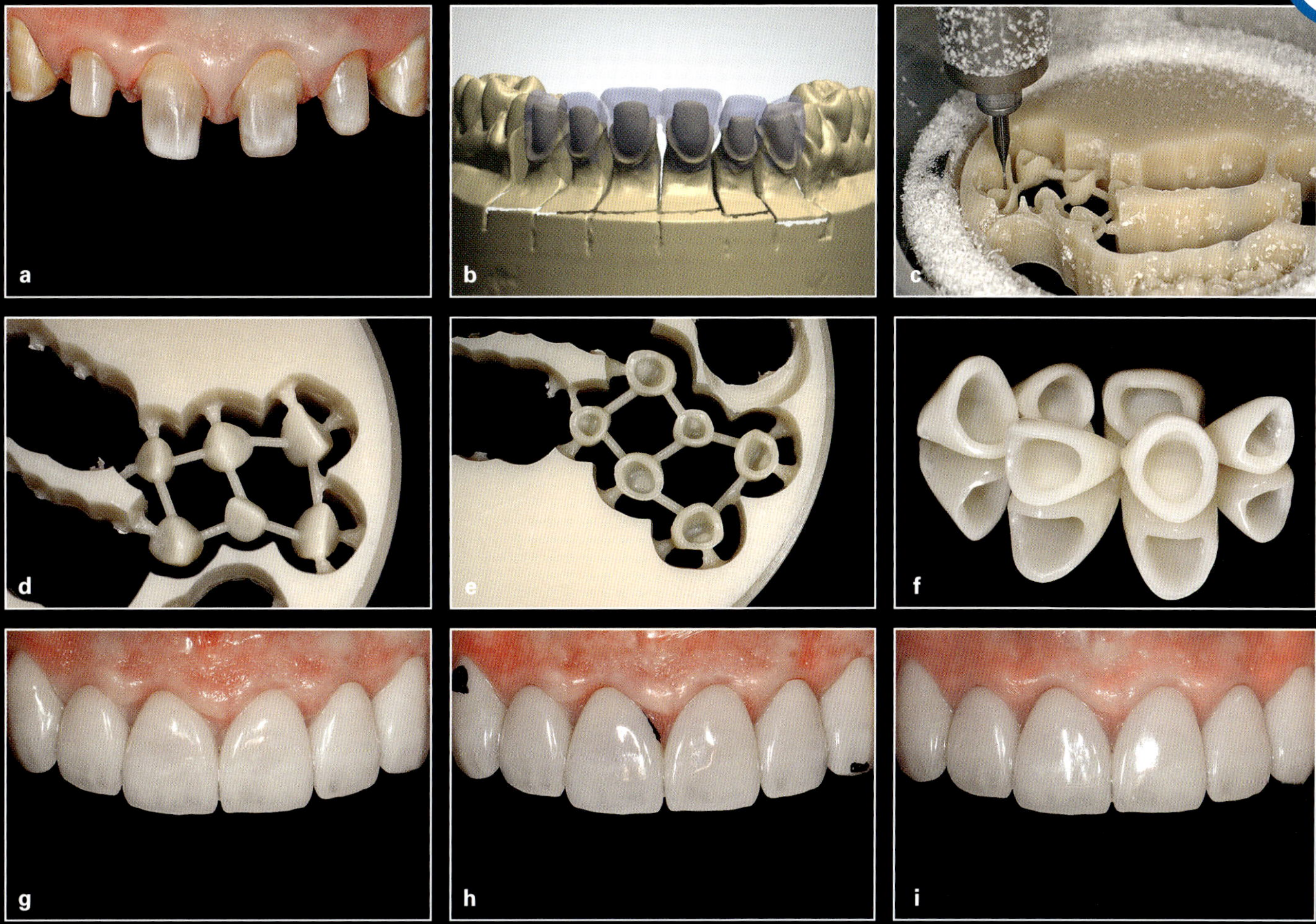

Fig 3-7 *(a)* Facial view of the final tooth preparation for zirconia-based ceramic crowns. *(b)* A master impression of the tooth preparations was made and poured. A removable wax-up was made on the definitive cast. The definitive cast was scanned with and without a complete-contour wax-up made based on the initial provisional restoration. Digitized data of the definitive cast and the diagnostic wax-up were superimposed for the fabrication of the complete provisional restorations. *(c)* The provisional restorations are milled from a block of PMMA. *(d and e)* The cameo and intaglio surfaces of the milled restorations are complete. *(f)* A view of the single-unit individual provisional crowns demonstrates well-defined margins. *(g and h)* A try-in of the provisional restorations demonstrates the need for minor cervical, interproximal, and incisal contour adjustments as marked with a black marker. *(i)* The complete individualized provisional crowns after adjustment of contours and delivery.

high-quality provisional restoration with the desired axial and occlusal cameo contours is placed in the patient's mouth immediately on the day of tooth preparation, and no second provisional restoration is usually required. The same limitations of the traditional indirect-direct combination technique arise with a CAD/CAM PRES. However, enhanced control over restoration contours with precisely digitalized images minimizes the time required for chairside adjustments. As with the PRES indirect-direct combination technique, a relatively small amount of provisional material will polymerize in contact with the prepared abutment teeth and soft tissues, resulting in decreased exothermic reaction and less polymerization shrinkage and contact between the resin monomer and the soft tissues.

B

Continued from chapter 2

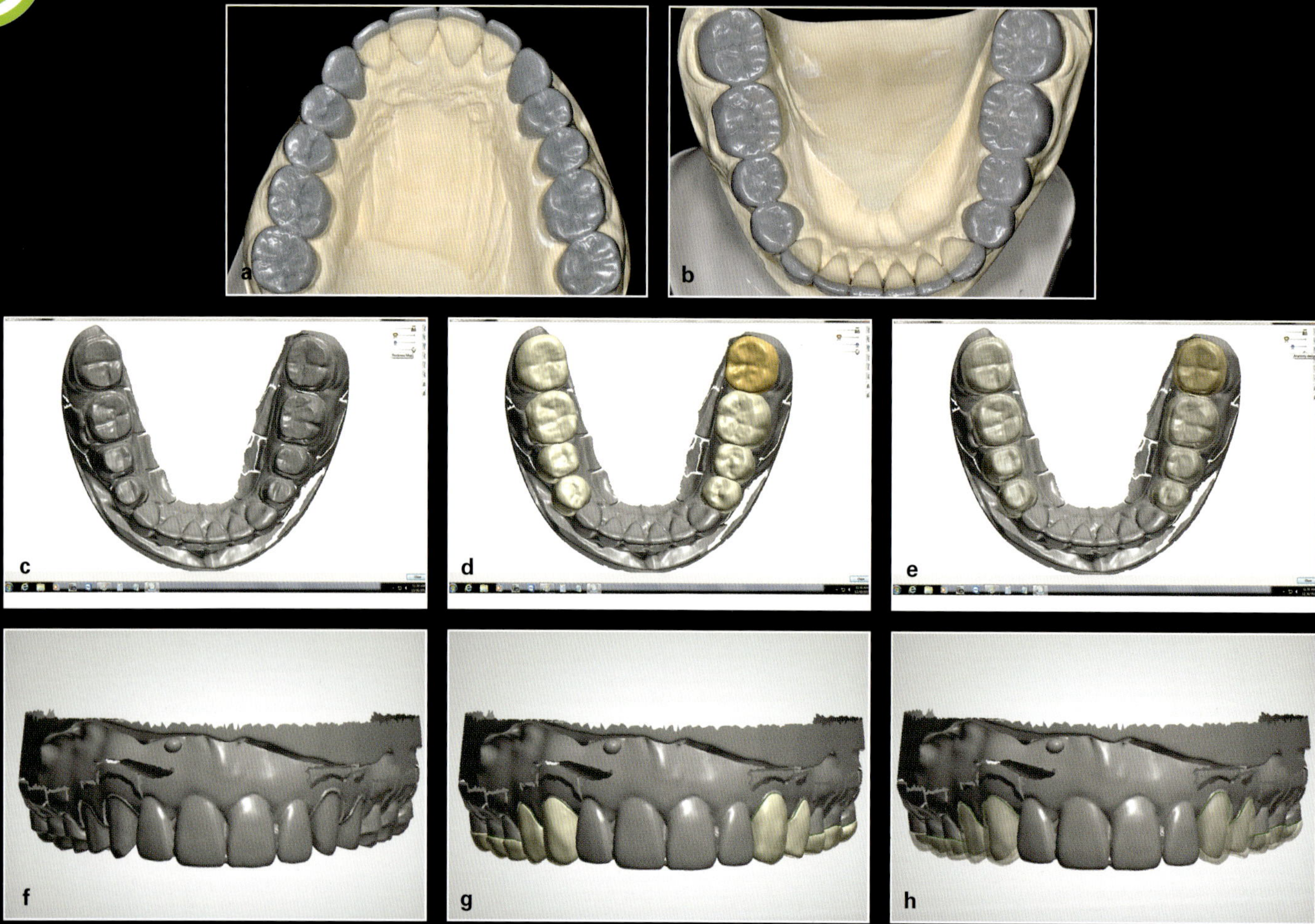

Fig 3-8 *(a and b)* Maxillary and mandibular diagnostic wax-ups. *(c to e)* A duplicate cast of the mandibular diagnostic wax-up for occlusal ceramic veneers and ceramic crowns is scanned. Subsequently, it is prepared and scanned again. Digitized data of both scans is superimposed for the fabrication of a PRES for a mandibular provisional restoration. *(e)* A semitranslucent view demonstrating the relationship between the prepped teeth on the cast and the PRES. *(f and g)* A duplicate cast of the maxillary diagnostic wax-up for occlusal ceramic veneers and ceramic crowns is scanned. Subsequently, it is prepared and scanned again. Digitized data of both scans is superimposed for the fabrication of a PRES for a maxillary provisional restoration. *(h)* A semitranslucent view demonstrating the relationship between the prepped teeth on the cast and the PRES. Each PRES is milled from a block of PMMA.

Procedures for Implant-Supported Provisional Restorations

As previously discussed, the role of implant-supported provisional restorations goes beyond providing an esthetic and functional replacement of the missing dentition. Such restorations also have the ability to mold and shape the soft tissue, with the goal of creating the desired emergence profile for the prospective definitive restorations at the space between the implant platform and the facial free gingival margins and the interproximal papillae. In terms of apicocoronal space, this area has also been defined as the sum of the critical contour, the area immediately apical to the free gingival margins (with a range of 1 mm), and the subcritical contour, the emergence area of the abutment from the implant platform to the critical contour (about 1 mm below the free gingival margins).[11]

There are two major clinical scenarios in terms of soft tissue management with implant-supported restorations in the esthetic zone. The first scenario is soft tissue preservation. This scenario pertains to immediate implant placement with immediate placement of a provisional restoration or a custom anatomical healing abutment, where the tissue may already be shaped and located close to its desired position.[96] In this instance, only a minor amount of site development

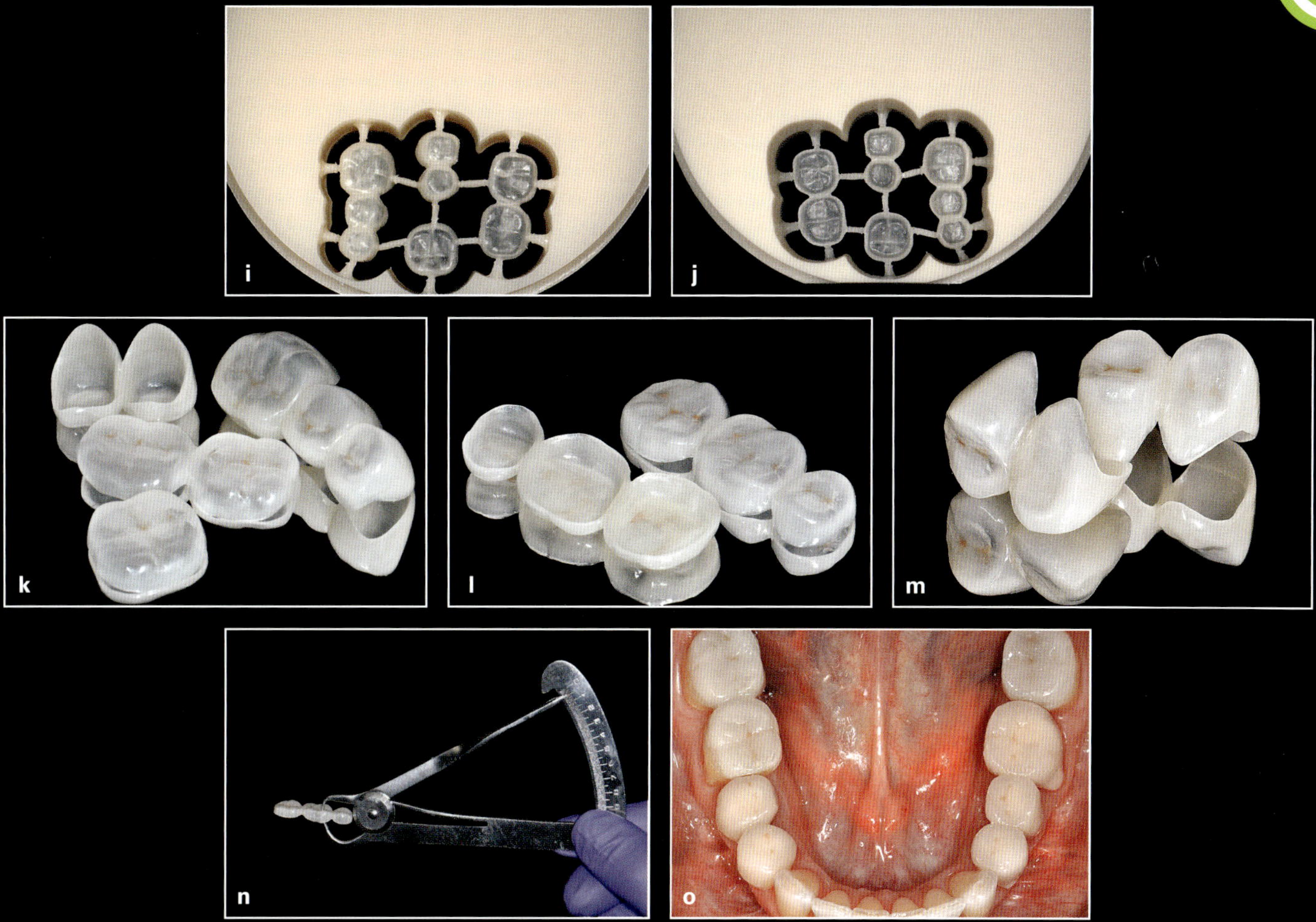

Fig 3-8 *(cont) (i and j)* The cameo and intaglio surfaces of the PRES once the milling of the PMMA block is complete. *(k to m)* Views of the finished and stained PRES for occlusal veneers and crowns. *(n)* Random measuring with a caliper of a maxillary PRES for occlusal veneers, demonstrating a thickness of 0.5 mm. *(o)* Occlusal view of the mandibular CAD/CAM PRES provisional restorations after reline delivery.

may be required. In such clinical scenarios, site preservation is the critical factor.[97,98] Randomized controlled clinical trials demonstrated that in the short-term, implant-supported restorations following immediate implant placement with immediate placement of a provisional restoration had better soft tissue stability on the labial aspect compared with implants restored with a delayed implant placement protocol.[99,100] However, it was also demonstrated in a study with a 4-year mean follow-up that even for immediate implant placement with immediate placement of a provisional restoration, gingival recession may proceed over time, and a thin gingival phenotype may significantly increase the extent of such facial recession.[12]

The other clinical scenario is soft tissue molding and augmentation. Such an approach is mainly required in delayed implant placement situations, where the hard and/or the soft tissue must be either preserved or augmented surgically and subsequently molded and shaped restoratively to create an ideal emergence profile with the desired levels of the facial free gingival margins and interproximal papillae.[9,75,101]

To allow for either the preservation or the development of an ideal emergence profile, an accurate and precise implant positioning is a prerequisite. The ability of clinicians to mold and shape this emergence profile is mainly related to apicocoronal placement of the implant platform, which is usually placed 3 to 4 mm below the prospective free gingival margins, depending on the implant platform diameter and design,[102] or 3 mm apical to the zenith of the prospective facial free gingival margin.[103] Prior to any procedures, clinicians must determine where the facial free gingival margin should be placed in relation to the prospective restoration and then plan the implant placement accordingly, letting the restoration be the guide.[104]

Smith and Zarb[105] described criteria for implant success that were mainly related to the implants' ability to survive without loss of osseointegration and their ability to be restored. However, with increased patient expectations for implants placed in areas where esthetics are critical, the restorative success in terms of soft tissue contours and health, the restoration's appearance, and its ability to function adequately are all equally significant. The pink esthetic score and the white esthetic score have been developed as tools to facilitate an objective assessment of implant-supported restorations' success in such clinical scenarios.[30,31] With soft tissue–related parameters such as papillae volume, the level and contours of the facial free gingival margins, root convexity, and soft tissue color and texture, a frame is created for receiving the implant-supported restoration that is further evaluated in terms of white esthetics as with conventional tooth-borne restorations.

Thus, the challenge clinicians face in the dental practice is to re-create that emergence profile from the implant platform (a cylinder) to the level of the free gingival margins while meeting the soft tissue esthetic parameters that have been previously described. Once the desired emergence profile and soft tissue contours have been achieved and stabilized, those soft tissue contours can be transferred to the definitive working cast or to a virtual model (see chapter 5). Subsequently, the cervical contours of a custom abutment and the cervical contours of the crown/retainer for a cement- or screw-retained implant-supported restoration can be designed and fabricated as a copy of the cervical contours of the provisional implant-supported restoration.

Consequently, the role of the provisional implant-supported restoration is to manage and shape that soft tissue over time and allow it to mature prior to making the master impression. Managing the restoration's cervical and intaglio contours goes hand in hand with shaping and molding the recipient site by selectively adding and reducing contours to different areas of the provisional restoration as needed with either PMMA or composite resin. The implant-supported provisional restoration can be selectively manipulated by adding or subtracting restorative material at different areas of the restoration to mold and shape the soft tissue contours and create the ideal emergence profile. Such an implant-supported provisional restoration is a powerful restorative tool. Several techniques for applying this approach have been described by different authors.[101,106,107] Generally, in terms of managing the critical and subcritical contours of the implant-supported provisional restoration, the definitive outcome may be achieved by selectively reducing or adding pressure/compression at the facial cervical area to minimize the likelihood of a facial recession and to facilitate the desired facial gingival margins (Fig 3-9). Pressure is applied at the interproximal papilla, and its contours are supported through the establishment of an interproximal contact point with the adjacent teeth. This can be achieved either with the provisional implant-supported restoration or with a custom anatomical healing abutment.[106–108] Thus, constant and continuous assessment of the soft tissue contours and health over time is required (see Figs 3-9e to 3-9g). In addition, the same esthetic and functional parameters for conventional crown and FDP provisional restorations are assessed as well.

As with definitive implant-supported restorations, clinicians have two options in terms of the retention mechanism for implant-supported provisional restorations: the cement-retained and the screw-retained provisional implant-supported restoration. For the fabrication of these provisional restorations, temporary abutment components made of either titanium or polymers (such as polyetheretherketone [PEEK] or PMMA with or without a titanium base) may be used. Both have their advantages and limitations, such as better mechanical properties for the titanium components and better esthetics and easier manipulation with the polymer components.[109,110] Currently, the difference between the two approaches of retention may not be as distinct if the provisional abutment used for the cement-retained provisional restoration is customized by adding direct composite resin restorative materials to form a custom anatomical provisional abutment.[111,112] This allows selective modification of the provisional abutment's contours and shape and facilitates the management of the finish line location of that custom provisional abutment following the scalloping of the soft tissue. Thus, the cervical contours of the custom anatomical provisional abutment are managed in a similar manner to the cervical contours of the screw-retained provisional restoration, and removal of residual excess temporary cement may be facilitated.

Screw-retained implant-supported provisional restorations

Screw-retained implant-supported provisional restorations have several advantages. With this type of provisional restoration, the soft tissue can be selectively pushed and molded as needed in a relatively quick and firm manner, which can sometimes be an issue in terms of patients' adaptation at delivery of the provisional restoration. If left unmonitored, the soft tissue may recede because it may not respond exactly as the stone cast did, which was scored to relatively arbitrary contours during the fabrication of the provisional restoration. In addition, a single interface exists between the provisional restoration and the implant, as compared with two interfaces for the cement-retained provisional restoration (crown/abutment and abutment/implant). One of the major features of the screw-retained provisional restoration is that any concerns with regard to retention of residual excess cement are eliminated.

However, screw-retained provisional restorations have several limitations as well. With implant-supported provisional restorations in the esthetic zone, the emergence profile may need to be modified. Thus, in addition to its removal for making the master impression and for delivery of the defini-

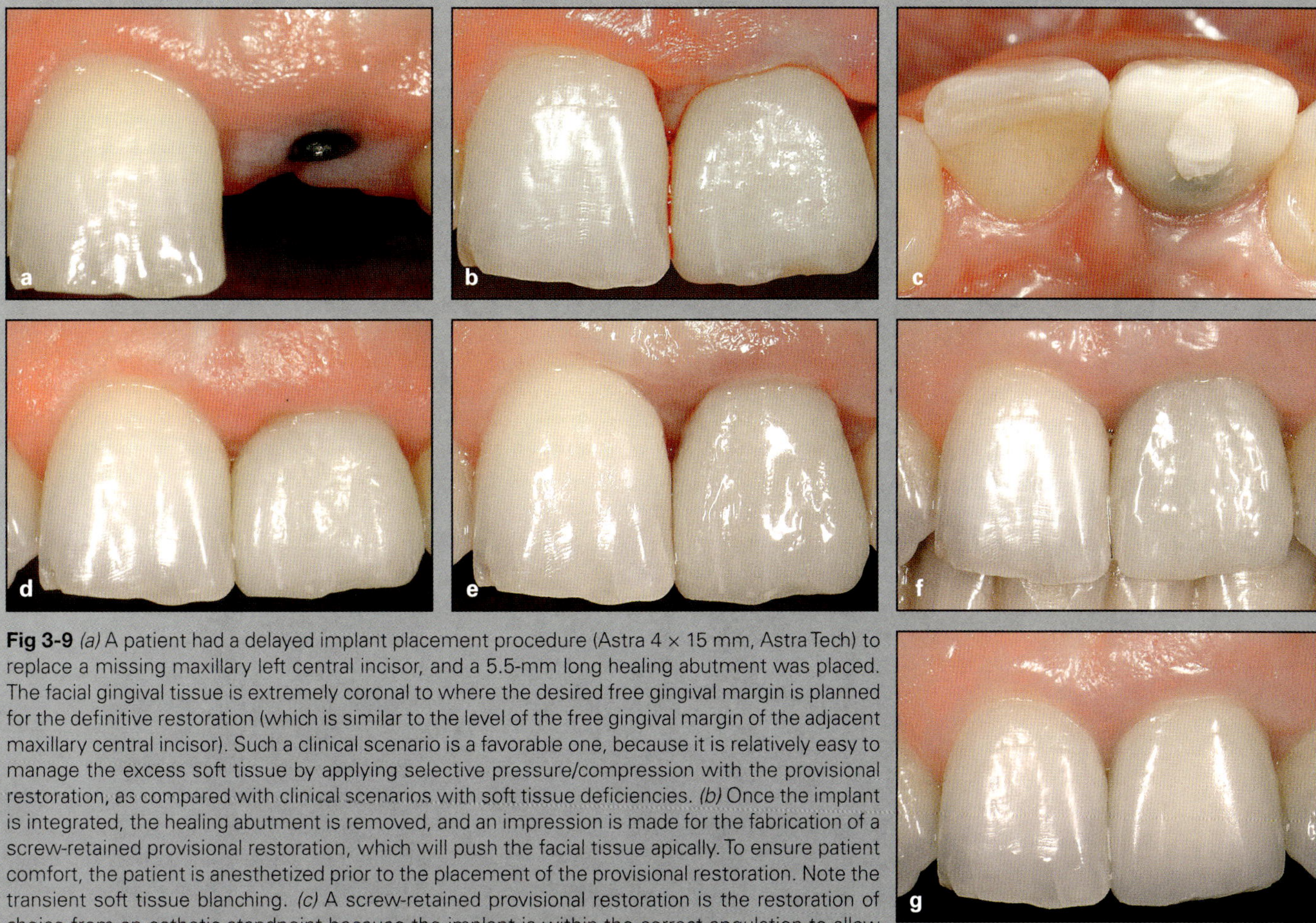

Fig 3-9 *(a)* A patient had a delayed implant placement procedure (Astra 4 × 15 mm, Astra Tech) to replace a missing maxillary left central incisor, and a 5.5-mm long healing abutment was placed. The facial gingival tissue is extremely coronal to where the desired free gingival margin is planned for the definitive restoration (which is similar to the level of the free gingival margin of the adjacent maxillary central incisor). Such a clinical scenario is a favorable one, because it is relatively easy to manage the excess soft tissue by applying selective pressure/compression with the provisional restoration, as compared with clinical scenarios with soft tissue deficiencies. *(b)* Once the implant is integrated, the healing abutment is removed, and an impression is made for the fabrication of a screw-retained provisional restoration, which will push the facial tissue apically. To ensure patient comfort, the patient is anesthetized prior to the placement of the provisional restoration. Note the transient soft tissue blanching. *(c)* A screw-retained provisional restoration is the restoration of choice from an esthetic standpoint because the implant is within the correct angulation to allow the screw access to emerge from the palatal aspect. In addition, retention of residual excess cement is prevented in a scenario where the implant platform is relatively apical to the free gingival margin. *(d)* The tissue is healed after 3 weeks. However, further shaping of the tissue cervically and interproximally is required. Changes in the cervical contours may be made gradually, with 2- to 3-week intervals between appointments, for evaluation and for performing modifications as needed until the desired soft tissue contours are achieved. *(e)* Additional composite resin material is added to the facial cervical aspect to move the soft tissue further apically. *(f)* Three weeks later, the tissue is maturing, and minor shaping at the cervical area and at the distal papilla is still required. *(g)* Note that once the desired cervical contours of the restoration and the soft tissue emergence profile are achieved, the soft tissue is stabilized for 3 months to confirm no further adverse changes. Without the support from the cervical contours of the provisional restoration, the soft tissue may creep back coronally. An esthetic and functional provisional restoration that allows the patient to function adequately reduces the need to complete the definitive restoration promptly. (Prosthodontics: Drs Lien-Feng Hsiao and Ariel J. Raigrodski; Periodontics: Dr Jim Janakievski.)

tive restoration, the provisional restoration may also have to be removed several times to allow for selective adding or removal of provisional restorative material. These multiple removals may cause irreversible trauma to the soft tissue, which may increase the likelihood of a soft tissue recession, as demonstrated in a study in dogs.[113] However, limited data in clinical studies demonstrated that several removals and reconnections of implant components as compared with placement of the definitive abutment on the day of surgery with no further removal in immediate implant placement scenarios may result in clinically negligible differences in tissue levels between the two approaches. Therefore, further research may be required to assess the clinical significance of placing the definitive abutment on the day of implant placement with no further removal.[114,115] Such a consideration is also relevant for the use of cement-retained provisional restorations that use provisional anatomical custom abutments. It is the author's opinion that placement of a definitive abutment on the day of implant placement, which takes away the clinician's ability to control the finish line levels of the abutment in relation to the prospective soft tissue scalloping and contour changes, may compromise not only soft tissue support but also residual excess cement removal, particularly at the interproximal area, where the finish line may be positioned too apically in relation to the interproximal papillae. In addition, placing the definitive abutment on the day of surgery means that clinicians make an informed decision not to use a screw-retained restoration.

Box 3-5 Clinical scenarios in which screw-retained implant-supported provisional restorations should be considered

- When the patient presents with excess soft tissue
- When the implant is placed with adequate inclination and the screw access presents no esthetic liability
- When the implant is placed too deep apicocoronally (although if the provisional abutment is anatomically customized, it may not make a considerable difference)
- When the patient presents with limited interocclusal distance
- When implants are being used for orthodontic anchorage to facilitate orthodontic movement[40]

Additionally, every time a screw-retained provisional restoration is removed and reseated, an adequate seating verification may be needed via a radiograph, and a concern over additional radiation may arise. Moreover, in the anterior maxillary segment, the implant may not be perfectly placed in terms of where the screw access emerges due to anatomical restrictions. Consequently, the screw access may emerge from the facial or incisal aspect of the provisional restoration, depending on the implant system used. (Recently, a new angulated screw channel concept was introduced by Nobel Biocare for their conical connection implant systems [NobelProcera Angulated Screw Channel abutment].) Generally, this may create an esthetic liability, and extra time and effort may be required in managing that provisional restoration each time it is removed and reseated.

Finally, with multiple-unit implant-supported provisional restorations, screw retention may be challenging due to a limited path of insertion, depending on the angulation of the implants. In such clinical scenarios, it may be easier to fabricate a cement-retained provisional restoration with custom anatomical provisional abutments that are prepared with an adequate path of insertion followed by the creation of a PRES, which can be subsequently relined on the provisional abutments. The author's personal preferences for using screw-retained implant-supported provisional restorations are presented in Box 3-5.

Cement-retained implant-supported provisional restorations

Cement-retained provisional restorations have several advantages. They may allow a gradual development of the soft tissue emergence profile. However, to date, with the use of custom anatomical provisional abutments with composite resin placed at the cervical subcritical and critical areas of the restoration, the soft tissue may be managed in a similar manner as for screw-retained provisional restorations. For minor contour modifications at the critical contour area, the removal of the custom anatomical provisional abutment may not be required, and if the changes in the emergence profile are 1 mm below the free gingival margin and coronally, those changes may be made by just removing and modifying the contours of the cement-retained provisional crown/FDP retainer. In such clinical scenarios, the likelihood of trauma to the soft tissue may be reduced because the custom anatomical provisional abutment may not have to be removed. In addition, the esthetics are easier to manage and maintain in those clinical scenarios in which the abutment screw access may penetrate through the incisal or facial aspect. Moreover, it may be easier to use this type of provisional restoration for multiple splinted units when the implants are severely divergent and when restoring teeth and implants simultaneously in the same arch for restorative convenience (see Case G).

Cement-retained provisional restorations have several limitations as well. Two interfaces exist with such a restoration: one between the custom anatomical provisional abutment and the implant platform, and one between the crown and the abutment. The most notable limitation is the need to manage residual excess temporary cement, although with custom anatomical provisional abutments the likelihood of such a complication may be reduced due to the ability to control the finish line location (Fig 3-10). The authors' personal preferences for using this type of provisional restorations are presented in Box 3-6. F

Fabrication procedures for a custom anatomical healing abutment G

The following steps are followed for the fabrication of a custom anatomical healing abutment to enhance soft tissue preservation (Figs 3-11a to 3-11d):

1. A provisional titanium abutment may be used for the fabrication of the custom anatomical healing abutment (Fig 3-11e).
2. Apply thread seal tape (Teflon) around the cervical subgingival area below the finish line of the abutment to protect it from the prospective airborne-particle abrasion procedure (Fig 3-11f).
3. Use airborne-particle abrasion to roughen the surface of the provisional abutment (with 50-micron aluminum-oxide particles) at the coronal aspect above the finish

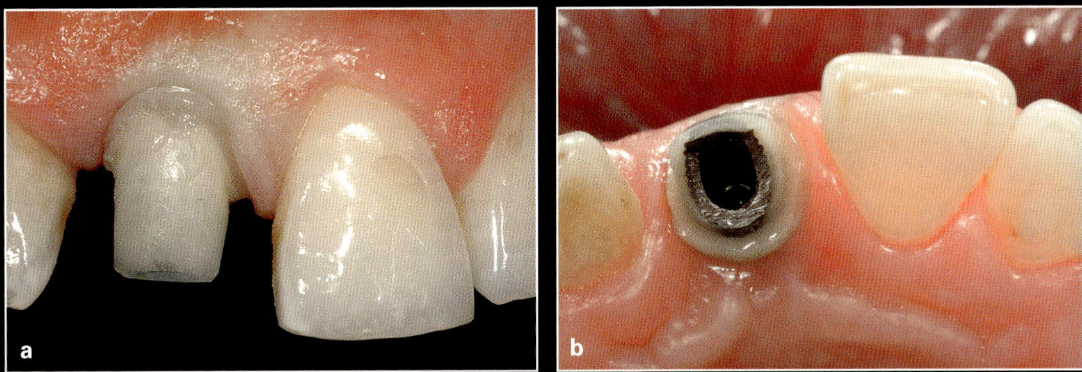

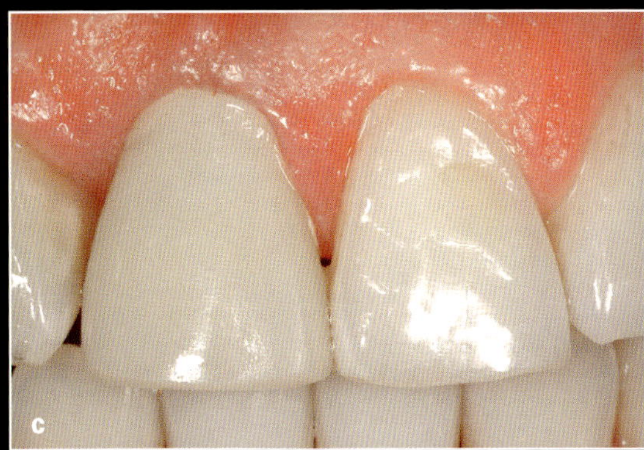

Fig 3-10 *(a)* Placement of a custom provisional abutment in the patient's mouth. Note the initial blanching due to the pressure created mainly interproximally by the addition of composite resin to the metal provisional abutment. *(b)* Occlusal view of the custom provisional abutment. Note that the finish line is placed above the free gingival margins to minimize the risk of residual excess cement complications. *(c)* Close-up facial view of the provisional restoration after placement of the provisional crown. Note that the initial blanching has vanished.

Box 3-6 **Clinical scenarios in which cement-retained provisional implant-supported restorations should be considered**

- When there is deficient to adequate soft tissue (mainly with a thinner tissue phenotype, which may require more gentle management)
- When there are severely malaligned, divergent implants that are planned to be splinted
- When the screw access emerges from the incisal or facial aspect
- When an extracted tooth is to be used for making the provisional restoration and is to be relined with a provisional restorative material such as PMMA
- When teeth and implants are being restored in the same arch for restorative convenience (such as a crown on a natural tooth next to an implant-supported crown)

line (Fig 3-11g). Subsequently, apply a bonding agent and light-polymerize it (Fig 3-11h). This procedure can be done prior to the patient's surgical visit.

4. Once the implant is placed, if a stock healing abutment was initially placed during surgery, remove it and secure the provisional abutment to the implant platform.
5. Inject light-polymerized direct composite resin restorative material circumferentially to the provisional abutment at the level of the free gingival margin and light-polymerize it.
6. Remove the modified provisional abutment from the patient's mouth and resecure the stock healing abutment to the implant platform. Evaluate the composite resin, which may appear in the form of a supragingival ring attached to the provisional abutment (Fig 3-11i).
7. Add additional light-polymerized composite resin to the provisional abutment at the area between the abutment's finish line and the composite resin ring (Figs 3-11j and 3-11k).
8. Modify the anatomical cervical contours in the patient's mouth as needed, and verify that cervical contours simi-

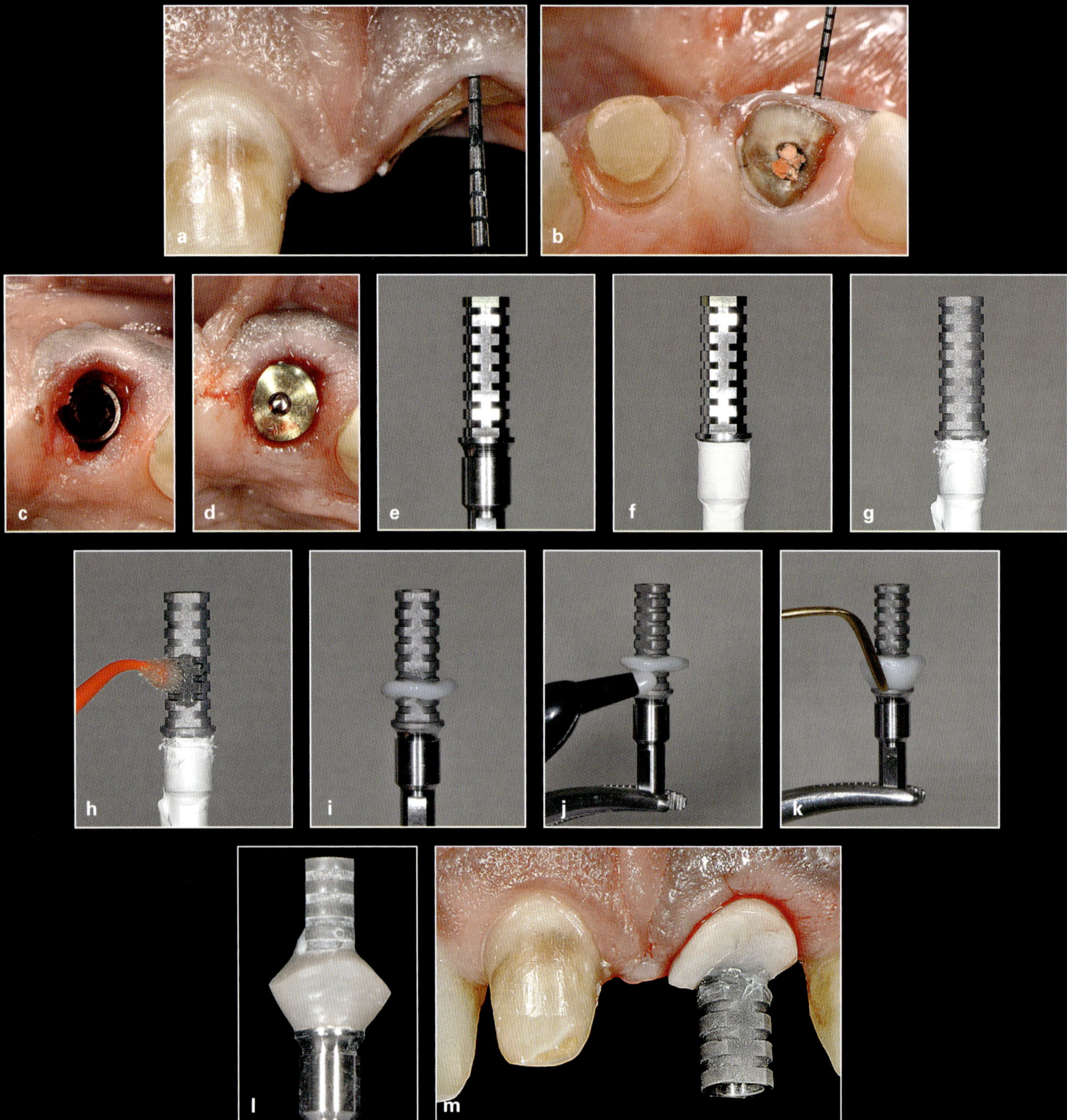

Fig 3-11 Custom anatomical healing abutment for soft tissue preservation. *(a and b)* A patient presented with a nonrestorable maxillary left central incisor with a thick soft tissue phenotype as reflected from the periodontal probe assessment. The tooth was planned to be extracted followed by immediate implant placement. *(c)* An atraumatic extraction was made to ensure that the existing labial plate remained intact. An implant with a conical connection (NobelActive 4.3 × 13 mm, Nobel Biocare) was immediately placed in the extraction socket, which was also grafted with a dental bone substitute (NuOss, ACE Surgical Supply). The goal was to facilitate the surgical site and the soft tissue contours by creating a custom anatomical healing abutment that would preserve the emergence profile of the soft tissue by mimicking the contours of the preexisting root of the maxillary left central incisor. *(d)* A standard stock healing abutment was subsequently placed. Note that the stock healing abutment does not support the tissue adequately to maintain the soft tissue emergence profile. The patient presented with the maxillary right central incisor prepared for a crown. Consequently, the surgical site was planned to be provisionalized with an FDP with a cantilever pontic off the right central incisor in conjunction with a custom anatomical healing abutment connected to the implant. *(e)* A titanium provisional abutment connected to the implant analog. *(f)* Thread seal tape is applied around the abutment below the finish line. *(g)* The titanium provisional abutment after airborne-particle abrasion with 50-micron aluminum-oxide particles. *(h)* The titanium provisional abutment connected to the implant analog during the application of a bonding agent. *(i)* The titanium provisional abutment connected to the implant analog with the circumferential ring of composite resin after removal from the patient's mouth. *(j and k)* Additional light-polymerized composite resin material is added circumferentially between the abutment finish line and the composite resin ring. *(l and m)* The modified provisional abutment is verified in the patient's mouth for adequate cervical contours and subsequently polished extraorally.

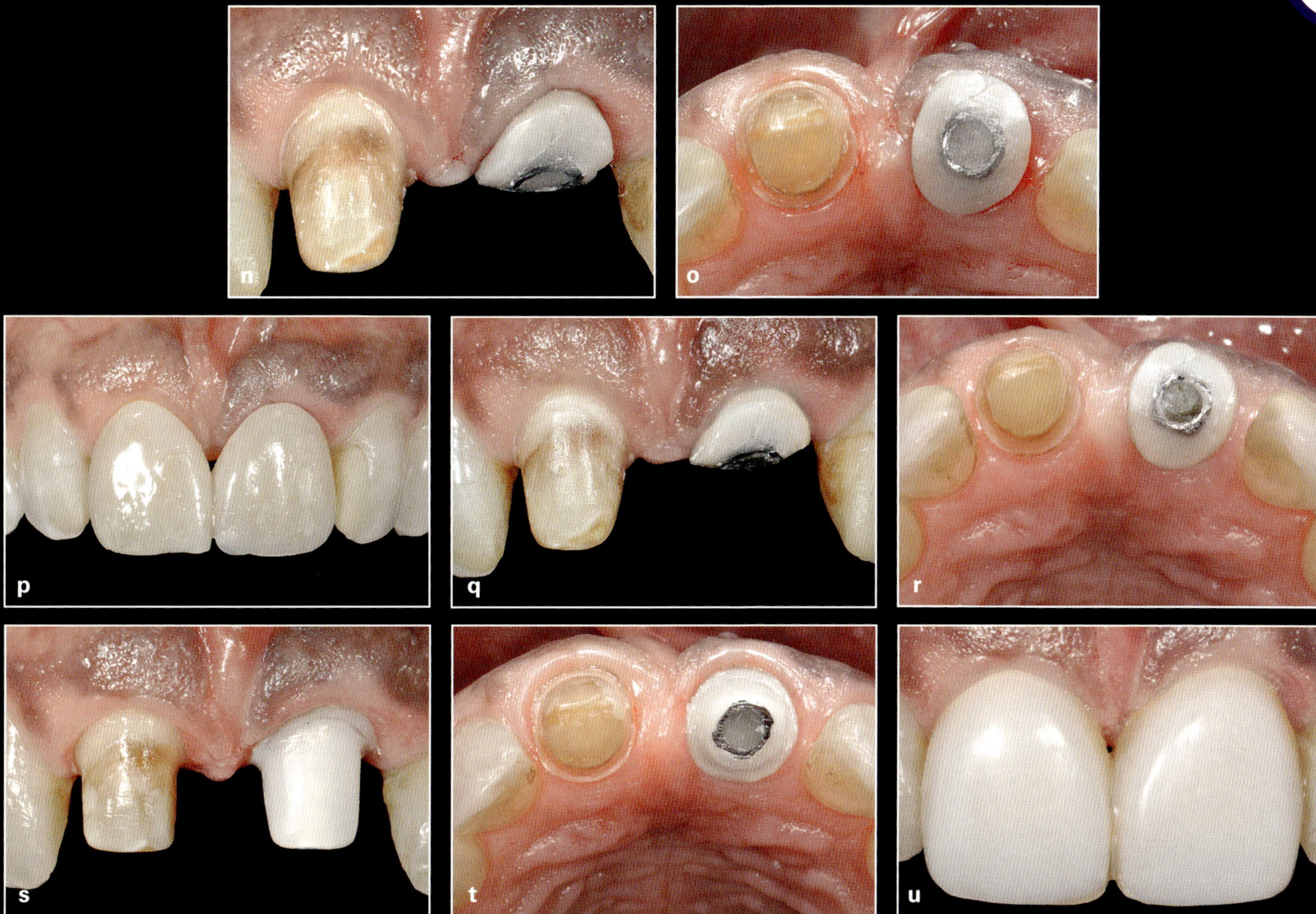

Fig 3-11 *(cont) (n and o)* The complete custom anatomical healing abutment with the desired cervical contours to preserve the soft tissue profile is secured to the implant platform. *(p)* A provisional FDP, with the maxillary left central incisor serving as a cantilever restoration, is placed. *(q and r)* The complete custom anatomical healing abutment several weeks after implant placement. Note the satisfactory soft tissue healing. *(s to u)* Three months later, a custom provisional implant abutment and a cement-retained provisional restoration are placed.

lar to those of the extracted root were created. Polish the composite resin attached to the modified provisional abutment (Figs 3-11l and 3-11m).

9. Ensure adequate support of the papillae and undercontour the facial cervical aspect of the provisional abutment to ensure reduced pressure at the level of the facial free gingival margins to minimize the risk of recession. In retrospect for this clinical scenario, it is the author's opinion that the distal part of the provisional abutment could have been further augmented with composite resin to provide better support for the interproximal papilla.
10. Once the cervical contours of the provisional abutment are finalized, section the excess coronal part of the modified titanium abutment. Secure the newly created custom anatomical healing abutment to the implant platform according to the manufacturer's instructions. Fill the screw access hole with temporary light-polymerized composite resin (Figs 3-11n to 3-11r).
11. Once the osseointegration of the implant is confirmed, the custom anatomical healing abutment is replaced with a custom provisional abutment and a cement-retained restoration (Figs 3-11s to 3-11u).

In summary, the cervical contours of the custom anatomical healing abutment, which simulates the cross section of the tooth to be restored, are different from the contours of a stock healing abutment or semi-anatomical healing abutment provided by most manufacturers. The cross section of the custom anatomical healing abutment should be comparable to the cross section of the apical aspect of an immediate implant-supported provisional restoration. Managing the critical and subcritical areas is fundamental to the

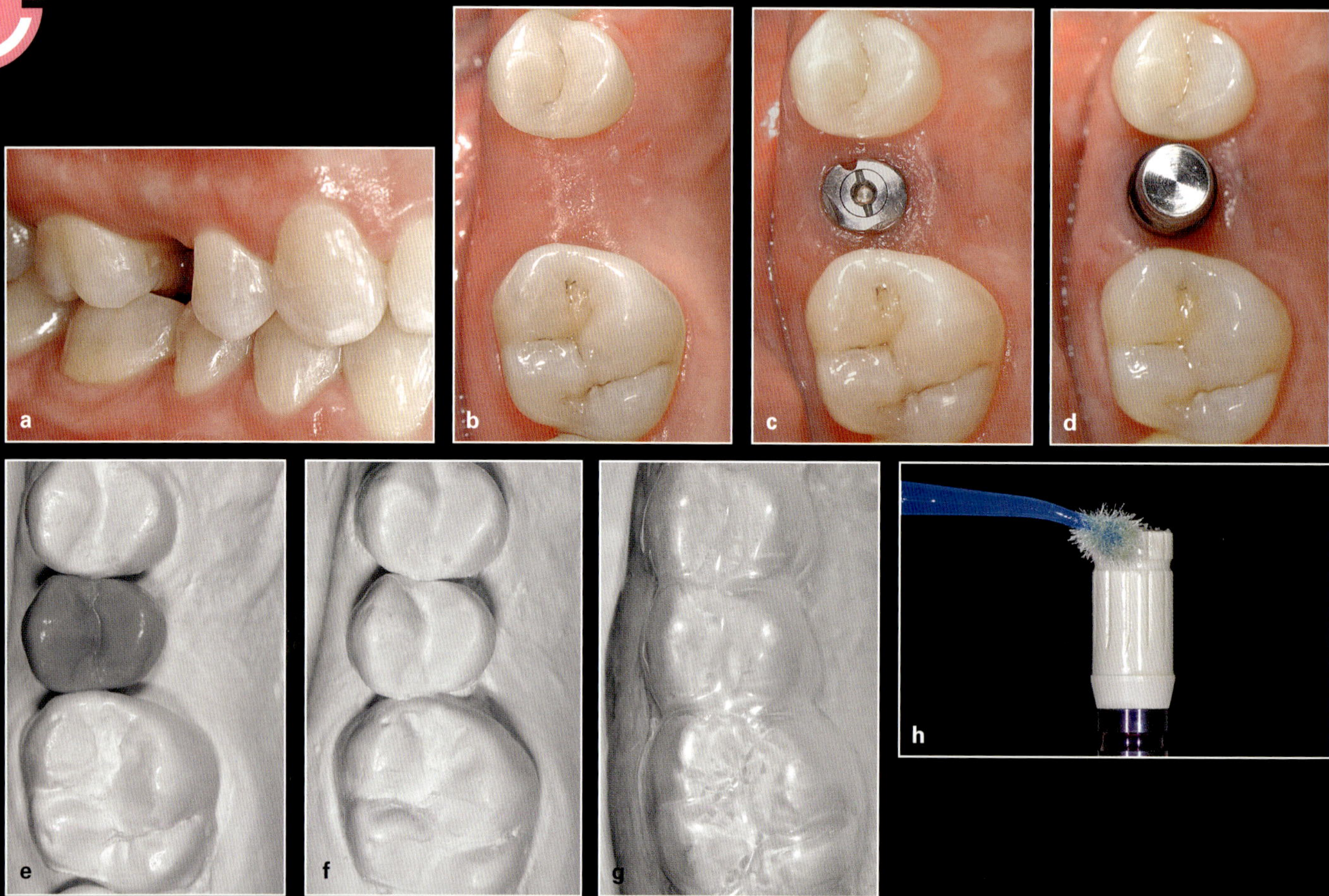

Fig 3-12 *(a and b)* A patient presented after orthodontic therapy had been completed to create adequate space to restore the missing maxillary right second premolar. The residual alveolar ridge was augmented. *(c)* After 6 months of healing, an osseointegrated implant with an internal connection (Osseotite Tapered Certain Prevail 4.3 × 11.5 mm, Biomet 3i) was placed following a one-stage surgical protocol. A modified and polished stock healing abutment was placed to create a gradual oval cross section with an undercontour at the facial area to minimize the likelihood of recession. *(d)* Three months after implant placement, an impression was made for the fabrication of a screw-retained provisional restoration with a PEEK provisional abutment. *(e to g)* The diagnostic wax-up was duplicated. A thermoplastic template was fabricated using the duplicate cast. *(h)* The provisional abutment was coated with a bonding agent, which was then light-polymerized.

creation of an essential foundation for the definitive restoration, which may be provided via either an immediate implant-supported provisional restoration (which was not necessary for the patient in Case G) or a custom anatomical healing abutment.

Fabrication procedures for a provisional implant-supported restoration

The following steps are followed for the fabrication of a provisional implant-supported restoration (Figs 3-12a to 3-12c):

1. Make an implant-level impression (Fig 3-12d).
2. Fabricate a diagnostic wax-up and duplicate it (Figs 3-12e and 3-12f).
3. Make a vacuum-formed thermoplastic template (Copyplast 1 mm, Great Lakes Orthodontics) to be later used for the fabrication of the provisional restoration (Fig 3-12g).
4. Treat the provisional abutment as needed prior to the fabrication of the provisional restoration. If using a PEEK abutment, apply a bonding agent and light-polymerize it. If using a titanium abutment, use airborne-particle abrasion with 50-micron aluminum-oxide particles and subsequently apply a bonding agent and light-polymerize it (Fig 3-12h).
5. Perforate the thermoplastic template at the central fossa area of the tooth to be restored, and place it on the working cast to assess the fit (Fig 3-12i).
6. Secure the provisional abutment to the analog on the working cast. The emergence area in this case was

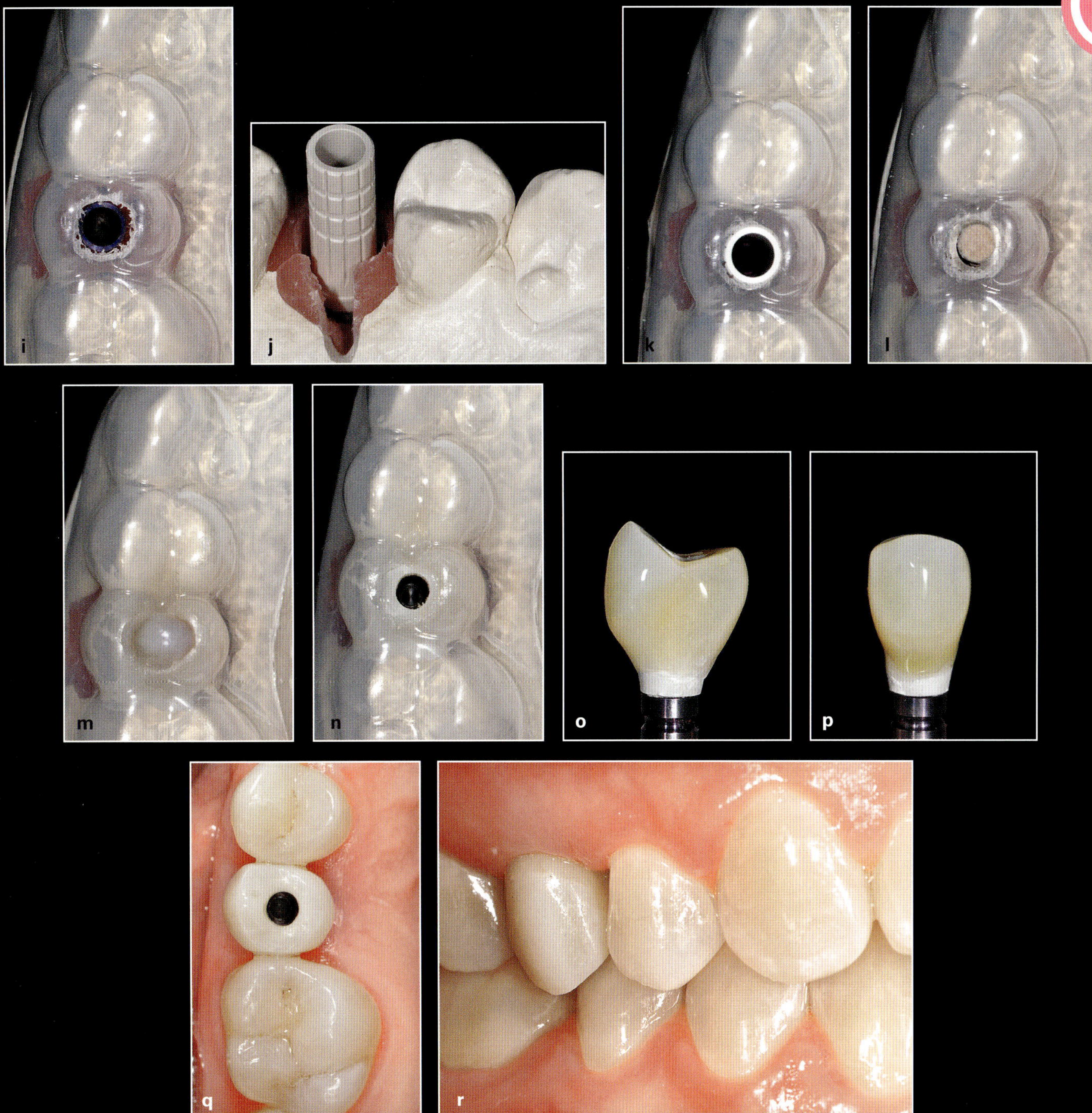

Fig 3-12 *(cont) (i)* View of the perforated thermoplastic template seated on the working cast. *(j and k)* The provisional abutment was secured to the analog on the working cast, and the thermoplastic template was seated on the cast and perforated with the abutment penetrating the perforation in the template. *(l)* A cotton swab was inserted through the screw access hole and through the perforation in the template. *(m and n)* The thermoplastic template filled with the bis-acryl material was seated on the working cast with excess coming out of the occlusal perforation. The excess material and cotton swab were removed. *(o and p)* Buccal and facial views of the completed screw-retained restoration. Note the critical and subcritical contours made with light-polymerized composite resin. *(q and r)* Occlusal and buccal views of the provisional restoration once delivered.

shaped to facilitate the creation of subcritical and critical contours of a maxillary second premolar (Fig 3-12j).

7. Verify that the provisional abutment penetrates the perforation at the central fossa of the thermoplastic template. Subsequently, remove the template and the provisional abutment from the cast. Cut the occlusal aspect of the provisional abutment 2 mm below the central fossa of the thermoplastic template (Fig 3-12k). Place a cotton swab through the perforation in the thermoplastic template and through the provisional abutment (Fig 3-12l). It will protect the screw access hole from being clogged with the material used for fabricating the provisional restoration.
8. Apply petroleum jelly to the cotton swab and on the cast at the areas surrounding the analog to prevent the provisional material from sticking to the cast. Block interproximal undercuts on the cast with wax, and insert the cotton swab on top of the abutment.
9. Fill the template at the occlusal, facial, and lingual areas of the tooth to be restored with bis-acryl material (Protemp Plus), and seat it on the working cast with the hole corresponding to the cotton swab penetrating through (Fig 3-12m).
10. Allow the bis-acryl material to set on the cast for at least 5 minutes. Gently tease and remove the cotton swab to gain access to the abutment screw (Fig 3-12n). Remove the template, unscrew the abutment screw, and remove the screw-retained provisional restoration.
11. Evaluate proximal contacts and adjust them as needed by adding or subtracting light-polymerized direct composite resin material.
12. Shape and finish the critical and subcritical cervical contours by hand using light-polymerized composite resin (Filtek Supreme), applying selective pressure at the interproximal papillae and reducing pressure by undercontouring the facial cervical area (Figs 3-12o and 3-12p). The provisional restoration is finished and polished in a similar manner as for tooth-borne provisional restorations.

The patient in Case H returned for the delivery of the provisional restoration. Minor adjustments were made in terms of the proximal contact point, occlusion, and cervical and interproximal contours, and the tissue was left to mature for 2 to 3 weeks prior to making any modifications (Figs 3-12q and 3-12r).

Summary

This chapter described the concepts and some of the practices for the fabrication of therapeutic provisional restorations for different treatment modalities using various techniques and materials. Emphasis was placed on soft tissue management and on techniques that may be applied in a relatively simple manner in the restorative dental clinic. In general, several fundamental concepts must be followed and met to ensure the delivery of a functional, therapeutic, diagnostic, and esthetic provisional restoration that will set the stage for an uneventful fabrication and delivery of an esthetic and functional definitive restoration. The following are key considerations for the successful design and fabrication of provisional restorations:

- With complex clinical scenarios in which the occlusal scheme and/or the vertical dimension of occlusion are to be modified when using the indirect-direct combination technique, use a reference or an index to orient a PRES so that it can be relined following the designed occlusal plane and incisal edge position while providing the desired vertical dimension of occlusion.
- To achieve excellent fit and excellent marginal integrity with the indirect-direct combination technique, use the multiple reline technique and inject the reline PMMA material onto the finish line of the tooth preparations using a disposable syringe.
- Careful trimming of the provisional restoration is crucial for the elimination of any overhangs created at the margins of the provisional restoration. It will also facilitate the elimination of any overcontoured areas and will ensure the creation of adequately open gingival embrasures, which tend to be closed due to a fear of black triangles and fractured connectors.
- Verify an adequate emergence profile and interproximal contours.
- Provide high polish to reduce plaque retention and to improve luster and esthetics.
- Verify that soft tissue trauma is minimized during the provisionalization procedure and after the delivery of the provisional restoration. Ensure that the patient can adequately maintain oral hygiene and gingival health, particularly in those scenarios in which the prospective definitive restorations are to be bonded, such as with ceramic veneers.
- Verify the design and execution of the desired occlusal scheme. This will also reduce the likelihood of fractures, microleakage, and cement wash that could further result in secondary caries and loss of retention.
- Ensure residual excess temporary cement removal to facilitate the health of the soft tissue.
- For implant-supported provisional restorations, the goal is to minimize pressure at the facial free gingival margins by undercontouring the cervical aspect of the restoration. This concept is to be used with ovate pontics as well, until the desired level of the free gingival margins is achieved.
- Create pressure interproximally at the papillae while creating an interproximal contact point with the adjacent teeth using the provisional restoration or a custom anatomical healing abutment. Depending on where the interproximal bone is located on the adjacent teeth and the distance between the implant and the adjacent teeth, this will either maintain those ideal interproximal contours (for immediate implant placement scenarios) or push and enhance the pa-

pillae coronally (for delayed implant placement scenarios). Adjust the design of the provisional restoration accordingly for scenarios of adjacent implants.

Acknowledgments

The author would like to thank Dr Yen-Wei Chen for his contribution to this chapter.

References

1. The Glossary of Prosthodontic Terms. Eighth edition. J Prosthet Dent 2005;94:46.
2. Patras M, Naka O, Doukoudakis S, Pissiotis A. Management of provisional restorations' deficiencies: A literature review. J Esthet Restor Dent 2012;24:26–38.
3. Besimo CR, Rochner HP. Three-dimensional treatment planning for prosthetic rehabilitation. Int J Periodontics Restorative Dent 2005;25:81–87.
4. Gratton DG, Aquilino SA. Interim restorations. Dent Clin North Am 2004;48:487–497.
5. Fradeani M, Barducci G. Creating and integrating the provisional restoration. In: Esthetic Rehabilitation in Fixed Prosthodontics, vol 2. Chicago: Quintessence, 2008:123–276.
6. Federick DR. The provisional fixed partial denture. J Prosthet Dent 1975;34:520–526.
7. Shavell HM. The periodontal-restorative interface in fixed prosthodontics: Tooth preparation, provisionalization, and biologic final impressions. Part I. Pract Periodontics Aesthet Dent 1994;6:33–44.
8. Shavell HM. The periodontal-restorative interface in fixed prosthodontics: Tooth preparation, provisionalization, and biologic final impressions. Part II. Pract Periodontics Aesthet Dent 1994;6:49–60.
9. Bichacho N. Achieving optimal gingival esthetics around restored natural teeth and implants. Rationale, concepts, and techniques. Dent Clin North Am 1998;42:763–780.
10. Dylina TJ. Contour determination for ovate pontics. J Prosthet Dent 1999;82:136–142.
11. Su H, Gonzalez-Martin O, Weisgold A, Lee E. Considerations of implant abutment and crown contour: Critical contour and subcritical contour. Int J Periodontics Restorative Dent 2010;30:335–343.
12. Kan JY, Rungcharassaeng K, Lozada JL, Zimmerman G. Facial gingival tissue stability following immediate placement and provisionalization of maxillary anterior single implants: A 2- to 8-year follow-up. Int J Oral Maxillofac Implants 2011;26:179–187.
13. Donovan TE, Cho GC. Diagnostic provisional restorations in restorative dentistry: The blueprint for success. J Can Dent Assoc 1999;65:272–275.
14. Bral M. Periodontal considerations for provisional restorations. Dent Clin North Am 1989;33:457–477.
15. Yuodelis RA, Faucher R. Provisional restorations: An integrated approach to periodontics and restorative dentistry. Dent Clin North Am 1980;24:285–303.
16. Koumjian JH, Holmes JB. Marginal accuracy of provisional restorative materials. J Prosthet Dent 1990;63:639–642.
17. Givens EJ Jr, Neiva G, Yaman P, Dennison JB. Marginal adaptation and color stability of four provisional materials. J Prosthodont 2008;17:97–101.
18. Hernandez EP, Oshida Y, Platt JA, Andres CJ, Barco MT, Brown DT. Mechanical properties of four methylmethacrylate-based resins for provisional fixed restorations. Biomed Mater Eng 2004;1:107–122.
19. Koumjian JH, Nimmo A. Evaluation of fracture resistance of resins used for provisional restorations. J Prosthet Dent 1990;64:654–657.
20. Pfeiffer P, Grube L. In vitro resistance of reinforced interim fixed partial dentures. J Prosthet Dent 2003;89:170–174.
21. Scherrer SS, Wiskott AH, Coto-Hunziker V, Belser UC. Monotonic flexure and fatigue strength of composites for provisional and definitive restorations. J Prosthet Dent 2003;89:579–588.
22. Ogawa T, Tanaka M, Koyano K. Effect of water temperature during polymerization on strength of autopolymerizing resin. J Prosthet Dent 2000;84:222–224.
23. Vahidi F. The provisional restoration. Dent Clin North Am 1987; 31:363–381.
24. Magne P, Magne M, Belser U. The diagnostic template: A key element to the comprehensive esthetic treatment concept. Int J Periodontics Restorative Dent 1996;16:560–569.
25. Small BW. Pretreatment wax-ups and provisionals for restorative dentistry. Gen Dent 2005;53:98–100.
26. Becker CM, Kaldahl WB. Current theories of crown contour, margin placement, and pontic design. J Prosthet Dent 1981;45:268–277.
27. Ackerman MB. The full coverage restoration in relation to the gingival sulcus. Compend Contin Educ Dent 1997;18:1131–1138.
28. Bichacho N. Cervical contouring concepts: Enhancing the dentogingival complex. Pract Periodontics Aesthet Dent 1996;8:241–254.
29. Edelhoff D, Spiekermann H, Yildirim M. A review of esthetic pontic design options. Quintessence Int 2002;33:736–746.
30. Fürhauser R, Florescu D, Benesch T, Haas R, Mailath G, Watzek G. Evaluation of soft tissue around single-tooth implant crowns: The pink esthetic score. Clin Oral Implants Res 2005;16:639–644.
31. Belser UC, Grütter L, Vailati F, et al. Outcome evaluation of early placed maxillary anterior single-tooth implants using objective esthetic criteria: A cross-sectional, retrospective study in 45 patients with a 2- to 4-year follow-up using pink and white esthetic scores. J Periodontol 2009;80:140–151.
32. Skurow HM, Nevins M. The rationale of the preperiodontal provisional biologic trial restoration. Int J Periodontics Restorative Dent 1988;8:8–29.
33. Sheets CG, Ono Y, Taniguchi T. Esthetic provisional restorations for porcelain veneer preparations. J Esthet Dent 1993;5:215–220.
34. Raigrodski AJ, Sadan A, Mendez AJ. Use of a customized rigid clear matrix for fabricating provisional veneers. J Esthet Dent 1999; 11:16–22.
35. Shavell HM. Mastering the art of tissue management during provisionalization and biologic final impressions. Int J Periodontics Restorative Dent 1988;8:24–43.
36. Waerhaug J. Effect of rough surfaces upon gingival tissue. J Dent Res 1956;35:323–325.
37. Magne P, Magne M, Belser U. The esthetic width in fixed prosthodontics. J Prosthodont 1999;8:106–118.
38. Rieder CE. Use of provisional restorations to develop and achieve esthetic expectations. Int J Periodontics Restorative Dent 1989; 9:122–139.
39. Spoor R. Predictable provisionalization: Achieving psychological satisfaction, form, and function. Pract Proced Aesthet Dent 2004; 16:433–440.
40. Smalley WM. Clinical and laboratory procedures for implant anchorage in partially edentulous dentitions. In: Higuchi K (ed). Orthodontic Applications of Osseointegrated Implants. Chicago: Quintessence, 2000:33–70.
41. Smalley WM. Comprehensive interdisciplinary management of patients with missing or abnormally proportioned teeth. In: Cohen M (ed). Interdisciplinary Treatment Planning: Principles, Design, Implementation. Chicago: Quintessence, 2008:343–382.
42. Edelhoff D, Beuer F, Schweiger J, Brix O, Stimmelmayr M, Güth JF. CAD/CAM-generated high-density polymer restorations for the pretreatment of complex cases: A case report. Quintessence Int 2012;43:457–467.
43. Osman YI, Owen CP. Flexural strength of provisional restorative materials. J Prosthet Dent 1993;70:94–96.

44. Scherrer SS, Wiskott AH, Coto-Hunziker V, Belser UC. Monotonic flexure and fatigue strength of composites for provisional and definitive restorations. J Prosthet Dent 2003;89:579–588.
45. Koumjian JH, Firtell DN, Nimmo A. Color stability of provisional materials in vivo. J Prosthet Dent 1991;65:740–742.
46. Ergün G, Mutlu-Sagesen L, Ozkan Y, Demirel E. In vitro color stability of provisional crown and bridge restoration materials. Dent Mater J 2005;24:342–350.
47. Doray PG, Li D, Powers JM. Color stability of provisional restorative materials after accelerated aging. J Prosthodont 2001;10:212–216.
48. Sham AS, Chu FC, Chai J, Chow TW. Color stability of provisional prosthodontic materials. J Prosthet Dent 2004;91:447–452.
49. Driscoll CF, Woolsey G, Ferguson WM. Comparison of exothermic release during polymerization of four materials used to fabricate interim restorations. J Prosthet Dent 1991;65:504–506.
50. Michalakis K, Pissiotis A, Hirayama H, Kang K, Kafantaris N. Comparison of temperature increase in the pulp chamber during the polymerization of materials used for the direct fabrication of provisional restorations. J Prosthet Dent 2006;96:418–423.
51. Stungis TE, Fink JN. Hypersensitivity to acrylic resin. J Prosthet Dent 1969;22:425–428.
52. Kanerva L, Estlander T, Jolanki R. Allergy caused by acrylics: Past, present and prevention. Curr Probl Dermatol 1996;25:86–96.
53. Fan PL, Meyer DM. FDI report on adverse reactions to resin-based materials. Int Dent J 2007;57:9–12.
54. Pfeiffer P, Grube L. In vitro resistance of reinforced interim fixed partial dentures. J Prosthet Dent 2003;89:170–174.
55. Verri FR, Pellizzer EP, Mazaro JV, de Almeida EO, Antenucci RM. Esthetic interim acrylic resin prosthesis reinforced with metal casting. J Prosthodont 2009;18:541–544.
56. Emtiaz S, Tarnow DP. Processed acrylic resin provisional restoration with lingual cast metal framework. J Prosthet Dent 1998;79:484–488.
57. Waerhaug J. Tissue reactions around artificial crowns. J Periodontol 1953;24:172–185.
58. Kurbad A. CAD/CAM-based polymer provisionals as treatment adjuncts. Int J Comput Dent 2013;16:327–346.
59. Güth JF, Almeida E Silva JS, Ramberger M, Beuer F, Edelhoff D. Treatment concept with CAD/CAM-fabricated high-density polymer temporary restorations. J Esthet Restor Dent 2012;24:310–318.
60. Duke ES. Provisional restorative materials: A technology update. Compend Contin Educ Dent 1999;20:497–500.
61. Young HM, Smith CT, Morton D. Comparative in vitro evaluation of two provisional restorative materials. J Prosthet Dent 2001; 85:129–132.
62. Castelnuovo J, Tjan AH. Temperature rise in pulpal chamber during fabrication of provisional resinous crowns. J Prosthet Dent 1997; 78:441–446.
63. Strassler HE, Lowe RA. Chairside resin-based provisional restorative materials for fixed prosthodontics. Compend Contin Educ Dent 2011;32:10,12,14.
64. Labban N, Song F, Al-Shibani N, Windsor LJ. Effects of provisional acrylic resins on gingival fibroblast cytokine/growth factor expression. J Prosthet Dent 2008;100:390–397.
65. Hammond BD, Cooper JR 3rd, Lazarchik DA. Predictable repair of provisional restorations. J Esthet Restor Dent 2009;21:19–24.
66. Lang R, Rosentritt M, Behr M, Handel G. Fracture resistance of PMMA and resin matrix composite-based interim FPD materials. Int J Prosthodont 2003;16:381–384.
67. Luthardt RG, Stössel M, Hinz M, Vollandt R. Clinical performance and periodontal outcome of temporary crowns and fixed partial dentures: A randomized clinical trial. J Prosthet Dent 2000;83:32–39.
68. Regish KM, Sharma D, Prithviraj DR. Techniques of fabrication of provisional restorations: An overview. Int J Dent 2011;12:1–5.
69. Gürel G. Predictable, precise, and repeatable tooth preparation for porcelain laminate veneers. Pract Proced Aesthet Dent 2003; 15:17–24.
70. Magne P, Belser UC. Novel porcelain laminate preparation approach driven by a diagnostic mock-up. J Esthet Restor Dent 2004;16:7–16.
71. Kois DE, Schmidt KK, Raigrodski AJ. Esthetic templates for complex restorative cases: Rationale and management. J Esthet Restor Dent 2008;20:239–248.
72. Higginbottom FL. Quality provisional restorations: A must for successful restorative dentistry. Compend Contin Educ Dent 1995; 16:442,444–447.
73. Crispin BJ, Watson JF, Caputo AA. The marginal accuracy of treatment restorations: A comparative analysis. J Prosthet Dent 1980; 44:283–290.
74. Malone M. Smile design and advanced provisional fabrication. Gen Dent 2008;56:238–242.
75. Lewis S, Parel S, Faulkner R. Provisional implant-supported fixed restorations. Int J Oral Maxillofac Implants 1995;10:319–325.
76. Amsterdam M, Fox L. Provisional splinting—Principles and techniques. Dent Clin North Am 1959;4:73–99.
77. Chiche G. Improving marginal adaptation of provisional restorations. Quintessence Int 1990;21:325–329.
78. Harrison JD, Chiche GJ, Pinault A. Tissue management for the maxillary anterior region. In: Chiche GJ, Pinault A (eds). Esthetics of Anterior Fixed Prosthodontics. Chicago: Qunitessence, 1994:143–160.
79. Aviv I, Himmel R, Assif D. A technique for improving the marginal fit of temporary acrylic resin crowns using injection of self-curing acrylic resin. Quintessence Int 1986;17:313–315.
80. Kurtz KS. Constructing direct porcelain laminate veneer provisionals. J Am Dent Assoc 1995;126:653–656.
81. Kano P, Xavier C, Ferencz JL, Van Dooren E, Silva RFA. The anatomical shell technique: An approach to improve the esthetic predictability of CAD/CAM restorations. Quintessence Dent Technol 2013;36:27–36.
82. Chang SW, Cho BH, Lim RY, et al. Effects of blood contamination on microtensile bond strength to dentin of three self-etch adhesives. Oper Dent 2010;35:330–336.
83. Magne P, Kim TH, Cascione D, Donovan TE. Immediate dentin sealing improves bond strength of indirect restorations. J Prosthet Dent 2005;94:511–519.
84. Grajower R, Shaharbani S, Kaufman E. Temperature rise in pulp chamber during fabrication of temporary self-curing resin crowns. J Prosthet Dent 1979;41:535–540.
85. Nealon FH. Acrylic restorations by the operative nonpressure procedure. J Prosthet Dent 1952;2:513–527.
86. Kim TH, Cascione D, Knezevic A. Simulated tissue using a unique pontic design: A clinical report. J Prosthet Dent 2009;102:205–210.
87. Rosenstiel SF, Gegauff AG. Effect of provisional cementing agents on provisional resins. J Prosthet Dent 1988;59:29–33.
88. Fujisawa S, Kadoma Y. Action of eugenol as a retarder against polymerization of methyl methacrylate by benzoyl peroxide. Biomaterials 1997;18:701–703.
89. Lewinstein I, Stoleru-Baron J, Block J, Kfir A, Matalon S, Ormianer Z. Antibacterial activity and tensile strength of provisional cements modified with fluoride containing varnish. Quintessence Int 2013; 44:107–112.
90. Lewinstein I, Block J, Melamed G, Dolev E, Matalon S, Ormianer Z. Fluoride ion release and solubility of fluoride enriched interim cements. J Prosthet Dent 2014;112:188–193.
91. Featherstone JD, Singh S, Curtis DA. Caries risk assessment and management for the prosthodontic patient. J Prosthodont 2011; 20:2–9.
92. Alt V, Hannig M, Wöstmann B, Balkenhol M. Fracture strength of temporary fixed partial dentures: CAD/CAM versus directly fabricated restorations. Dent Mater 2011;27:339–347.
93. Stawarczyk B, Ender A, Trottmann A, Özcan M, Fischer J, Hämmerle CH. Load-bearing capacity of CAD/CAM milled polymeric three-unit fixed dental prostheses: Effect of aging regimens. Clin Oral Investig 2012;16:1669–1677.

94. Güth JF, Zuch T, Zwinge S, Engels J, Stimmelmayr M, Edelhoff D. Optical properties of manually and CAD/CAM-fabricated polymers. Dent Mater J 2013;32:865–871.
95. Beuer F, Schweiger J, Edelhoff D, Sorensen JA. Reconstruction of esthetics with a digital approach. Int J Periodontics Restorative Dent 2011;31:185–193.
96. Garber DA, Salama MA, Salama H. Immediate total tooth replacement. Compend Contin Educ Dent 2001;22:210–216,218.
97. Chu SJ, Salama MA, Salama H, et al. The dual-zone therapeutic concept of managing immediate implant placement and provisional restoration in anterior extraction sockets. Compend Contin Educ Dent 2012;33:524–532,534.
98. Rodriguez AM, Rosenstiel SF. Esthetic considerations related to bone and soft tissue maintenance and development around dental implants: Report of the Committee on Research in Fixed Prosthodontics of the American Academy of Fixed Prosthodontics. J Prosthet Dent 2012;108:259–267.
99. De Rouck T, Collys K, Wyn I, Cosyn J. Instant provisionalization of immediate single-tooth implants is essential to optimize esthetic treatment outcome. Clin Oral Implants Res 2009;20:566–570.
100. Block MS, Mercante DE, Lirette D, Mohamed W, Ryser M, Castellon P. Prospective evaluation of immediate and delayed provisional single tooth restorations. J Oral Maxillofac Surg 2009;67(11 suppl):89–107.
101. Raigrodski AJ, Block MS. Clinical considerations for enhancing the success of implant-supported restorations in the aesthetic zone with delayed implant placement. Pract Proced Aesthet Dent 2002;14:21–28.
102. Kois JC, Kan JY. Predictable peri-implant gingival aesthetics: Surgical and prosthodontic rationales. Pract Proced Aesthet Dent 2001;13:691–698.
103. Priest GF. The esthetic challenge of adjacent implants. J Oral Maxillofac Surg 2007;65(7 suppl 1):2–12.
104. Garber DA. The esthetic dental implant: Letting restoration be the guide. J Am Dent Assoc 1995;126:319–325.
105. Smith DE, Zarb GA. Criteria for success of osseointegrated endosseous implants. J Prosthet Dent 1989;62:567–572.
106. Priest G. Esthetic potential of single-implant provisional restorations: Selection criteria of available alternatives. J Esthet Restor Dent 2006;18:326–338.
107. Wittneben JG, Buser D, Belser UC, Brägger U. Peri-implant soft tissue conditioning with provisional restorations in the esthetic zone: The dynamic compression technique. Int J Periodontics Restorative Dent 2013;33:447–455.
108. Pow EH, McMillan AS. A modified implant healing abutment to optimize soft tissue contours: A case report. Implant Dent 2004;13:297–300.
109. Santing HJ, Meijer HJ, Raghoebar GM, Özcan M. Fracture strength and failure mode of maxillary implant-supported provisional single crowns: A comparison of composite resin crowns fabricated directly over PEEK abutments and solid titanium abutments. Clin Implant Dent Relat Res 2012;14:882–889.
110. Agustín-Panadero R, Serra-Pastor B, Roig-Vanaclocha A, Román-Rodriguez JL, Fons-Font A. Mechanical behavior of provisional implant prosthetic abutments. Med Oral Patol Oral Cir Bucal 2015;20:e94–e102.
111. Hirayama H, Kang KH, Oishi Y. The modification of interim cylinders for the fabrication of cement-retained implant-supported provisional restorations. J Prosthet Dent 2003;90:406–409.
112. Kourtis S, Psarri C, Andritsakis P, Doukoudakis A. Provisional restorations for optimizing esthetics in anterior maxillary implants: A case report. J Esthet Restor Dent 2007;19:6–17.
113. Abrahamsson I, Berglundh T, Lindhe J. The mucosal barrier following abutment dis/reconnection. An experimental study in dogs. J Clin Periodontol 1997;24:568–572.
114. Canullo L, Bignozzi I, Cocchetto R, Cristalli MP, Iannello G. Immediate positioning of a definitive abutment versus repeated abutment replacements in post-extractive implants: 3-year follow-up of a randomized multicentre clinical trial. Eur J Oral Implantol 2010;3:285–296.
115. Koutouzis T, Koutouzis G, Gadalla H, Neiva R. The effect of healing abutment reconnection and disconnection on soft and hard peri-implant tissues: A short-term randomized controlled clinical trial. Int J Oral Maxillofac Implants 2013;28:807–814.

Impression Making: A Clinical Perspective

4

Ariel J. Raigrodski | Sami Dogan

Master impressions capture not only the tooth preparations and finish lines but also the area apical to the finish line of the tooth preparation, with a fin of impression material penetrating into the sulcus (Fig 4-1). It is this excess impression material that allows the dental technician to easily identify and mark the finish line on a definitive die or at the computer-aided design (CAD) unit. Consequently, the restoration can be predictably designed and fabricated either traditionally or via CAD/computer-assisted manufacturing (CAM) technology with excellent fit and excellent marginal integrity. Major considerations for enhancing a superior master impression include tooth preparation design (particularly at the finish line, as discussed in chapter 2), soft tissue management during preparation and provisionalization procedures (see chapters 2 and 3), tray selection, tissue retraction techniques, impression material, and impression techniques. This chapter shares concepts and procedures that may facilitate the fabrication of a successful master impression, whether conventional or digital, while minimizing trauma and irreversible damage to the soft tissue.

Making adequate and accurate master impressions is not a simple proposition, especially for multiple-unit restorations (crowns and fixed dental prostheses [FDPs]) with subgingival finish lines, which are placed as such due to esthetic and biomechanical requirements or preexisting restorations with margins already placed in the gingival crevice (Fig 4-2). In such clinical scenarios, it may not be possible to predictably make a successful impression. Thus, achieving healthy soft tissue prior to this procedure is critical in facilitating an accurate reproduction of the tooth preparation and finish line as well the soft tissue contours (see chapter 5).

Continued from chapter 3

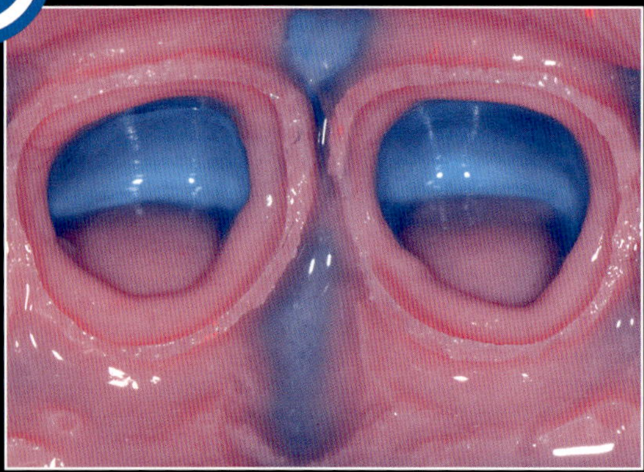

Fig 4-1 A master impression of tooth preparations for ceramic crowns (Imprint 4, 3M ESPE). Note the fin of the impression material extended into the gingival sulcus beyond the finish line. Such a fin ensures a clear reading of the finish line and subsequently facilitates the fabrication of a restoration with excellent marginal integrity.

Continued from chapter 3

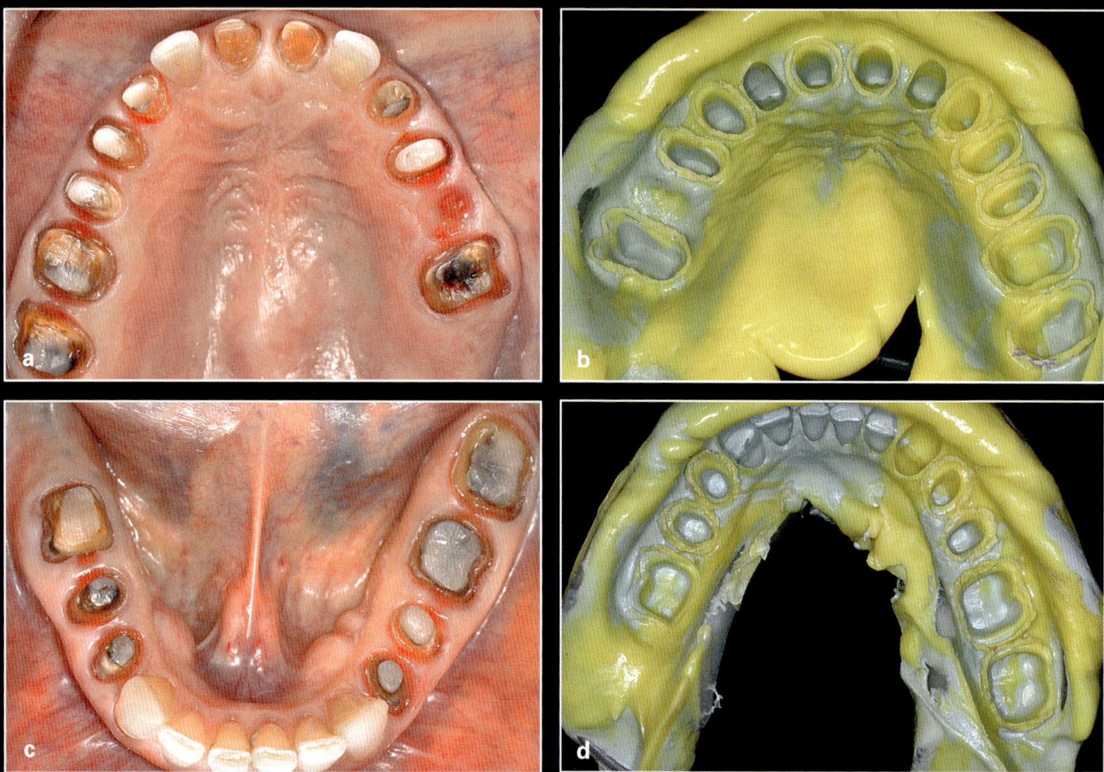

Fig 4-2 *(a and b)* Occlusal view of the definitive maxillary tooth preparations, with the finish lines mostly placed below the free gingival margins due to the preexisting indirect restorations, and the corresponding master impression made with the one-step/two-viscosity technique with a putty (tray material) and light-body consistencies. *(c and d)* Occlusal view of the definitive mandibular tooth preparations, with the finish lines mostly placed below the free gingival margins due to the preexisting indirect restorations, and the corresponding master impression made using the one-step/two-viscosity technique with a putty (tray material) and light-body consistencies.

Considerations for a Successful Impression

Soft tissue management

A critical factor in ensuring a successful impression is soft tissue health. If excellent soft tissue health is achieved during the preceding clinical steps (ie, adequate oral hygiene; adequate tooth preparation with acceptable finish line design and placement; and well-contoured, sealed, and polished provisional restorations), the probability of making an accurate master impression is increased dramatically. If, during the tooth preparation procedure, the patient is diagnosed with deep cervical caries, deep preexisting restorations, or cracks in the tooth extending to the bone crest, the finish line of the tooth preparation may extend beyond the epithelial and connective tissue attachment. In such cases, a provisional restoration must be placed without making a master impression. Surgical crown lengthening with osseous recontouring is indicated to ensure that the biologic width is reestablished in a controlled manner, and adequate healing time is allowed prior to making the master impression (see chapter 1). It was shown that in 12% of sites, 2 to 4 mm of recession occurred between 6 weeks and 6 months after surgical crown lengthening.[1] Therefore, in areas where soft tissue esthetics is critical, it is advised to delay impression procedures until the biologic width is reestablished and the stability of the free gingival margin is established as well.[2]

Trauma to the soft tissue should be minimized during impression procedures not only because it can compromise the success of the impression but also because, more importantly, irreversible trauma to the soft tissue could result in recession and free gingival margin level disparities, which can compromise the esthetic outcome. The combination of uncontrolled gingival inflammation and a subgingivally placed finish line may further augment the risk of a gingival recession after impression making.[3-5] Furthermore, crevicular fluid and heme from inflamed gingivae may displace the impression material, which can cause voids and indistinct finish line reproduction and result in an unsuccessful master impression. If signs of gingival inflammation are visible, an antimicrobial rinse (chlorhexidine gluconate 0.12%) can be prescribed for 2 weeks prior to the impression-making appointment as an adjunct measure to enhance soft tissue health.[6] In the authors' experience, daily use by the patient of an end-tufted toothbrush impregnated with chlorhexidine gluconate 0.12% may be beneficial in reducing gingival inflammation prior to impression making while minimizing adverse effects such as staining. Such a technique requires excellent patient compliance; the bristles of the toothbrush must be meticulously placed at a 45-degree angle into the gingival sulcus while applying slight mechanical pressure (Fig 4-3).

Tray selection

The next important step is the impression tray selection, which has to fit adequately in the mouth to allow for uniform thickness of the impression material without traumatizing the hard and soft tissues. Rigid custom trays should be designed with adequate spacing to allow sufficient thickness of at least 3 mm of impression material, which should be able to resist undue stress and strain upon removal from undercut areas. Among the impression materials, polyvinyl siloxane (PVS) requires the least time for recovery from viscoelastic deformation upon removal from undercut areas.[7] Although custom trays have been recommended to produce more accurate impressions, the improved physical properties of PVS impression materials make rigid stock trays a more convenient and cost-effective choice in clinical practice.[8,9]

A well-adapted impression tray must prevent the impression material from flowing away from critical areas and must not induce impression drags, which are usually seen on the distal aspects of teeth adjacent to edentulous spaces and in large undercut regions.[10] Invisible impression flaws, resulting in an apparently good fit of the restoration on the die but a poor fit on the tooth, may also occur because of tray and impression recoil. It was demonstrated that the use of nonrigid plastic stock trays with the one-step/two-viscosity technique (described later) using a putty tray impression material can result either in outward flexion of the tray wall or the incorporation of residual stresses within the impression material. Upon removal of the tray from the mouth, the tray walls may rebound, resulting in buccolingually undersized dies.[11] Therefore, the tray has to be well fitted and rigid to minimize the likelihood of such a complication.

In addition to recoil, detachment of impression material from the tray may occur, causing permanent deformation of the impression material and resulting in gross distortion of the definitive cast.[12] Detachment of the impression from the tray can occur upon removal of the impression from the mouth and may often go unnoticed. Prevention of detachment relies on the proper use of tray adhesives and using trays with adequate retentive features such as perforations and undercuts designed to lock the impression material in the tray.[13,14] Tray adhesives form a chemical bond between the tray and the impression material. After application of the tray adhesives, 7 to 15 minutes of waiting time is recommended prior to impression making.[15] Adhesive-coated intaglio surfaces of trays that become contaminated have demonstrated a significant drop in their bond strength to the impression material. Therefore, the common practice is to try in the tray first and only then, once the fit is confirmed, paint the tray with the tray adhesive.[16] To date, visible light-polymerized tray materials made of urethane dimethacrylate–based materials can be successfully used for custom tray fabrication. They are considered to be a better choice than polymethyl methacrylate–based materials due to their better bond to PVS adhesives and their superior dimensional stability.[17,18]

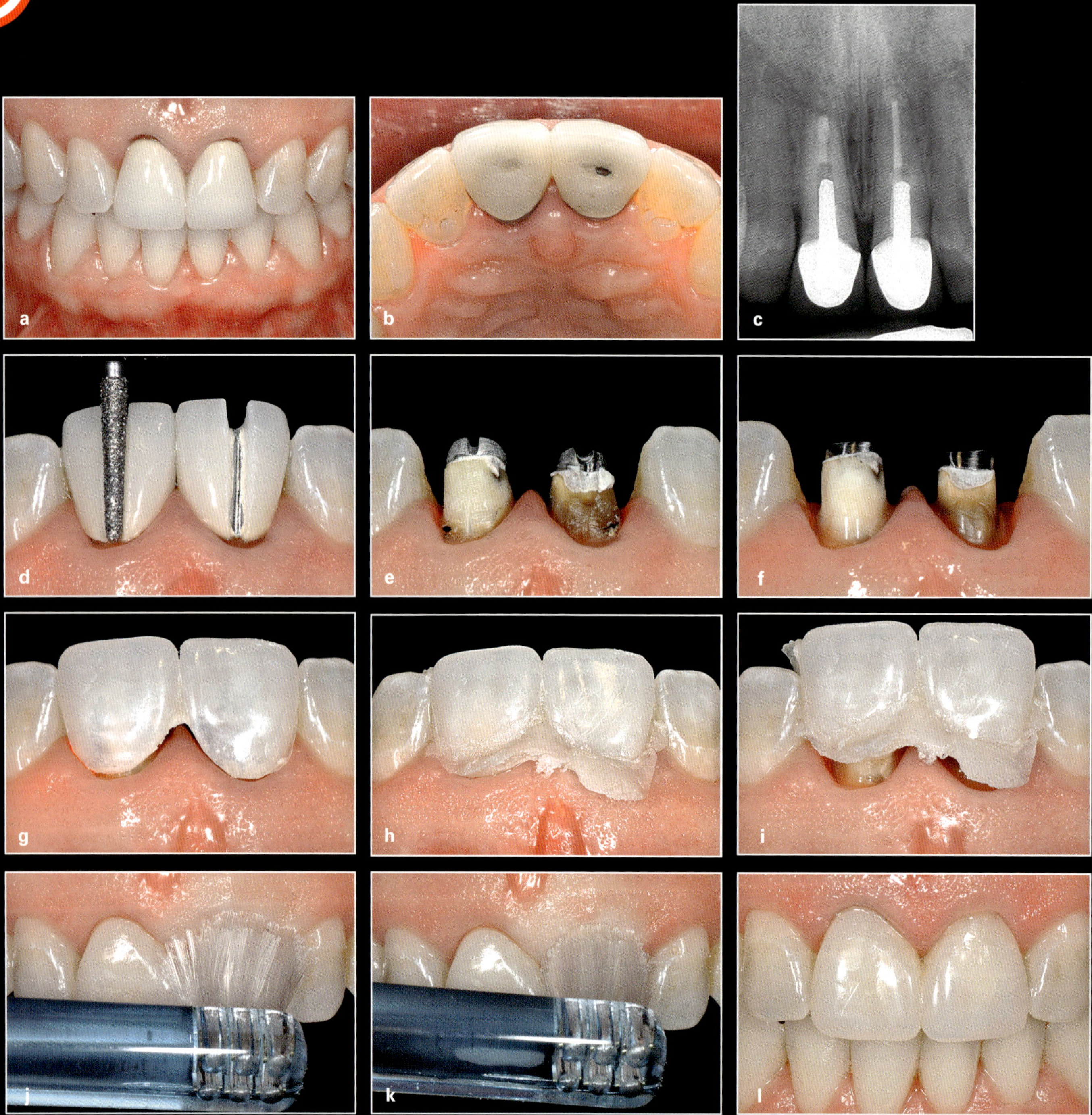

Fig 4-3 *(a and b)* Facial and occlusal views of a patient with esthetically failing metal-ceramic crowns on the maxillary central incisors. *(c)* Periapical radiograph demonstrating less than satisfactory endodontic therapy. *(d and e)* The restorations were sectioned and removed. Note the less than ideal fit of the cast post and cores and the thick cement layer present between the post and cores and the tooth structure, as well as the discoloration of the maxillary right central incisor. *(f)* Facial view of the refined tooth preparations. *(g to i)* A provisional restoration eggshell (PRES) was tried in and relined in the patient's mouth following the procedures described in chapter 3. The patient was referred for endodontic retreatment of the maxillary right central incisor. *(j and k)* The patient used an end-tufted toothbrush impregnated with chlorhexidine gluconate 0.12%, with the bristles inserted into the gingival sulcus at 45 degrees. While performing this procedure, the patient must ensure that the bristles of the brush are not placed around the gingiva *(incorrect way, j)* but are inserted into the sulcus *(correct way, k)*, creating a slight pressure and blanching and thereby reducing gingival inflammation. *(l)* Facial view of the provisional restorations prior to impression making.

Impression materials

It is important to use an impression material with adequate properties. Impression materials should be selected based on the specific needs of each clinical scenario, taking into account the advantages and limitations of each class of impression materials. The accuracy of impression materials is influenced by shrinkage caused by polymerization, the byproducts of chemical reactions, thermal changes, and incomplete elastic recovery from deformation.[19] In addition, factors such as impression disinfection, pouring time, and the impression technique used will also impact the accuracy of the master impression.[20,21]

With the advent of CAD/CAM systems, digital impressions are becoming more widely available, accurate, and affordable.[22,23] However, the use of conventional impressions is still considered the gold standard mainly for extensive, complex clinical scenarios. The same considerations of soft tissue health and accurate impression making apply to both digital and conventional impressions.

It is the authors' preference to use PVS impression materials, but prior to selecting a PVS impression material, its physical and chemical characteristics must be considered. According to the American Dental Association (ADA) specification #19, elastomeric impression materials used to fabricate precision castings must be able to reproduce fine detail of 25 μm or less. PVS impression materials can reproduce details of 1 to 2 μm. These materials require the least time for recovery from viscoelastic deformation because of their creep compliance.[7]

The yield strength, strain at yield point, and tear energy are important clinical and mechanical properties of elastomeric impression materials.[24] The *yield strength* determines the ability of the impression to withstand stress without permanent deformation; the *strain at yield point* indicates the amount of undercut an impression material can overcome without permanent elastic deformation; and the *tear energy* indicates the resistance to tear of the material after setting. A well-performing impression material should display high tear energy and adequate elastic recovery and should require the expenditure of large amounts of energy to initiate and propagate tearing.

PVS impression materials have demonstrated sufficient strength to sustain tear with a complete elastic recovery.[25] PVS and polyethers tear before the limit of permanent deformation. However, polyethers present with higher rigidity. Therefore, the clinical use of PVS is more suitable when undercuts are present, because the material will deform in the range of its yield strength. Although blocking out embrasure spaces and undercuts will prevent impression deformation, it is important to use an impression material flexible enough to overcome such undercuts on adjacent teeth and other intraoral structures such as mandibular tori, pontics, open gingival embrasures, or any additional space with undercuts.[25]

The assorted viscosities of the materials also play an important role in the accuracy of impressions. Light-body materials possess excellent flow characteristics and detail reproduction. However, in general, light-body materials also tend to flow away from the area to be impressed and demonstrate higher changes in their linear coefficient of thermal contraction due to their lower filler content, which translates to higher shrinkage during setting.[26] To facilitate accurate impression making, the optimal combination of different viscosities consists of the use of the smallest amount of light-body material possible to capture the fine detail of the prepared tooth, in particular at the finish line, while the mass of the impression material should be made with a high-viscosity impression material to minimize shrinkage. Several techniques are commonly used with PVS impression materials of varying viscosities, including the one-step/two-viscosity impression technique; the monophase/single-viscosity impression technique; and the two-step/two-viscosity putty-wash impression technique.The general rule is to combine a low-viscosity material with a high-viscosity material when using a two-step/two-viscosity technique.

Different opinions have been expressed with regard to these various impression techniques. Some investigators have demonstrated no significant difference in accuracy between the one-step/two-viscosity technique and the two-step/two-viscosity putty-wash impression technique.[27] Others have claimed that the impression technique has a greater influence on accuracy than the material itself. The main concern with the one-step/two-viscosity technique using a medium-body, low-viscosity tray material is the uncontrolled bulk of the light-body material.[28]

Impression materials must have adequate viscosity to avoid slumping when loaded into an impression tray. A convenient and reliable way of making an impression is with a PVS putty and a corresponding light-body material with the one-step/two-viscosity technique using rigid metal trays or rigid plastic trays. If the putty consistency is used as the tray material with the one-step/two-viscosity technique, a horseshoe channel should be made in the tray material and subsequently filled with light-body material. This will minimize the displacement of the light-body material at the tooth preparation (particularly at the finish line), because that channel is filled with light-body impression material. Also, it will facilitate the reproduction of the surface texture of the adjacent dentition, which is critical for the fabrication of a restoration with adequate light reflection, facilitating a better match between the prospective restoration and the adjacent teeth. The advantage of using putty consistency is subjective in terms of creating a definitive seating of the tray. If a heavy-body material is used, more movement of the tray is expected, and the likelihood of touching the cusp tips of the teeth or the preparations (depending on the type of case) is increased, which may compromise adequate mounting of the definitive and opposing casts on the articulator and the prospective occlusion. In addition, the tray material can push the light-body impression material into the gingival sulcus, thus facilitating the reproduction of the finish line and beyond (the subgingival fin area) (see Fig 4-1).

Continued from page 86

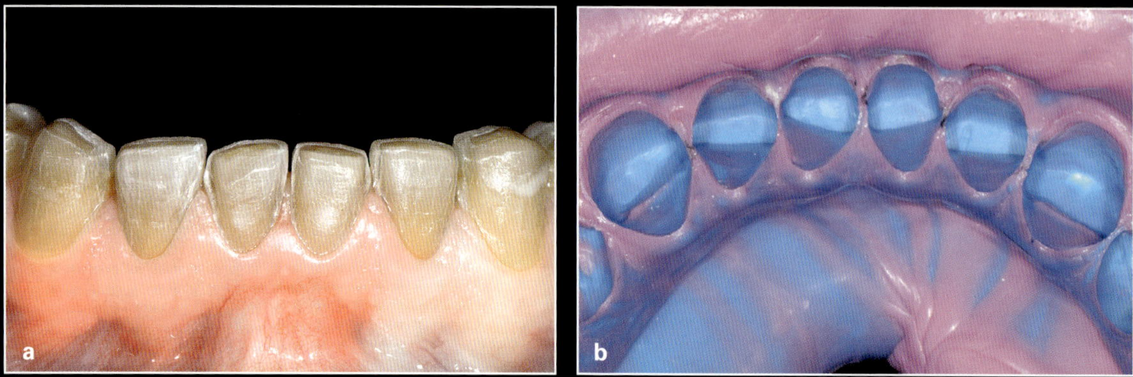

Fig 4-4 *(a)* Facial view of the definitive preparations for ceramic labial veneers. *(b)* An impression made for six ceramic veneer preparations. Note the interproximal areas, where the contact was slightly broken with a metal strip, and the thin impression material between the teeth, which is essential for marginal integrity of the prospective restorations at the interproximal areas, for adequate sectioning of individual dies, and for adequate fabrication of the ceramic labial veneers.

The putty (type 0) or heavy-body (type 1) impression material can be combined with a low-viscosity silicone when making master impressions using a procedure known as the *two-step putty-wash technique*. However, this technique has its limitations in terms of accuracy. If undercuts are not removed, displacement of the first impression material will occur through the pressure of the light-body wash material during the second step of the impression, which may cause inaccuracies within the impression.[10,29]

Some of the newest "hydrophilic" PVS materials have an excellent tear strength and toughness, which is critical for reproducing the finish line area and subgingival fin area. It is more critical when impressing preparations for ceramic veneers where the proximal contact points are gently broken and a thin sliver of light-body impression material must be maintained between the tooth preparations to ensure accurate separation between the teeth on the definitive cast for easier sectioning of the dies (Fig 4-4).

Polyethers are the only true hydrophilic elastomeric impression materials[30] and have been very popular with many clinicians. It is the authors' preference to use polyethers when good control of the soft tissue cannot be achieved and crevicular fluid and heme are of concern during the impression-making procedure. However, the tear strength of this material is inferior in comparison with some of the new PVS materials. In the authors' experience, PVS materials in general are excellent impression materials with excellent detail reproduction, relative hydrophilicity, and high tear strength and toughness, as demonstrated in clinical studies.[4,31–33]

A minimum thickness of light-body impression material is required for both optimal accuracy and adequate tear resistance of the material. A light-body thickness of 2 mm was the most accurate for the fabrication of stone dies in some studies using the putty-wash technique.[34,35] However, the results of these studies are related to the specific brands and impression technique used and therefore may not have universal application. From a clinical perspective, if the tissue is healthy and well controlled with the provisional restorations, the brand of material to be used is secondary, and some clinicians may express a personal preference of one over another.

Retraction techniques

A major factor to be considered in the impression-making procedure is the tissue retraction technique and its clinical application. Management of the gingival tissues is essential for obtaining accurate impressions for the fabrication of fixed restorations, particularly when the finish line is placed at, or just within, the gingival sulcus.[36–40] The goal of the retraction procedure is to expose the finish line of the tooth preparation in a manner that will allow the impression material to penetrate beyond the finish line. It was demonstrated that in order to achieve adequate bulk of light-body impression material below the free gingival margins, a minimum sulcular width of 0.2 mm is needed to facilitate accurate impressions with no distortion and no tear.[41,42] The other goal of the retraction procedure is to ensure that such a retraction is reversible and avoids permanent trauma. Some techniques advocate the use of retraction cords, while others use injectable retraction materials. Materials used for gingival retraction must be effective and should not cause significant tissue damage. Contemporary techniques used to accomplish gingival retraction can be classified as mechanical, chemical, surgical, or combinations of these.[43,44]

Retraction cords

The *single-cord technique* is indicated when an impression is being made for a small number of abutments with healthy tissues and no hemorrhage and with a shallow sulcus that is not deep enough to accommodate a second cord.[45] This technique has been described as the simplest and least traumatic retraction option.[46] The *double-cord technique* is beneficial when the finish line is located relatively deep below the free gingival margins and when cords can be placed and accommodated into the sulcus. With this technique, a narrow-diameter cord is placed first in the sulcus, followed by a larger-diameter cord usually impregnated with a hemostatic agent. The latter is removed prior to the impression-making procedure, as discussed later. This technique has been described as the most consistent in achieving accurate impressions of subgingivally placed finish lines.[39] This approach also helps control gingival heme and assists in overcoming the problem of impression material tearing in the sulcus due to inadequate bulk remaining there. It reduces the tendency of the gingival cuff to recoil/rebound and displace the impression material. The single-cord and double-cord techniques are the most widely accepted methods of gingival retraction for making master impressions for natural dentition.[38] Both techniques can traumatize the delicate sulcular epithelial lining and may lead to an average postoperative gingival recession of 0.2 mm ± 0.1 mm.[47] Therefore, retraction cords should be placed carefully using a sustained and controlled force while displacing the soft tissue horizontally.

Either braided or knitted cords may be used. The highly fibrous, highly organized periodontal complex surrounding natural teeth provides support for the gingival tissues when they are retracted, thus reducing the collapse of the tissues when the retraction cords are removed prior to impression making. The amount of time that cord should be allowed to remain in the sulcus has been evaluated by several authors to range from 1 minute to 30 minutes, as demonstrated in one study in dogs.[48] However, the latter may jeopardize gingival health, potentially causing irreversible recession, also depending on the type of hemostatic agent used.[42,48–52] From a clinical perspective, the cord has to be left long enough to create adequate displacement of the gingiva. However, to preserve the gingival health and contours, it is important not to leave the cord for longer than is necessary. Depending on the cord's diameter, adequate tissue displacement can be achieved by retracting the gingiva for at least 4 minutes. In a study by Baharav et al,[51] placing retraction cords for longer than 4 minutes provided no further advantage. However, placing the retraction cords for less time caused a significant reduction in the retraction effect.[51]

The precise use of instruments for cord placement has not been described in an objective manner in the literature, and the required forces involved in cord placement remain undetermined as well. Placement of retraction cords can cause injury to the sulcular epithelium and underlying connective tissues.[47] Therefore, use of minimal force is necessary when placing cords to protect the Sharpey's fibers.[53] In contrast, the application of excessive force may cause crevicular bleeding, gingival inflammation,[54] and shrinkage of marginal tissues. No prolonged adverse effects of the epithelial attachment were observed when the cords were placed in a cautious manner. However, if the cords are placed dry, then they may tear the crevicular epithelium and induce a wound-healing reaction.[3,55] Healing of the sulcus can take 7 to 10 days.[48,56] When the double-cord technique is used, once the impression is made, the first narrow-diameter cord must be removed carefully. The sulci have to be flushed with water to remove any possible residue from the cord itself, which may contain debris resulting from the manufacturing or packaging process,[57] or from any hemostatic agent used in conjunction with the cord.

Hemostatic agents

A variety of hemostatic agents are available for use with gingival retraction procedures. Epinephrine may be used for impregnating retraction cords because it provides effective vasoconstriction and hemostasis during retraction. However, it may be associated with significant local and systemic side effects.[58] Thus, clinicians should avoid applying high concentrations of epinephrine in large areas of lacerated or abraded gingival tissues.[59] Several popular alternatives to epinephrine are currently used successfully in practice. Synthetic sympathomimetic agents that mimic the actions of epinephrine are shown to be more effective and safer than epinephrine.[60]

Aluminum sulfate and aluminum potassium sulfate prevent capillary bleeding by causing minimal vasoconstriction, by precipitating tissue proteins with tissue contraction, and by inhibiting the transcapillary movement of plasma proteins.[61] Both astringents are hemostatic and retractive and cause minimal postoperative inflammation at therapeutic concentrations.

The action of aluminum chloride is similar to that of aluminum sulfate, causing precipitation of tissue proteins but less vasoconstriction than epinephrine. However, it might disturb the setting of PVS impression materials, so testing is recommended for any new brands of impression materials prior to using them for making master impressions.[42] Concentrated aluminum chloride solutions of more than 0.33% can cause severe inflammation and tissue necrosis.[62]

Ferric sulfate is another astringent used for impregnating retraction cords. However, the iron in ferric sulfate stains gingival tissues and tooth structure with a yellow-brown to black color for several days after a clinician has used it as a hemostatic agent. The accuracy of surface detail reproduction during impressions can also be adversely modified by ferric sulfate, and it may disturb the setting reaction of PVS impression materials. Thus, it is important for clinicians to carefully remove all traces of hemostatic agents from the surfaces of tooth preparations as well as from the soft tissues prior to impression making.[63]

In general, there are two main limitations of using hemostatic agents in conjunction with retraction cords. The first is the occurrence of rebound hyperemia that often occurs after cord removal, which may determine how effective and accurate the master impression is. The second is the inflammatory reaction induced by these chemicals, which can affect the subepithelial connective tissue and may subsequently cause gingival recession.[64]

Injectable matrices/pastes

In addition to mechanical retraction with cord (in conjunction with hemostatic agents), cordless systems have been introduced as means of retraction without the need for a cord. It has been reported that all cordless systems produce less traumatic pressure in the sulcus area during retraction when compared with traditional mechanical retraction with cords.[65–67] Careful, atraumatic application of the cordless systems is still paramount for gingival health because of the possible temporary gingival inflammation during application.[67]

Gingival retraction pastes (3M ESPE Astringent Retraction Paste; Expasyl, Kerr; Traxodent, Premier Dental) combine kaolin for gingival displacement and 15% aluminum chloride for generating hemostasis. It is claimed that the procedure is not time-consuming and does not cause patient discomfort or gingival trauma. Injecting 15% aluminum chloride in a kaolin matrix opens the sulcus, providing significant mechanical retraction.[68] Its effectiveness in reducing the flow of crevicular fluid and heme is similar to that of epinephrine-soaked cords.[69] It is hydrophilic and can be rinsed away relatively easily from the gingival crevice. As with any foreign materials introduced into the oral cavity, there remains a small risk of residue persisting in the gingival crevice. The viscosity of the injectable matrix may not be enough to provide sufficient retraction for deeper subgingival preparations, and the aluminum chloride can inhibit the set of polyether and PVS impression materials if clinicians do not rinse it away properly before impression making.[68,69]

A silicone polymer retraction material (Magic FoamCord, Coltène/Whaledent) was recently proposed to facilitate access to the tooth preparation finish line using a potentially less traumatic and less time-consuming procedure than traditional retraction cord placement. This material is an expanding two-component PVS silicone without a hemostatic agent. During setting, the polymerization reaction of the PVS generates hydrogen gas. The released hydrogen gas creates bubbles and transforms the polymerized material into a spongelike texture. The material has to be syringed around the finish line of the tooth preparation and maintained under pressure prior to impression making. A clinical study demonstrated that in cases of equigingival and subgingival finish line placement of less than 2.0 mm, the silicone polymer retraction material was shown to be a less traumatic alternative to gingival retraction. However, when the finish line was placed more than 2.0 mm apical to the free gingival margins, and when the finish line design was a bevel, this technique was less effective than the single-cord retraction technique.[5]

Lasers

Diode lasers with a wavelength of 980 nm and neodymium: yttrium-aluminum-garnet (Nd:YAG) lasers with a wavelength of 1,064 nm were shown to be less aggressive, caused less bleeding, and resulted in less recession around natural teeth compared with mechanical retraction with cord and sulcus conditioning with electrosurgery.[70] However, the use of Nd:YAG lasers is contraindicated near implant surfaces, owing to the effects of this laser's wavelength on metal, because implants tend to absorb energy, which causes them to heat up and transmit the heat to bone.[71]

Erbium:yttrium-aluminum-garnet (Er:YAG) lasers with a wavelength of 2,940 nm are reflected by metal implant surfaces[71] and minimally penetrate the soft tissues, so they are relatively safe to use. The hemostasis achieved with the Er:YAG laser, however, is not as effective as that achieved with the carbon dioxide (CO_2) laser. The CO_2 laser has a wavelength of 10,600 nm and reflects off metal surfaces. When used near metallic implant surfaces, CO_2 lasers absorb little energy, with only small temperature increases ($< 3°C$) and minimal collateral damage. CO_2 lasers do not alter the structure of the implant surface.[71]

Although CO_2 lasers may be significantly useful in some impression situations, they are invasive, thus failing to meet the ideal objective of a truly conservative technique. For the applications in which esthetics is critical, it may not be desirable to create a trough in the soft tissue around the finish line, as it may have a detrimental effect on the patient's appearance by causing soft tissue defects.[71]

Electrosurgery

Clinicians may choose to use electrosurgery to effectively widen the gingival sulcus around natural teeth before placing the cord and to provide hemostasis by coagulation.[56,72] However, electrosurgery is not recommended around dental implants. The concentrated electrical current at the tip of electrodes can generate heat, which may cause osseous or mucosal necrosis. In addition, it was demonstrated that the use of electrosurgery as a means of retraction may cause more recession as compared with the use of retraction cord with a hemostatic agent.[47]

Rotary curettage

Rotary curettage involves the use of a high-speed turbine to excise the gingival tissue quickly and create a trough around the margins. For healthy, disease-free tissue around natural teeth, rotary curettage has little effect on gingival margin heights if adequate keratinized gingiva is present.[73] In the absence of keratinized gingiva, rotary curettage could lead to an exaggerated response, including deepening of the sulcus and recession.[74] In a dog study, gingival recession was found to be greater with rotary curettage techniques than with electrosurgery and mechanical retraction with cord.[56]

Copper-band retraction

For decades copper-band retraction has been used in conjunction with a corresponding impression technique. However, the technique is not described here because currently it is not widely used. The use of copper bands precludes the need for gingival retraction with retraction cords and hemostatic agents. On the basis of wound healing and gingival recession, the copper-band retraction method was shown to be satisfactory.[47]

Summary

In summary, clinically acceptable impressions require clinical expertise and appropriate materials and techniques. Properly managing tissues and following proper protocols are important to consider before making impressions. Gingival retraction is essential for soft tissue management before an impression is made. There are limitations with any retraction technique, and the choice of technique and material depends on the operator's judgment of the clinical situation. Mechanical retraction with cord is still accepted as standard compared with the cordless systems. With the progress of CAD/CAM systems, digital impressions will become more widely available because of their speed, efficiency, and acceptance by the patients. However, the use of conventional impression techniques is still the gold standard for dentists until digital impressions become a common procedure for all clinical scenarios—from the single veneer impression to the complete-mouth rehabilitation impression with or without implants.

Translation to Procedures

Cord placement with the double-cord technique

J Case J illustrates procedures for making a master impression using the double-cord technique (Fig 4-5). Once the provisional restoration is removed and the tooth preparation, gingiva, and sulcus are gently cleaned (see Figs 4-5a to 4-5e), the cord is placed. Cord placement is a technique-sensitive procedure. Consequently, it should be performed gently and prudently. When the double-cord technique is used in the anterior segment, the first cord, which is typically a triple zero in size (Ultrapak, Ultradent), should be placed without a hemostatic agent to minimize the likelihood of recession. The cord is placed on the facial aspect first, and then it is condensed gently while the tissue is displaced horizontally in an attempt to minimize the likelihood of bleeding (see Figs 4-5f and 4-5g). A plain cord packer (N122PN Cord Packer PN, Brasseler USA) is used for the purpose of compressing the cord mesiodistally and displacing the tissue horizontally. Therefore, the instrument is moved circumferentially around the tooth preparation while the tissue is displaced laterally with minimal pressure in the occlusogingival direction.

The cord packer preferred by the authors has no serrations. It is the authors' opinion that such serrations may compromise the integrity of such a braided cord by pulling its fibers. In certain clinical situations in which the teeth are triangular and close together with extensive soft tissue scalloping and the tissue is thick and fibrous, the use of a flat periodontal probe (Goldman-Fox/Williams Probe, Hu-Friedy) may be helpful for facilitating a relatively atraumatic cord placement (Fig 4-6). If localized bleeding occurs during the A cord placement, a microbrush dipped in aluminum chloride can be used to blot the traumatized area to stop the heme. The first cord is placed 360 degrees circumferentially without overlapping or any excess coming out of the sulcus. This cord compresses the tissue horizontally to prevent seepage from the sulcus (see Fig 4-5h).

Once the first cord placement is completed without any excess coming out of the sulcus, the second cord, a zero in diameter (Ultrapak), impregnated with 25% aluminum chloride (ViscoStat Clear, Ultradent), is placed with excess cord coming out of the palatal aspect (see Fig 4-5i) to deflect the tissue in a similar manner while promoting hemostasis (see Fig 4-5i). Once the second, coronal cord placement is complete, the entire finish line of the tooth preparation should be exposed from an occlusal view. If at this stage it appears as if the tissue may have receded (see Fig 4-5j), clinical judgment must be carefully exercised with regard to the definitive finish line position. Some may consider dropping the finish line apically to the newly positioned free gingival margin to ensure that the soft tissue–restorative interface is concealed. However, major considerations such as the distance between the free gingival margin and the crest of the bone, the gingival health after tooth preparation and placement of the provisional restoration, the thickness of the tissue and its translucency, and the gingival levels from an esthetic standpoint, must all be weighed in making such a critical decision (see chapter 1). Once the cord is placed, the tissue tends to be displaced horizontally as well as vertically, so exposure of the finish line is expected. Therefore, the question to be asked is this: Is the tissue going to rebound once the impression is made? Further dropping of the finish line may result in biologic width violation and in disparate gingival levels, both of which will compromise the definitive clinical outcome. If the levels of the free gingival margins have been adequate and the gingiva is healthy, clinicians should move forward with making the impression as is (without further dropping the finish line apically), which is a reversible procedure. The master impression can be poured, and if, 2 weeks later, the tissue does not rebound coronally and an esthetic liability is of concern, the clinician can always see the patient, drop the

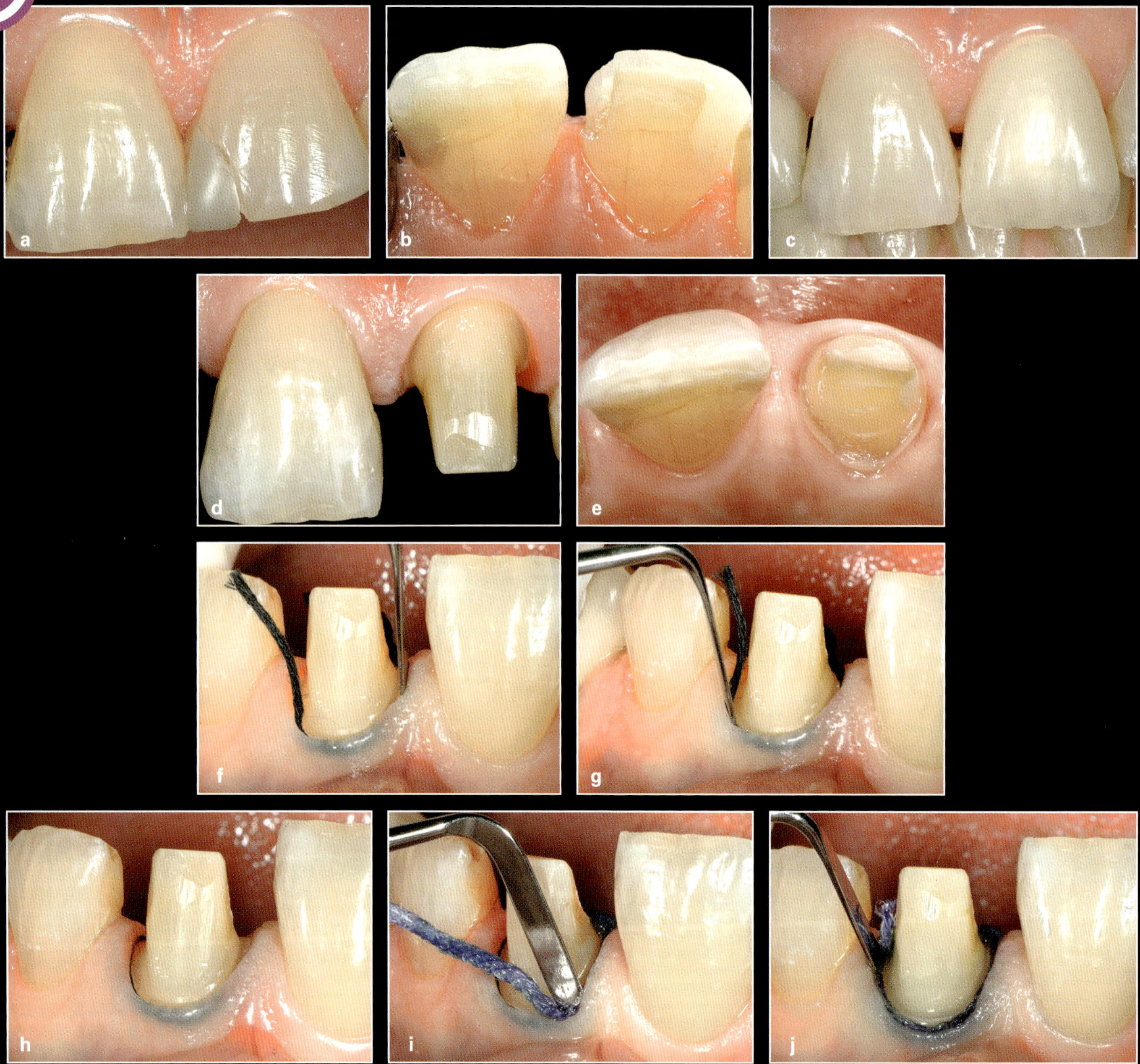

Fig 4-5 *(a and b)* Facial and occlusal views of maxillary central incisors. The maxillary left central incisor was planned to be restored with a zirconia-based ceramic crown due to dental caries and failing extensive direct composite resin restorations. *(c)* The tooth has been prepared using the concepts and techniques described in chapter 2, and a provisional restoration was fabricated and placed using the concepts described in chapter 3. Note the gingival health 4 weeks after tooth preparation. *(d and e)* Facial and occlusal views of the prepared tooth after removal of the provisional restoration. All remnants of temporary cement were cleaned from the tooth preparation and the gingival sulcus. Note the gingival health. *(f and g)* The first (cervical) cord (Ultrapak #000) was placed without a hemostatic agent to minimize the likelihood of recession. The cord was placed gently while the tissue was displaced horizontally in an attempt to minimize the likelihood of bleeding. A plain cord packer with no serrations (N122PN Cord Packer PN) was used with the purpose of compressing the cord mesiodistally and the tissue horizontally. *(h)* The first cord placement was completed without any excess cord coming out of the sulcus. Note that it is visually reflected through the tissue. Thus, the tissue may be characterized to have a thin phenotype and high translucency, which is risky in terms of increased probability of recession. *(i and j)* A second cord (Ultrapak #0), impregnated with aluminum chloride (ViscoStat Clear), was subsequently placed with excess coming out of the palatal aspect of the gingival sulcus. Note that the tissue seems to have receded.

A

Continued from page 90

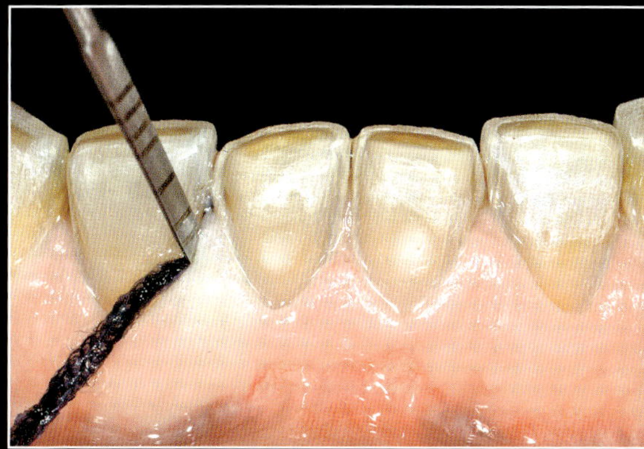

Fig 4-6 Because the mandibular incisors presented with a triangular shape and a narrow root with extensive soft tissue scalloping, root proximity, and thick and fibrous surrounding tissue, the use of a flat periodontal probe (Goldman-Fox/Williams Probe) rather than a conventional cord packer facilitated a relatively atraumatic cord placement prior to impression making.

C

Continued from chapter 3

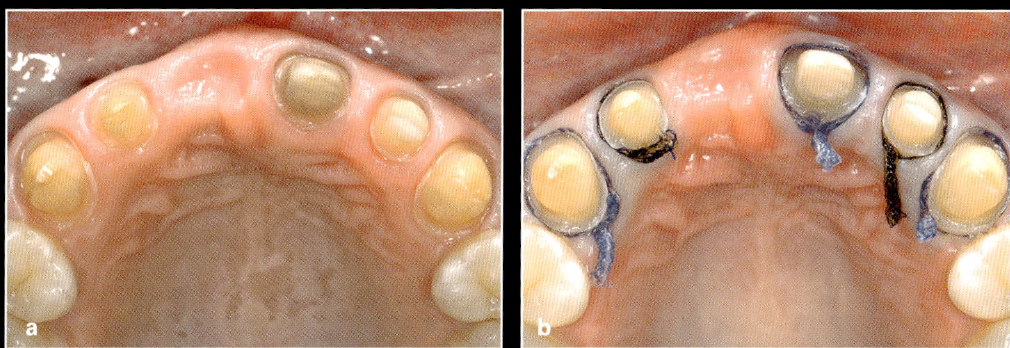

Fig 4-7 *(a)* Occlusal view of the definitive tooth preparations and the matured and healed soft tissue prior to impression making. *(b)* Occlusal view demonstrating cord placement with the edges of the cord toward the palatal aspect. These aspects generally require less extensive retraction compared with the facial and interproximal areas, and cord removal is easily facilitated. *(c)* A view of the master impression demonstrating a clear reproduction of the tooth preparations, finish lines, and surrounding tissue contours.

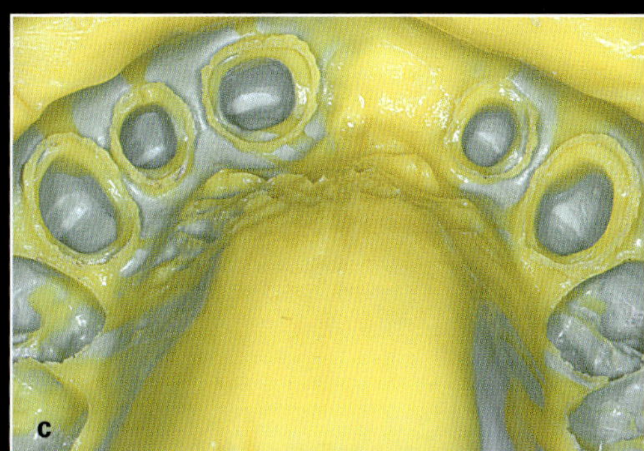

finish line further apically, and make a new impression. If, on the other hand, the tissue rebounds, the definitive cast can be used for fabricating the definitive restoration.

With regard to the placement of the coronal (second) cord with the double-cord technique or the single cord with the single-cord technique, enough excess cord should be available at the palatal area, where the finish line is often placed supragingivally and tissue retraction may not be critical. Therefore, it is recommended to place the cord with the edges toward the palatal/lingual aspect, which is less likely to need extensive retraction compared with the facial and interproximal areas (Fig 4-7). Too much excess cord may be detrimental, however, because the cord may cover the tooth preparation and contaminate it with hemostatic agent, which may adversely affect the impression's accuracy, especially when polyethers are used. Consistency in terms of cord length and position in relationship to the tooth preparation may facilitate its removal at the time of impression making. This is crucial, especially when multiple units are to be impressed and when working time is valuable.

One must consider that during the impression procedure, when the coronal cord is removed, the tissue may start to collapse. Therefore, the role of the first cervical cord is to prevent gingival fluid and heme from contaminating the tooth preparation and to keep the sulcus open. In certain clinical scenarios in which the soft tissue is thin and narrow, or with crown preparations for mandibular incisors and maxillary lateral incisors (where the soft tissue tends to be thin and fragile), triple-zero cord is still used as the cervical cord while double-zero cord is used as the coronal cord to reduce the risk of irreversible recession. For ceramic labial veneers, the approach may be more conservative; in general, a single cord is used, usually triple zero in diameter. However, because there are so many clinical variations with ceramic labial veneer preparations, clinicians must use sound clinical judgment and modify the procedure as needed to ensure adequate impressions while minimizing soft tissue trauma.

Impression material application/delivery

Regarding the accuracy and stability of the gingival sulcus area in a normal setting, both the one-step/two-viscosity and the two-step/two-viscosity techniques result in acceptable accuracy for the finish line and the gingival sulcular area.[75] Both techniques resulted in accuracy measurements of less than 0.5%, as described by the ADA specification standard, and these results were therefore not clinically significant.[27] Variables with significant influence were the impression technique, heme at the impression, and probing depths.[76]

One crucial factor for impression accuracy is the quality of the mix of impression material for both the tray and the syringe material if the two-step/two-viscosity technique is used. The formation of a uniform mix, with no air voids, will facilitate optimal and uniform working and setting times. Such a uniform mix has been available for most heavy, monophase, and light-body impression materials. However, it has limited availability for impression materials with a putty consistency. With some of the materials available in the market (Imprint 3 and Imprint 4 Penta Putty, 3M ESPE), the ability to use an automixed putty consistency tray material is extremely advantageous.[77,78]

Another critical factor is the technique used to deliver the light-body impression material to the tooth preparation, particularly at the finish line. Single-use, disposable automix intraoral syringes are available from multiple companies (3M ESPE Intra-oral Syringe; Extrude Intra-oral Syringe, Kerr) (Fig 4-8). Using such ergonomic automix syringes, which allow access at different angles without incorporating air bubbles into the light-body impression mix, will extend the working time for multiple units and facilitate an adequate, detailed impression.[79] These syringes also facilitate a hygienic procedure with minimal cleanup in the dental practice. Less impression material is put to waste, and chair time is saved.

Isolation

Once the provisional restoration is removed, attention should be given not only to cleaning of the tooth preparation but also to removal of any excess cement and other contaminants from the gingival sulcus. Dry angles or tips, cotton rolls, salivary ejectors, and high-volume evacuation tips are all critical for effective moisture control prior to and during impression making. Dry angles or tips should be used in the buccal vestibule instead of cotton rolls where possible; cotton rolls can slip and interfere with the placement of the impression material in the buccal vestibule. Salivary ejectors and high-volume evacuation tips should be kept away from the sulcus in order to avoid displacing the dental cords in the area. During the impression procedure, the placement of cheek retractors allows the operator better control of the operating field.

Impression-making procedure

The technique described in this chapter is the one-step/two-viscosity technique. Prior to impression making, the prepared tooth is cleaned with wet cotton pellets (impregnated in water) or with a surface cleanser (B4 Pre-Impression Surface Optimizer, Dentsply Caulk; Detail Pre-Impression Cleansing Gel, Clinician's Choice Dental) to remove any hemostatic agent from the tooth surface that could compromise the integrity and accuracy of the impression (Fig 4-9). Subsequently, the cords are left in the sulcus for 5 to 7 minutes. The goal is to leave the cord long enough to ensure adequate retraction, yet briefly enough so as not to cause recession. As previously mentioned, 4 minutes of retraction with a triple-zero cord and a number-one cord impregnated with aluminum chloride (Hemodent Liquid, Premier Dental) is adequate to achieve this goal.[51] The duration of cord retraction can be easily controlled for one or two teeth. However, it would be impossible to control the duration of cord retraction in the sulcus for multiple teeth. Consequently, the sequence of cord placement may become critical in reducing the likelihood of a recession in esthetically critical areas. If a complete arch requires an impression, then a preferable cord-placement sequence would be to place the cord first at the molars followed by the premolars, proceeding with the canines and the central incisors, and finishing the procedure with the lateral incisors, which may be more susceptible to recession. This will result in longer duration of retraction on the posterior teeth than the anterior teeth, thus reducing the risk of a recession in the areas where esthetics is crucial.

The next step prior to impression making is to gently rinse the teeth and cords with water to ensure that the cords are moist. Dry cords may increase the risk of epithelium tear and hemorrhage during removal of the coronal cord.[80] Once all of the coronal cords have been removed, the tooth prepara-

I

Continued from page 88

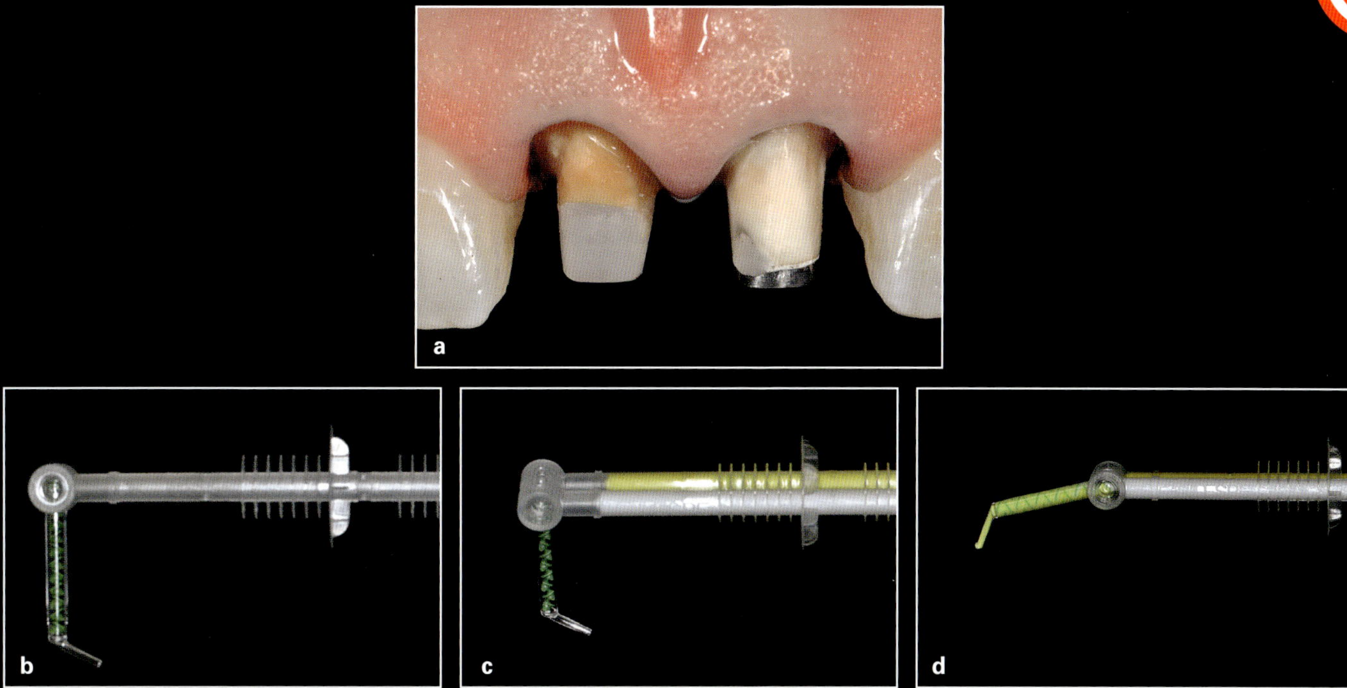

Fig 4-8 *(a)* Facial view of the definitive tooth preparations. Internal bleaching was performed on the maxillary right central incisor, followed by the placement of a prefabricated post and composite resin core. Subsequently, the tooth preparations were refined. *(b to d)* A disposable automix intraoral syringe (3M ESPE Intra-oral Syringe) was attached to the light-body impression cartridge and then filled with base and catalyst of the impression material. Once the master impression was ready to be made, the angle of the tip was modified at 90 degrees, and the impression was automixed as it was syringed.

J

Continued from page 94

Fig 4-9 Prior to impression making, the prepared tooth is cleaned with agitating wet cotton pellets on the tooth preparation, adjacent teeth, and adjacent soft tissue to ensure removal of any hemostatic agent from the tooth surface that could compromise the integrity and accuracy of the impression.

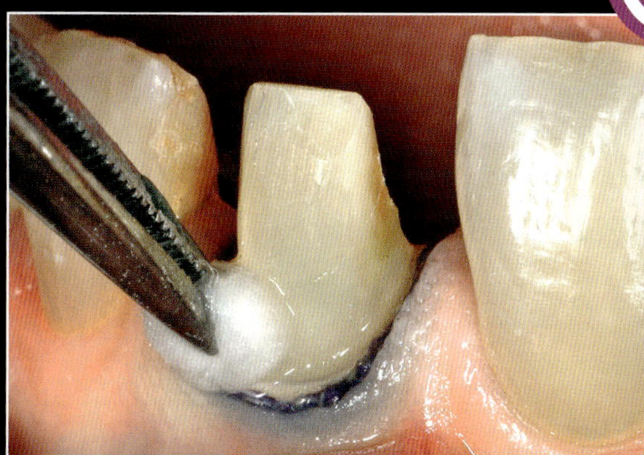

tions, sulci, and surrounding tissues should be dried with a gentle stream of air.

Subsequently, the impression tray is filled (in a horseshoe configuration) with a tray material of the selected viscosity (either heavy-body or putty consistency) by the dental assistant. Once the tray is filled with the viscous tray material, the assistant forms a horseshoe-shaped channel within the impression tray material and fills it with the light-body material. Simultaneously, the light-body impression material is syringed on the finish line circumferentially while the tip of the syringe is maintained on the finish line. As previously described, automixing syringes are great adjuncts for such

Continued from page 97

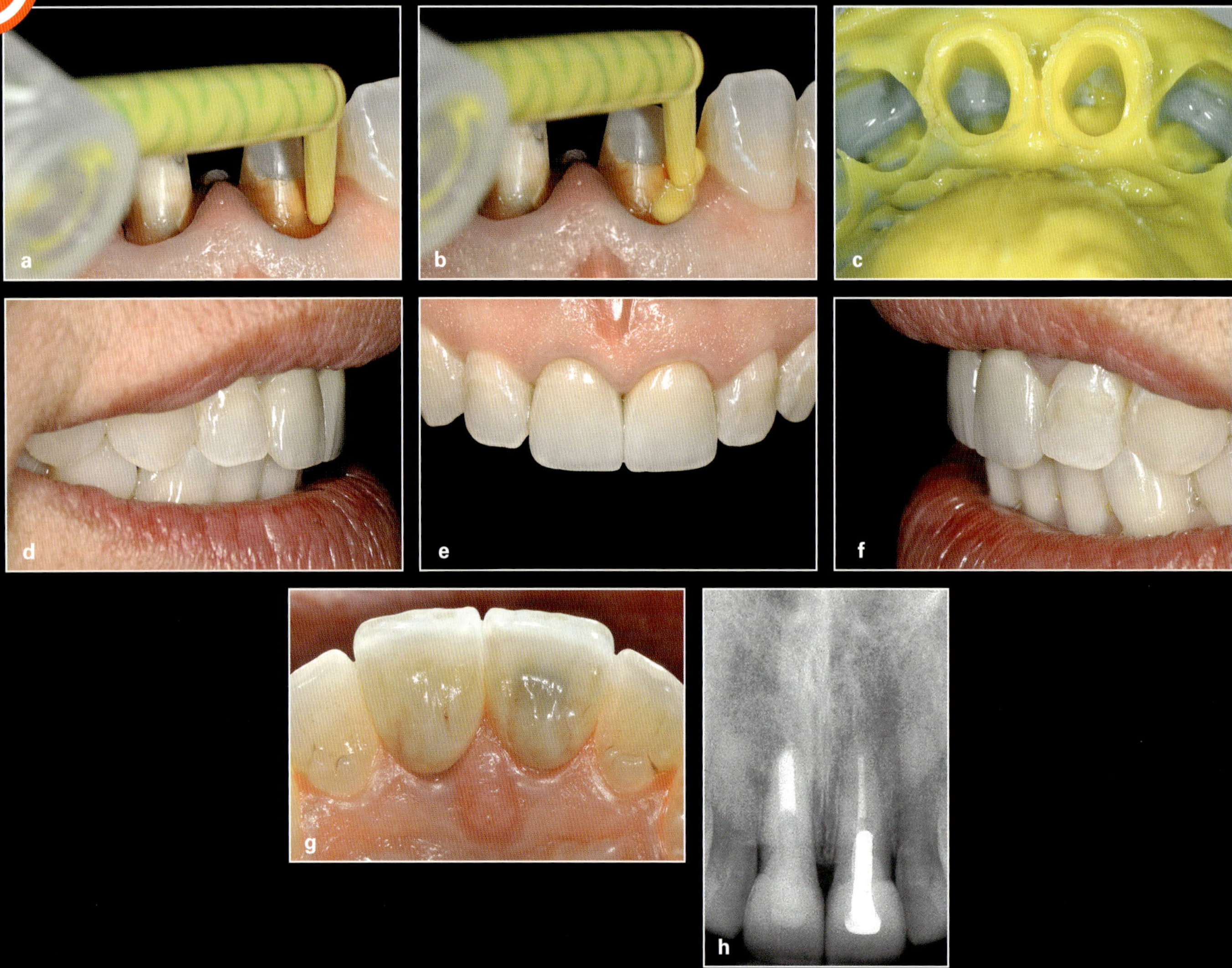

Fig 4-10 *(a and b)* The tip of the automixed syringe is placed on the finish line, and the light-body impression material is carefully automixed as the material is syringed circumferentially on the finish line to ensure an adequate master impression. *(c)* View of the master impression. *(d to f)* Facial and lateral views of the definitive lithium-dislicate (e.max, Ivoclar Vivadent) ceramic crowns. *(g)* Occlusal view of the definitive restorations. Note that the metal post reflects through the palatal aspect of the maxillary left central incisor. *(h)* Periapical radiograph of the definitive restorations.

a procedure, particularly for multiple units. The material is automixed as it is dispensed on the prepared teeth. The tip of the syringe is small and angled, which facilitates the delivery of the impression material at the finish line (Figs 4-10a and 4-10b). Leaving the tip of the syringe on the finish line (to facilitate adequate reproduction of the finish line in the impression) may prove to be clinically challenging in certain scenarios such as posterior teeth and limited mouth opening. Syringing should start from the most difficult area (usually distolingual areas) by expression of the material into the sulcus and should progress 360 degrees at the finish line without any discontinuation. Depending on the number of tooth preparations involved and if working time permits, an air syringe may be used to gently force the light-body impression material into the gingival sulcus. Another round of light-body syringing at the finish line should follow. Syringing the light-body impression material onto the occlusal surface of the tooth preparation should be the final step in the placement of light-body impression material. Finally, the impression tray is seated in the patient's mouth with minimal horizontal movement to avoid voids and drags (Figs 4-10c to 4-10h).

Impressions for implant-supported restorations

With impressions that also include dental implants, additional considerations must be weighed; several options, such as the use of open and closed tray impression copings, are available. In the case of multiple-unit, splinted implant-supported restorations, open tray impression copings may be preferred and used in a splinted or nonsplinted manner.[81–83] This topic is discussed in detail in chapter 7. When multiple implants are placed at different angles, the likelihood of distortion of the impression material upon removal of the impression from the mouth may increase. This effect may be further compounded by the presence of more than four implants.[84] It has been reported that angulation does not affect the accuracy of impressions for up to two to three implants.[85,86] It is the authors' preference to make impressions with closed tray impression copings for single units and splinted posterior units when patients present with a limited interocclusal distance (Fig 4-11a). Also, in clinical scenarios in which both implants and natural teeth within the same arch must be impressed, the use of closed tray impression copings will allow for immediate making of a second impression to ensure that all finish lines and prepared teeth are accurately reproduced. Such an approach may be helpful particularly for multiple units or complete arches or when implants are not placed too deep occlusogingivally (Figs 4-11b and 4-11c).

In addition, it is critical to impress the soft tissue profile created with the provisional restoration to facilitate the dental technician's accurate design of the restoration at the intaglio surface, from the level of the implant platform to the level of the free gingival margins. This is discussed in detail in chapter 5.

Impression evaluation and soft tissue recovery

Once the impression is made (Fig 4-12a), clinicians should do all they can to facilitate the tissue's ability to rebound and recover. When the double-cord technique is used, it is critical to remove the cervical cord (Fig 4-12b) and subsequently rinse the sulcus to remove as much of the residual hemostatic agent as possible (Figs 4-12c and 4-12d). As the tissue continues to rebound, the provisional restoration is cemented, and care should be taken to ensure that all excess cement is removed (Figs 4-12e and 4-12f). The master impression should be carefully assessed for drags, voids, air bubbles, and tears, particularly at the finish line. Ultimately, however, the evaluation of the dental definitive cast might be more clinically relevant than the evaluation of the impression to ensure a successful restoration (Figs 4-12g and 4-12h). Studies have shown that ratings of dies demonstrated more voids, bubbles, and tears compared with ratings of impressions.[21,32,75,87]

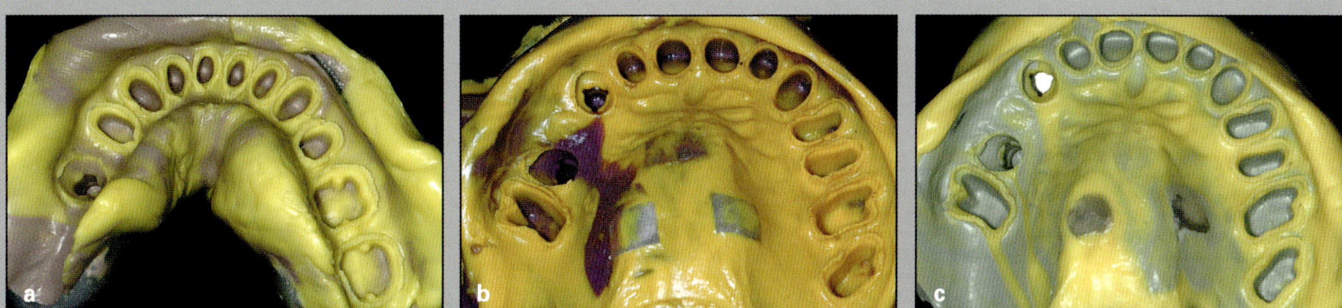

Fig 4-11 *(a)* A complete-arch master impression for both teeth and an implant-supported crown on the mandibular right first molar. Note that due to limited interocclusal distance, a closed tray impression coping was used. *(b and c)* Master impressions made for the complete-arch rehabilitation. The closed tray impression copings allowed for immediate making of a second impression to ensure that all finish lines and prepared teeth were accurately reproduced. Even though two different impression materials (Aquasil Ultra XLV, Medium Body and Light Body, Dentsply *[b]*; Imprint 3, Putty and Light Body *[c]*) were used, the impression outcome is similar due to the soft tissue health and the performance of the procedure. (Prosthodontics: Drs Yen-Wei Chen and Ariel J. Raigrodski.)

Continued from page 97

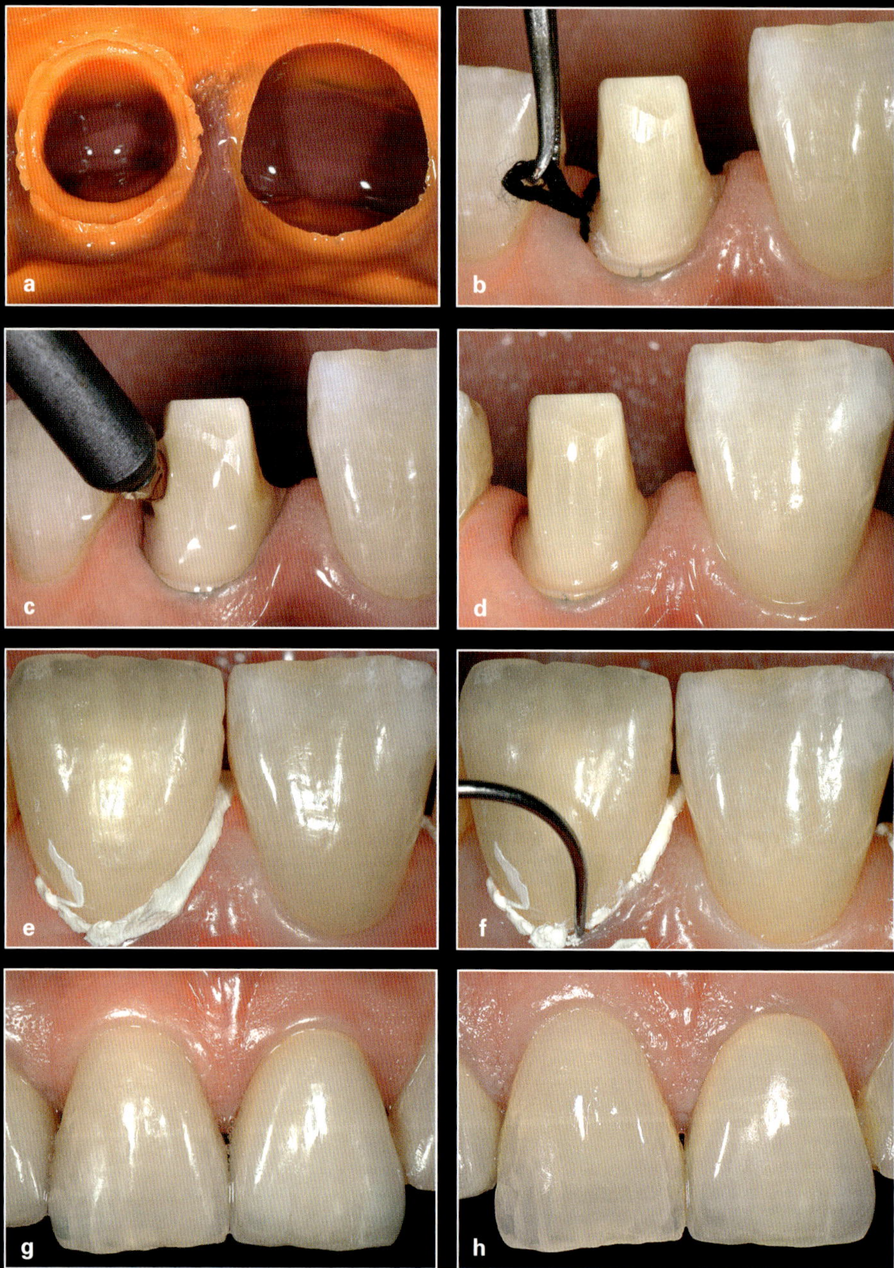

Fig 4-12 *(a)* The master impression was made. Note the fin of impression material extended circumferentially into the gingival sulcus beyond the finish line. *(b)* Once the master impression was complete, the first cervical cord was removed from the sulcus. *(c and d)* The sulcus and the tooth were rinsed to remove any residual hemostatic agent. The tissue started to rebound immediately after the cervical cord was removed. Further dropping of the finish line apically prior to impression making would have created a risk of biologic width violation and disparate gingival levels. *(e and f)* The provisional restoration was cemented, and residual excess cement was removed with a sickle-shaped explorer and a knotted floss to facilitate soft tissue recovery. *(g and h)* Facial views of the definitive restoration 2 weeks and 5 years after delivery, respectively. After the impression procedure, the tissue blended perfectly with the provisional restoration, and the definitive restoration was delivered without compromise at the soft tissue–restorative interface, which still demonstrated stability after 5 years.

References

1. Brägger U, Lauchenauer D, Lang NP. Surgical lengthening of the clinical crown. J Clin Periodontol 1992;19:58–63.
2. Ingber FJS, Rose LF, Coslet JG. The "biologic width"—A concept in periodontics and restorative dentistry. Alpha Omegan 1977; 10:62–65.
3. Anneroth G, Nordenram A. Reaction of the gingiva to the application of threads in the gingival pocket for taking impressions with elastic material. An experimental histologic study. Odontol Revy 1969; 20:301–310.
4. Beier US, Grunert I, Kulmer S, Dumfahrt H. Quality of impressions using hydrophilic polyvinyl siloxane in a clinical study of 249 patients. Int J Prosthodont 2007;20:270–274.
5. Beier US, Kranewitter R, Dumfahrt H. Quality of impressions after use of the Magic FoamCord gingival retraction system—A clinical study of 269 abutment teeth. Int J Prosthodont 2009;22:143–147.
6. Van Strydonck DA, Slot DE, Van der Velden U, Van der Weijden F. Effect of a chlorhexidine mouthrinse on plaque, gingival inflammation and staining in gingivitis patients: A systematic review. J Clin Periodontol 2012;39:1042–1055.
7. Blomberg PA, Mahmood S, Smales RJ, Makinson OF. Comparative elasticity tests for elastomeric (non-putty) impression materials. Aust Dent J 1992;37:346–352.
8. Tjan AH, Nemetz H, Nguyen LT, Contino R. Effect of tray space on the accuracy of monophasic polyvinylsiloxane impressions. J Prosthet Dent 1992;68:19–28.
9. Carrotte PV, Johnson A, Winstanley RB. The influence of the impression tray on the accuracy of impressions for crown and bridgework. Br Dent J 1998;185:580–585.
10. Chai J, Pang IC. A study of the "thixotropic" property of elastomeric impression materials. Int J Prosthodont 1994;7:155–158.
11. Abuasi HA, Wassell RW. Comparison of a range of addition silicone putty-wash impression materials used in the one-stage technique. Eur J Prosthodont Restor Dent 1994;2:117–122.
12. Saunders WP, Sharkey SW, Smith GM, Taylor WG. Effect of impression tray design and impression technique upon the accuracy of stone casts produced from a putty-wash polyvinyl siloxane impression material. J Dent 1991;19:283–289.
13. MacSween R, Price RB. Peel bond strengths of five impression material tray adhesives. J Can Dent Assoc 1991;57:654–657.
14. Sulong MZ, Setchell DJ. Properties of the tray adhesive of an addition polymerizing silicone to impression tray materials. J Prosthet Dent 1991;66:743–747.
15. Cho GC, Donovan TE, Chee WW, White SN. Tensile bond strength of polyvinyl siloxane impressions bonded to a custom tray as a function of drying time: Part I. J Prosthet Dent 1995;73:419–423.
16. Chai JY, Jameson LM, Moser JB, Hesby RA. Adhesive properties of several impression material systems: Part II. J Prosthet Dent 1991;66:287–292.
17. Payne JA, Pereira BP. Bond strength of three nonaqueous elastomeric impression materials to a light-activated resin tray. Int J Prosthodont 1992;5:55–58.
18. Dixon DL, Breeding LC, Bosser MJ, Nafso AJ. The effect of custom tray material type and surface treatment on the tensile bond strength of an impression material/adhesive system. Int J Prosthodont 1993;6:303–306.
19. Chee WW, Donovan TE. Polyvinyl siloxane impression materials: A review of properties and techniques. J Prosthet Dent 1992; 68:728–732.
20. Rios MP, Morgano SM, Stein RS, Rose L. Effects of chemical disinfectant solutions on the stability and accuracy of the dental impression complex. J Prosthet Dent 1996;76:356–362.
21. Schelb E, Cavazos E, Troendle KB, Prihoda TJ. Surface detail reproduction of type IV dental stones with selected polyvinyl siloxane impression materials. Quintessence Int 1991;22:51–55.
22. Lee SJ, Gallucci GO. Digital vs. conventional implant impressions: Efficiency outcomes. Clin Oral Implants Res 2013;24:111–115.
23. Yuzbasioglu E, Kurt H, Turunc R, Bilir H. Comparison of digital and conventional impression techniques: Evaluation of patients' perception, treatment comfort, effectiveness and clinical outcomes. BMC Oral Health 2014;30;14:10.
24. Chai J, Takahashi Y, Lautenschlager EP. Clinically relevant mechanical properties of elastomeric impression materials. Int J Prosthodont 1998;11:219–223.
25. Hondrum SO. Tear and energy properties of three impression materials. Int J Prosthodont 1994;7:517–521.
26. Anusavice KJ, Phillips RW, Shen C, Rawls HR (eds). Phillips' Science of Dental Materials, ed 12. St Louis: Elsevier/Saunders, 2013:151–181.
27. Levartovsky S, Zalis M, Pilo R, Harel N, Ganor Y, Brosh T. The effect of one-step vs. two-step impression techniques on long-term accuracy and dimensional stability when the finish line is within the gingival sulcular area. J Prosthodont 2014;23:124–133.
28. Caputi S, Varvara G. Dimensional accuracy of resultant casts made by a monophase, one-step and two-step, and a novel two-step putty/light-body impression technique: An in vitro study. J Prosthet Dent 2008;99:274–281.
29. Wassell RW, Ibbetson RJ. The accuracy of polyvinyl siloxane impressions made with standard and reinforced stock trays. J Prosthet Dent 1991;65:748–757.
30. Michalakis KX, Bakopoulou A, Hirayama H, Garefis DP, Garefis PD. Pre- and post-set hydrophilicity of elastomeric impression materials. J Prosthodont 2007;16:238–248.
31. Blatz MB, Sadan A, Burgess JO, Mercante D, Hoist S. Selected characteristics of a new polyvinyl siloxane impression material—A randomized clinical trial. Quintessence Int 2005;36:97–104.
32. Raigrodski AJ, Dogan S, Mancl LA, Heindl H. A clinical comparison of two vinyl polysiloxane impression materials using the one-step technique. J Prosthet Dent 2009;102:179–186.
33. Dogan S, Schwedhelm ER, Mancl L, Heindl H. Comparison of new self-warming impression material to gold standard PVS [abstract]. Presented at the 43rd Annual Meeting of the AADR, Charlotte, NC, 19–22 March 2014.
34. Nissan J, Laufer BZ, Brosh T, Assif D. Accuracy of three polyvinyl siloxane putty-wash impression techniques. J Prosthet Dent 2000;83:161–165.
35. Nissan J, Rosner O, Bukhari MA, Ghelfan O, Pilo R. Effect of various putty-wash impression techniques on marginal fit of cast crowns. Int J Periodontics Restorative Dent 2013;33:e37–e42.
36. Hansen PA, Tira DE, Barlow J. Current methods of finish-line exposure by practicing prosthodontists. J Prosthodont 1999;8:163–170.
37. Goldberg PV, Higginbottom FL, Wilson TG. Periodontal considerations in restorative and implant therapy. Periodontol 2000 2001;25:100–109.
38. Donovan TE, Chee WW. Current concepts in gingival displacement. Dent Clin North Am 2004;48:433–444.
39. Perakis N, Belser UC, Magne P. Final impressions: A review of material properties and description of a current technique. Int J Periodontics Restorative Dent 2004;24:109–117.
40. Rosenstiel SF, Land MF, Fujimoto J. Contemporary Fixed Prosthodontics, ed 4. St Louis: Mosby/Elsevier, 2006:431–465.
41. Laufer BZ, Baharav H, Cardash HS. The linear accuracy of impressions and stone dies as affected by the thickness of the impression margin. Int J Prosthodont 1994;7:247–252.
42. Laufer BZ, Baharav H, Langer Y, Cardash HS. The closure of the gingival crevice following gingival retraction for impression making. J Oral Rehabil 1997;24:629–635.
43. Donovan TE, Gandara BK, Nemetz H. Review and survey of medicaments used with gingival retraction cords. J Prosthet Dent 1985;53:525–531.
44. Wassell RW, Barker D, Walls AW. Crowns and other extra-coronal restorations: Impression materials and technique. Br Dent J 2002; 192:679–690.

45. Baba NZ, Goodacre CJ, Jekki R, Won J. Gingival displacement for impression making in fixed prosthodontics: Contemporary principles, materials, and techniques. Dent Clin North Am 2014;58:45–68.
46. Chiche G, Pinault A. Esthetics of Anterior Fixed Prosthodontics. Chicago: Quintessence, 1994:161–175.
47. Ruel J, Schuessler PJ, Malament K, Mori D. Effect of retraction procedures on the periodontium in humans. J Prosthet Dent 1980; 44:508–515.
48. Harrison JD. Effect of retraction materials on the gingival sulcus epithelium. J Prosthet Dent 1961;11:514–521.
49. Benson BW, Bomberg TJ, Hatch RA, Hoffman W Jr. Tissue displacement methods in fixed prosthodontics. J Prosthet Dent 1986; 55:175–181.
50. Fischer DE. Tissue management: A new solution to an old problem. Gen Dent 1987;35:178–182.
51. Baharav H, Laufer BZ, Langer Y, Cardash HS. The effect of displacement time on gingival crevice width. Int J Prosthodont 1997; 10:248–253.
52. Baharav H, Kupershmidt I, Laufer BZ, Cardash HS. The effect of sulcular width on the accuracy of impression materials in the presence of an undercut. Int J Prosthodont 2004;17:585–589.
53. Löe H, Silness J. Tissue reactions to a new gingivectomy pack. Oral Surg Oral Med Oral Pathol 1961;14:1305–1314.
54. de Gennaro GG, Landesman HM, Calhoun JE, Martinoff JT. A comparison of gingival inflammation related to retraction cords. J Prosthet Dent 1982;47:384–386.
55. Parker S. The use of lasers in fixed prosthodontics. Dent Clin North Am 2004;48:971–998.
56. Azzi R, Tsao TF, Carranza FA Jr, Kenney EB. Comparative study of gingival retraction methods. J Prosthet Dent 1983;50:561–565.
57. Ferrari M, Cagidiaco MC, Ercoli C. Tissue management with a new gingival retraction material: A preliminary clinical report. J Prosthet Dent 1996;75:242–247.
58. Weir DJ, Williams BH. Clinical effectiveness of mechanical-chemical tissue displacement methods. J Prosthet Dent 1984;51:326–329.
59. Woycheshin FF. An evaluation of the drugs used for gingival retraction. J Prosthet Dent 1964;14:769–776.
60. Bowles WH, Tardy SJ, Vahadi A. Evaluation of new gingival retraction agents. J Dent Res 1991;70:1447–1449.
61. Jokstad A. Clinical trial of gingival retraction cords. J Prosthet Dent 1999;81:258–261.
62. Shaw DH, Krejci RF, Cohen DM. Retraction cords with aluminum chloride: Effect on the gingiva. Oper Dent 1980;5:138–141.
63. Nowakowska D, Raszewski Z, Saczko J, Kulbacka J, Więckiewicz W. Polymerization time compatibility index of polyvinyl siloxane impression materials with conventional and experimental gingival margin displacement agents. J Prosthet Dent 2014;112:168–175.
64. Csillag M, Nyiri G, Vag J, Fazekas A. Dose-related effects of epinephrine on human gingival blood flow and crevicular fluid production used as a soaking solution for chemo-mechanical tissue retraction. J Prosthet Dent 2007;97:6–11.
65. Bennani V, Aarts JM, He LH. A comparison of pressure generated by cordless gingival displacement techniques. J Prosthet Dent 2012; 107:388–392.
66. Bennani V, Inger M, Aarts JM. Comparison of pressure generated by cordless gingival displacement materials. J Prosthet Dent 2014; 112:163–167.
67. Al Hamad KQ, Azar WZ, Alwaeli HA, Said KN. A clinical study on the effects of cordless and conventional retraction techniques on the gingival and periodontal health. J Clin Periodontol 2008; 35:1053–1058.
68. Poss S. An innovative tissue-retraction material. Compend Contin Educ Dent 2002;23(1 suppl):13–17.
69. Shannon A. Expanded clinical uses of a novel tissue-retraction material. Compend Contin Educ Dent 2002;23(1 suppl):3–6.
70. Gherlone EF, Maiorana C, Grassi RF, Ciancaglini R, Cattoni F. The use of 980-nm diode and 1064-nm Nd:YAG laser for gingival retraction in fixed prostheses. J Oral Laser Applications 2004;4:183–190.
71. Martin E. Lasers in dental implantology. Dent Clin North Am 2004;48:999–1015.
72. Wilhelmsen NR, Ramfjord SP, Blankenship JR. Effects of electrosurgery on the gingival attachment in rhesus monkeys. J Periodontol 1976;47:160–170.
73. Brady WF. Periodontal and restorative considerations in rotary gingival curettage. J Am Dent Assoc 1982;105:231–236.
74. Kamansky FW, Tempel TR, Post AC. Gingival tissue response to rotary curettage. J Prosthet Dent 1984;52:380–383.
75. Thongthammachat S, Moore BK, Barco MT 2nd, Hovijitra S, Brown DT, Andres CJ. Dimensional accuracy of dental casts: Influence of tray material, impression material, and time. J Prosthodont 2002;11:98–108.
76. Luthardt RG, Walter MH, Weber A, Koch R, Rudolph H. Clinical parameters influencing the accuracy of 1- and 2-stage impressions: A randomized controlled trial. Int J Prosthodont 2008;21:322–327.
77. Nam J, Raigrodski AJ, Townsend J, Lepe X, Mancl LA. Assessment of preference of mixing techniques and duration of mixing and tray loading for two viscosities of vinyl polysiloxane material. J Prosthet Dent 2007;97:12–17.
78. Dogan S, Raigrodski AJ, Mancl L. Assessing tray filling with various mixing techniques and impression materials [abstract 3207]. Presented at the 86th General Session of the International Association for Dental Research, Toronto, 2–5 July 2008.
79. Dogan S, Raigrodski AJ, Spiekerman C. Comparison of new intraoral syringe versus automatic handgun cartridge dispenser [673]. Presented at the Sixth International Assocation for Dental Research Pan European Regional Meeting, Helsinki, 12–15 September 2012.
80. Pelzner RB, Kempler D, Stark MM, Lum LB, Nicholson RJ, Soelberg KB. Human blood pressure and pulse rate response to racemic epinephrine retraction cord. J Prosthet Dent 1978;39:287–292.
81. Naconecy MM, Teixeira ER, Shinkai RS, Frasca LC, Cervieri A. Evaluation of the accuracy of 3 transfer techniques for implant-supported prostheses with multiple abutments. Int J Oral Maxillofac Implants 2004;19:192–198.
82. Vigolo P, Fonzi F, Majzoub Z, Cordioli G. An evaluation of impression techniques for multiple internal connection implant prostheses. J Prosthet Dent 2004;92:470–476.
83. Kim S, Nicholls JI, Han CH, Lee KW. Displacement of implant components from impressions to definitive casts. Int J Oral Maxillofac Implants 2006;21:747–755.
84. Assuncao WG, Filho HG, Zaniquelli O. Evaluation of transfer impressions for osseointegrated implants at various angulations. Implant Dent 2004;13:358–366.
85. Conrad HJ, Pesun IJ, DeLong R, Hodges JS. Accuracy of two impression techniques with angulated implants. J Prosthet Dent 2007;97:349–356.
86. Choi JH, Lim YJ, Yim SH, Kim CW. Evaluation of the accuracy of implant-level impression techniques for internal-connection implant prostheses in parallel and divergent models. Int J Oral Maxillofac Implants 2007;22:761–768.
87. Brosky ME, Pesun IJ, Lowder PD, Delong R, Hodges JS. Laser digitization of casts to determine the effect of tray selection and cast formation technique on accuracy. J Prosthet Dent 2002;87:204–209.

Accurate Transfer of Soft Tissue Contours to the Dental Laboratory

5

Ariel J. Raigrodski | Motoaki Ishibe

As described in chapter 4, the primary goal of a master impression is to accurately capture the tooth preparation with the finish line as well as its position in the dental arch. When implant-supported restorations are to be fabricated, the master impression must capture the implant's tridimensional position in the arch. However, with both tooth-borne and implant-supported restorations, it is imperative to facilitate the dental technician's ability to fabricate restorations that integrate functionally and esthetically with the supporting tissues in a healthy manner. Once all needed surgical procedures (eg, implant placement, osseous crown lengthening, hard and soft tissue augmentation) have been completed and the supporting tissues have healed and matured, shaping and sculpting of the soft tissue is performed with the provisional restorations for crowns and fixed dental prosthesis (FDP) retainers,[1–5] ovate pontics,[6–9] and implant-supported restorations[10–13] as a prerequisite for achieving the desired integration with the supporting tissues.

In terms of soft tissue esthetics, studies have identified mean gingival zenith locations and levels as well as papillae heights in the anterior dentition. Such objective data may affect the design of the facial and interproximal topography of bone and soft tissue during surgical procedures, thus leading to the desired soft tissue contours and a matching cervical and interproximal design for the corresponding restorations. In one study, the location of the gingival zenith was assessed in a mediolateral position relative to the vertical tooth axis of the maxillary anterior teeth.[14] Gingival zenith positions were measured from the vertical bisected midline along the long axis of each individual maxillary anterior tooth. Mean values were 1.1 mm to the distal of the vertical bisected midline for maxillary central incisors, 0.4 mm to the distal for maxillary lateral incisors, and almost identical to the vertical bisected midline for maxillary canines. The gingival zenith levels of maxillary lateral incisors relative to the adjacent central incisors and canines were more coronal by approximately 1.0 mm. In another study, interdental papilla length measurements were made from the level of the gingival zenith to the coronal tip of the papilla.[15] Mean values for maxillary anterior teeth were 4.0 mm for mesial papillae and 4.1 mm for distal papillae. The mean mesial papilla proportion (mesial papilla height ÷ crown length × 100%) was 42%, and the mean distal papilla proportion (distal papilla height ÷ crown length × 100%) was 43%, with no significant difference for the maxillary incisors. Canines demonstrated a trend toward increased distal papilla heights. Papillae proportions were approximately 40% for all tooth groups.

Several studies have evaluated gingival display in different areas of the dentition for different sets of populations. One study demonstrated visual display of interdental papillae during maximum smiling in 380 (91%) of 420 study participants.[16] Note that 87% of the participants were diagnosed with a low gingival smile line. Another study evaluated soft tissue display during smiling in white people,[17] while another looked at soft tissue display during smiling in a Chinese population.[18] The first study assessed photographs of 66 participants and measured tooth, gingival, and papillary display; it revealed that over 90% of the participants displayed papillae in the anterior teeth and first premolars during extensive smiling regardless of sex.[17] The latter study demonstrated that out of 62 Chinese participants, 43.5% (n = 27) displayed papillae from the central incisor to the first molar.[18] Another study assessed 203 participants for gingival display during smiling in the premolar area.[19] The participants demonstrated gingival display at the first and second premolars at rates of 44% and 49%, respectively, with more gingival display recorded in female and younger participants.

This data regarding gingival contours, gingival facial interproximal contours, and gingival display can be used with other subjective and objective esthetic parameters during all phases of therapy. One phase of therapy includes the design of ideal cervical and interproximal contours of the restoration and the subsequent creation of the soft tissue profile, as these areas may be visible especially during smiling.

Various authors have outlined objective parameters of assessment for soft tissue esthetics around implant-supported restorations, and descriptive indexes have been introduced for soft tissue evaluation around implant-supported restorations. The Crown Aesthetic Index evaluates both the crown itself and the soft tissue in terms of the labial margin of the peri-implant mucosa, the position of the mucosa and the interproximal embrasure, the contours of the labial surface of the mucosa, and the color and surface texture of the labial mucosa.[20] Another index is the pink esthetic score (PES), which focuses on soft tissue esthetics exclusively and evaluates the mesial and distal papillae, soft tissue level and contour, soft tissue color and texture, and alveolar process deficiency as related to the presence or lack of root proximity.[21] Several clinical studies have demonstrated the feasibility of using the PES as an objective tool for soft tissue assessment for implant-supported restorations,[22,23] and one study demonstrated that the PES data reflect the degree of patient satisfaction with the soft tissue clinical outcome.[24] It is the authors' opinion that such a tool can also be used for assessing the soft tissue esthetics around crowns, FDP retainers, and ovate pontics.

To enhance the probability of soft tissue esthetics following the above-mentioned parameters, once the desired soft tissue contours have been obtained and stabilized via the provisional restoration, clinical and laboratory steps should be taken to ensure a methodical and accurate transfer of the soft tissue contours from the patient's mouth to the dental cast. A copy or a replica of the clinical soft tissue contours on the definitive cast will facilitate the fabrication of restorations with the desired cervical and interproximal contours. Accurate transfer of the soft tissue contours from the patient's mouth to the definitive cast will enhance the ability of the dental technician to design the contours of the restorations in terms of their intaglio surfaces and the cervical and interproximal aspects. Such a proper design will facilitate soft tissue esthetics, cleansability, and soft tissue health surrounding the definitive restorations. Over the years, different methods and procedures of soft tissue transfer have been described for different treatment modalities such as conventional crowns and FDP retainers, ovate pontics, implant-supported crowns, and implant-supported ovate pontics. The concept of methodical and accurate transfer of soft tissue contours is discussed for each of these types of restoration.

Conventional Crowns and FDP Retainers

To achieve esthetic integration and avoid a black triangle at the interproximal areas when the interproximal papillae are slightly deficient, convex interproximal extensions (mini-wings or mini-pontics) with a higher chroma (to minimize the wide appearance) may be added to the definitive restoration to lengthen the interproximal contact.[25,26] This can also be achieved with the provisional restoration. Therefore, achieving a definitive cast with accurate cervical and interproximal soft tissue contours around the crown preparation and the adjacent teeth is critical for facilitating the ceramist's ability to manage the contours of the restoration. Such contours should mirror the soft tissue contours on the cast. However, these contours become distorted during impression procedures when the tissue is retracted.

In conjunction with the definitive cast, which is sectioned to fabricate trimmed working dies, solid unsectioned casts, which may have significantly distorted soft tissue contours because of retraction procedures, have been used as an adjunct for establishing adequate cervical and interproximal contours for the definitive restoration with the goal of mimicking those of the provisional restoration. Consequently, the resulting restoration may be either over- or undercontoured in both the cervical and interproximal areas. Therefore, several techniques have been described to address this challenge in the context of crowns and FDP retainers.

A popular technique is the pickup transfer impression made during the framework try-in procedure. The use of a minimal amount of temporary cement or light-body silicone at the intaglio surface of the crown coping or FDP framework may be helpful for maximizing stability during this procedure[27,28] (Figs 5-1a to 5-1d). This technique has been used with cast restorations and can now be used with computer-aided design/computer-assisted manufacturing (CAD/CAM)–generated ceramic copings and FDP frameworks, due to their improved fit[29–32] (Figs 5-1e and 5-1f).

The historical copper-band impression technique has allowed the clinician to capture the soft tissue contours using a pickup impression with resin pickup copings; in this technique, the resin pickup copings may be splinted together to further stabilize them during the pickup impression procedure.[33–35] Others have used minimal retraction when possible and repoured the impression with a silicone material. However, such a technique may not provide an accurate reproduction of the soft tissue contours prior to applying retraction procedures, no matter how conservative these procedures may be.[36]

Continued from chapter 4

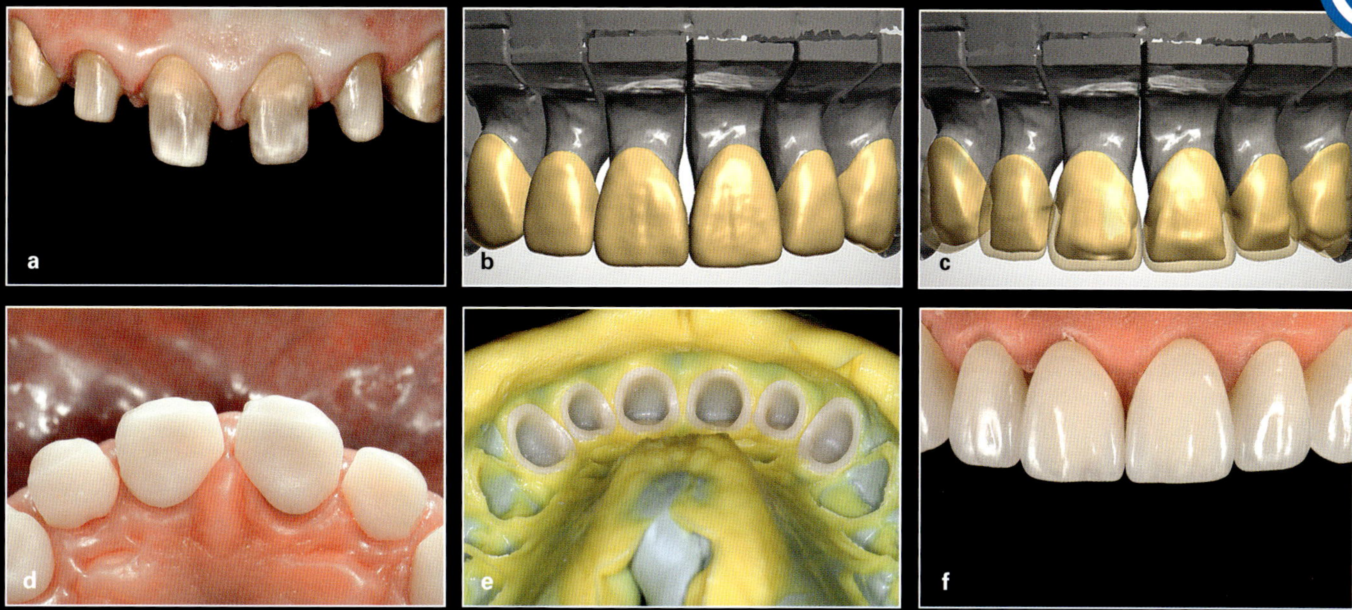

Fig 5-1 *(a)* Facial view of the completed definitive tooth preparations for anterior maxillary ceramic zirconia-based crowns. *(b and c)* Frontal views of the definitive virtual wax-up and the definitive virtual coping design for the ceramic zirconia-based crowns. Note that the copings have been designed to allow for adequate space for veneering porcelain on the facial and incisal aspects and are similar to labial veneer preparations. *(d)* Occlusal view of the copings during try-in in the patient's mouth. Note the complete contour of the palatal aspect of the copings, made of monolithic zirconia. *(e)* View of the pickup impression of the copings, which was made to allow for the refined design and fabrication of the cervical contours of the restorations. *(f)* Facial view of the complete restorations on the new soft tissue cast. Note that the cervical contours of the restorations follow the contours of the soft tissue simulation in its natural location because no retraction cord was used while making the pickup impression.

Others advocate first making an impression without retraction for accurate transfer of the soft tissue contours and then making a master impression with retracted tissue for the fabrication of the definitive cast and dies. Later, the first impression and the definitive cast are integrated to fabricate a removable silicone soft tissue simulation on the definitive cast.[37] A variation of this technique advocates making an impression of the soft tissue contours and the prepared teeth prior to placing the finish line subgingivally. Subsequently, the finish line is placed below the free gingival margins as needed, the gingival tissue is retracted, and the master impression is made. The master impression is then poured, and the working dies are sectioned and trimmed. The first soft tissue impression is trimmed to allow accurate seating of the sectioned and trimmed definitive dies from the master impression. The dies are inserted into the first nonretracted soft tissue impression, and the space between the dies and the impression is injected with soft tissue simulation silicone to generate a removable soft tissue model.[38] Noh et al[39] used a modified Geller model and a provisional restoration to record the soft tissue profile for single crowns. However, seating of the provisional restoration on the definitive cast may prove to be not as precise as the seating of a definitive coping or a definitive restoration, which may jeopardize an accurate soft tissue transfer to the cast.

Implant-Supported Crowns

Meticulously designed and contoured implant-supported restorations must allow subgingival and equigingival contour design, with a morphologic transition from a circular circumference at the level of the implant platform to the cross section of the tooth to be restored at the level of the prospective free gingival margins. Developing and confirming such contours at the provisional phase will facilitate adequate replication of critical and subcritical cervical and interproximal soft tissue contours for the definitive restoration.[40] Therefore, the role of the master impression for implant-supported restorations is not only to capture the tridimensional positions of implants in the dental arch but also to accurately capture and transfer the subgingival and equigingival emergence as well as the soft tissue contours at and below the level of the free gingival margins. Thus, accurate transfers of the critical and subcritical areas of the provisional restorations must be incorporated into the impression technique from the level of the free gingival margins apically to the implant platform.

However, once the provisional restoration is removed, the soft tissue collapses due to lack of support. Therefore, the emergence profile and soft tissue contours developed with the provisional restoration are temporarily lost. Thus, the use of stock impression copings secured to the implant platform, which may not support the soft tissue contours adequately, will enhance a master impression with an inaccurate replica of the soft tissue contours. The resulting definitive cast will facilitate a restoration design that may not coincide with the clinical emergence area, which may subsequently lead to compromised soft tissue contours at the cervical and interproximal areas, further compromising the definitive soft tissue esthetics.

Direct technique

Several techniques have been described for recording and transferring subgingival and equigingival soft tissue contours from the patient's mouth to the definitive cast. With direct techniques in general, once the provisional restoration is removed, the impression coping is connected intraorally to the implant platform, and the space left between the soft tissue and the impression coping is filled with light-body elastomeric impression material, autopolymerized acrylic resin (polymethyl methacrylate [PMMA]), or light- or autopolymerized composite resin material.[41,42]

The step-by step procedure for the direct technique is as follows (Fig 5-2):

1. Prior to the patient visit, take the impression coping and make horizontal serrations at the cervical aspect with a high-speed diamond bur (see Fig 5-2a). These serrations will enhance the mechanical retention of the resin to be used in the following procedures. If a light-body elastomeric impression material is to be used instead of a resin, apply the corresponding silicone adhesive on the impression coping to enhance the retention of the silicone to the impression coping. In addition, use a different type of silicone (eg, polyvinyl siloxane [PVS] if polyether is used for the syringing and vice versa) for making the master impression (see Fig 5-2b).
2. Remove the provisional restoration or the custom anatomical healing abutment (see Figs 5-2c to 5-2e), and immediately secure an impression coping to the implant platform intraorally.
3. Ensure that the impression coping is seated adequately, and verify its seating with a radiograph.
4. Immediately mix autopolymerized acrylic resin or light-polymerized composite resin (less polymerization shrinkage), and place it in a disposable syringe with a curved tip (Monoject, Tyco/Healthcare-Kendall; 1.2-mL Syringe, Ultradent). Alternatively, a light-body elastomeric material may be used.
5. Inject the material while it is still runny into the remaining space between the impression coping and the soft tissue "socket" at the space between the implant and the free gingival margins. If autopolymerized acrylic resin is used, spray water on the material to reduce increases in temperature due to the exothermic reaction. If light-polymerized composite resin is used, inject the material directly from the original cartridge/syringe in increments and light-polymerize. If elastomeric impression material is used, choose a fast-setting, hydrophilic light-body material (see Figs 5-2f to 5-2h).
6. Make the master impression, and then pour the definitive cast with dental stone and silicone soft tissue simulation at the soft tissue area around the implant analog. The critical and subcritical contours around the implant analog on the definitive cast should replicate those of the corresponding area in the patient's mouth.

Although the chairside appointment is relatively short, the downside of the direct technique is that after the provisional restoration has been removed, by the time the impression coping is seated and its seating is verified, the soft tissue may have partially collapsed, so the material injected into the space may not accurately capture the soft tissue profile created with the provisional restorations. Therefore, the accuracy of emergence profile replicas generated on the definitive casts may be compromised.

Indirect techniques

Indirect techniques may require a longer clinical appointment because they also require the use of the provisional restoration in the dental laboratory while the patient is waiting in the dental chair. However, indirect techniques allow for a more accurate reproduction and transfer of the clinical emergence profile to the definitive cast. A number of authors advocate making an impression of the provisional restoration and using it as either a closed tray impression coping[43,44] or an open tray pickup impression.[45,46] The provisional restorations are then connected to implant analogs, soft tissue simulation silicone material is poured around the cervical contours of the provisional restoration, and the rest of the cast is poured in dental stone, generating a definitive cast with an adequate emergence profile. Elian et al[44] suggested pouring such an impression completely with a soft tissue simulation silicone for making an emergence profile cast and, at the same time, making a standard implant-level impression with an impression coping to generate a standard definitive cast. Others have advocated the use of a standard implant platform impression, which involves pouring the impression in dental stone, trimming the stone around the implant analog, and then seating the provisional restoration and injecting light-body silicone around the cervical contours of the provisional restoration. Once the silicone soft tissue simulation material is set and the provisional restoration is removed, a replica of the emergence profile is generated on the definitive cast.[47] Still others describe a technique that requires a CAD/CAM laboratory scanner in close proximity. Once the contours of the soft tissue and the provisional restoration are approved, the provisional abutment of a cement-retained provisional restoration is removed from the patient's mouth. It is immediately scanned with a CAD/CAM unit to copy its design and to fabricate a replica definitive custom abutment out of the material of choice.[48] Currently, with the emerging use

Continued from chapter 3

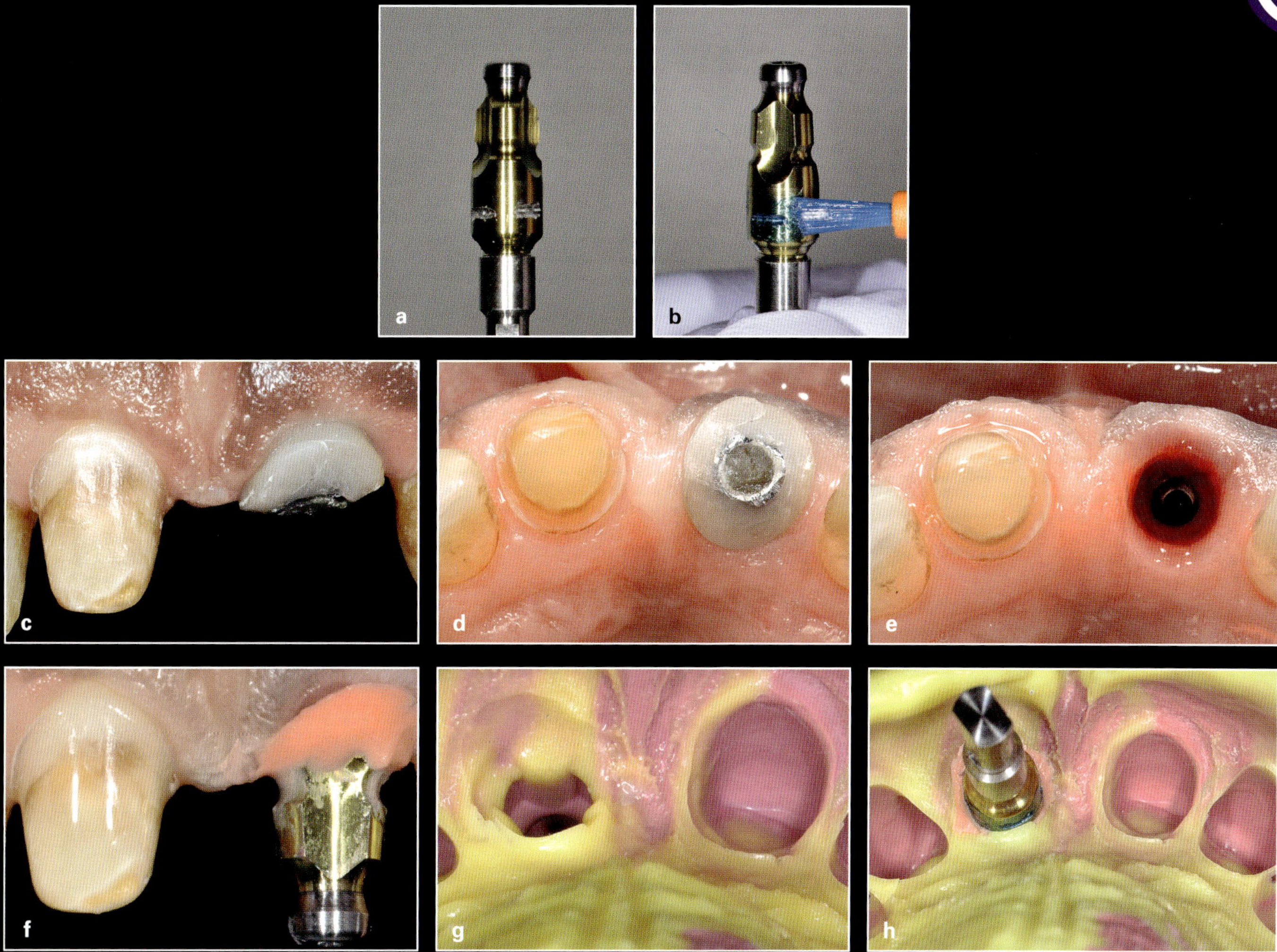

Fig 5-2 *(a)* View of a closed tray impression coping (NobelActive RP, Nobel Biocare) with a horizontal serration made with a high-speed bur to facilitate the retention of the material to be used to modify the impression coping. *(b)* A polyether adhesive (Polyether Adhesive, 3M ESPE) was applied to enhance the retention of the light-body polyether to be used during the procedure to modify the impression coping. *(c and d)* Occlusal and facial views of the custom anatomical healing abutment on the implant at the site of the maxillary left central incisor after 3 months of healing. *(e)* Occlusal view of the implant and the soft tissue at the area of the maxillary left central incisor after the anatomical healing abutment was removed. *(f)* The impression coping was secured to the implant platform, and light-body polyether impression material (Permadyne, 3M ESPE) was syringed to the remaining sulcus. This material was selected because of its hydrophilicity and because a PVS would be used to make the master impression (these materials do not adhere to each other). A custom impression coping was created. *(g and h)* Views of the impression (Imprint 3, 3M ESPE) for an implant-supported provisional restoration with and without the custom impression coping inserted. Note the cross section of the custom impression coping at the implant site, which is similar to the cross section of the cervical area of the adjacent maxillary central incisor.

of digital impressions to capture the position of implants, some authors have used implant scan bodies to make an implant-level master impression. Devices and software to accomplish this are available for different systems.[49,50] However, such scan bodies are generally circular in form, and their use may result in the collapse of the soft tissue and inaccurate recordings of soft tissue contours. To address this challenge, some authors suggest removal of the soft tissue areas around the implant analogs on models generated from a digital image. The provisional restoration is then removed from the patient's mouth, disinfected, and secured to the implant analogs on the CAD/CAM-generated model. Soft tissue simulation silicone is then injected around the cervical contours of the implant-supported provisional restoration to generate an accurate replica of the soft tissue contours as in the patient's mouth.[51]

Indirect-direct technique

Some authors have described an indirect-direct technique for transferring and replicating the cervical contours of provisional restorations to a modified impression coping, which is then used to make an impression of both soft tissue contours and implant positions in the dental arch.[52,53] To transfer the emergence profile from the patient's mouth to the definitive cast in an accurate manner, the critical and subcritical areas of the provisional restoration are incorporated tridimensionally into the impression coping from the level of the implant platform coronally to the level of the free gingival margins. With such a modified custom impression coping (either a closed or an open tray impression coping), the tissue will be supported in the same manner as with the provisional restoration. The following custom impression coping indirect-direct technique can facilitate simultaneous impression making for both tooth-borne and implant-supported restorations in the same arch.

The step-by-step procedure for the indirect-direct technique is as follows (Figs 5-3 and 5-4):

Prior to the patient's appointment

1. Mix some dental plaster and place it inside a plastic medicine cup. Take an implant analog of the system and diameter used in the patient's mouth and place it in the cup with the apical two-thirds embedded into the plaster. Make some retention grooves in the plaster prior to its complete setting. Let the plaster set and ensure the stability of the analog (see Figs 5-3a and 5-4a).
2. Take the corresponding impression coping and make horizontal serrations with a high-speed diamond bur (see Figs 5-3b and 5-3c and Figs 5-4b and 5-4c).

At the patient's appointment

1. Remove the provisional restoration from the implant (see Figs 5-3d to 5-3f and Fig 5-4d).
2. To prevent the tissue from collapsing once the provisional restoration has been removed, inject fast-setting light-body PVS or light-body polyether into the socket space left between the implant platform and the free gingival margins to stabilize the soft tissue contours as formed by the provisional restoration.[54,55] An alternative is to place cotton pellets impregnated with chlorhexidine gluconate into this socket space (see Fig 5-3g).
3. Disinfect the provisional restoration and secure it to the analog in the plastic medicine cup (see Figs 5-3h and 5-3i and Fig 5-4e).
4. Inject light-body elastomeric impression material to fill the space between the walls of the medicine cup and the apical third of the provisional restoration circumferentially (see Figs 5-3j and 5-3k and Figs 5-4f and 5-4g).
5. Once the light-body elastomeric impression material is set, remove the provisional restoration (see Figs 5-3l and 5-3m and Fig 5-4h). Note the space left between the light-body elastomeric impression material and the platform of the implant analog. That space should be a replica of the soft tissue emergence profile and a negative of the cervical and interproximal subcritical and critical contours of the provisional restoration.
6. Secure the impression coping on top of the analog in the plastic cup (see Figs 5-3n and 5-4i). The serrations on the impression coping will enhance the mechanical retention of the autopolymerized acrylic resin or light- or autopolymerized composite resin to be used in the next step.
7. Mix the autopolymerized acrylic resin or light- or autopolymerized composite resin (less polymerization shrinkage), and place it in a disposable plastic syringe. Inject the material while it is still runny into the space between the impression coping and the light-body elastomeric impression material (see Figs 5-3o and 5-3p and Fig 5-4j).
8. Once the resin is set, remove the impression coping from the analog. Note that the resin retained by the impression coping is a copy of the cervical contours of the provisional restoration at the cervical and interproximal aspects, creating a replica of the provisional restoration contours as part of the custom impression coping.
9. Trim any areas of excess resin at the coronal aspect of the custom impression coping. If the custom impression coping used is for an open tray pickup impression, such trimming will ensure that excess resin does not compromise the retention features of the impression coping. If a closed tray impression coping is used, trimming excess resin will prevent morphologic compromise of the coping designed for definitive seating in the master impression prior to pouring (see Figs 5-3q and 5-4k).
10. Return to the patient, and remove the fast-setting light-body elastomeric impression material or the chlorhexidine gluconate–impregnated cotton pellets from the socket. Immediately secure the custom impression coping to the implant platform, and evaluate the soft tissue contours. Make any necessary adjustments to the resin as needed (see Fig 5-3r), and verify the adequate seating of the impression coping with a periapical radiograph (see Figs 5-3s to 5-3v and Figs 5-4l and 5-4m).
11. Make the master impression, and pour the definitive cast with dental stone and silicone soft tissue simulation at the soft tissue areas around the custom impression coping. The critical and subcritical contours around the implant analog on the definitive cast should be a replica of the corresponding area in the patient's mouth.

Continued from page 107

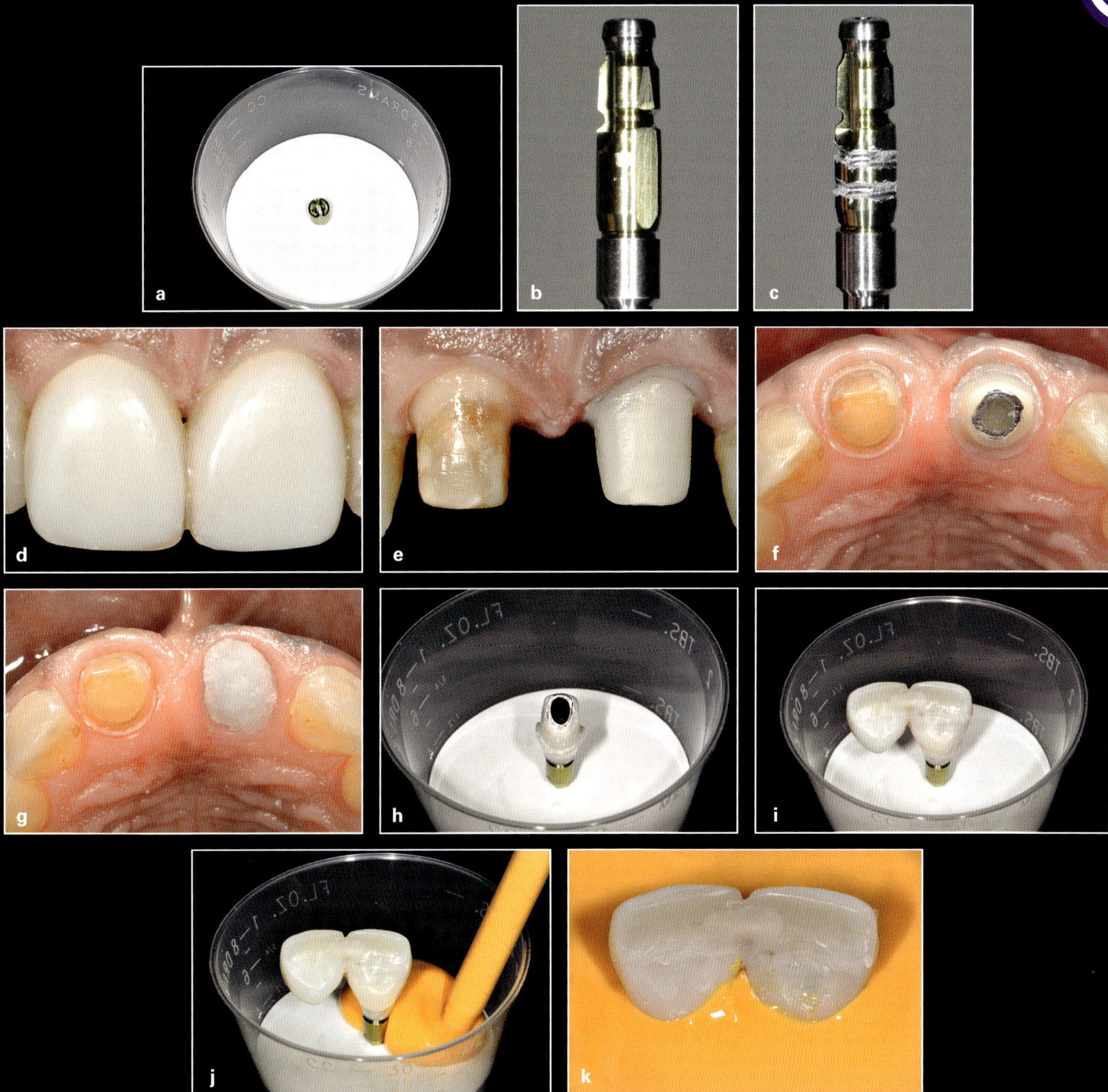

Fig 5-3 *(a)* View of the implant analog placed in a medicine cup with the apical two-thirds embedded in dental plaster. *(b and c)* The closed tray impression coping before and after horizontal serrations were made with a high-speed bur to facilitate the retention of the material to be used to modify the impression coping. *(d)* Facial view of the cement-retained provisional implant-supported restoration a few months after insertion. *(e and f)* Facial and occlusal views of the custom anatomical provisional abutment. Note the similarity in contours to the adjacent maxillary central incisor prepared for a zirconia-based ceramic crown, and note the corresponding gingival contours and gingival health. *(g)* Once the custom anatomical provisional abutment is removed from the implant platform, the socket contours are maintained and prevented from collapsing by placing cotton pellets impregnated with chlorhexidine gluconate into the socket. *(h)* Once disinfected, the custom anatomical provisional abutment was secured to the implant analog in the medicine cup. *(i)* Subsequently, the provisional FDP (including the adjacent provisional pontic) was placed on the provisional custom implant abutment. *(j and k)* Light-body PVS (Aquasil Ultra, Dentsply) was injected around the provisional restoration to the level of its apical third.

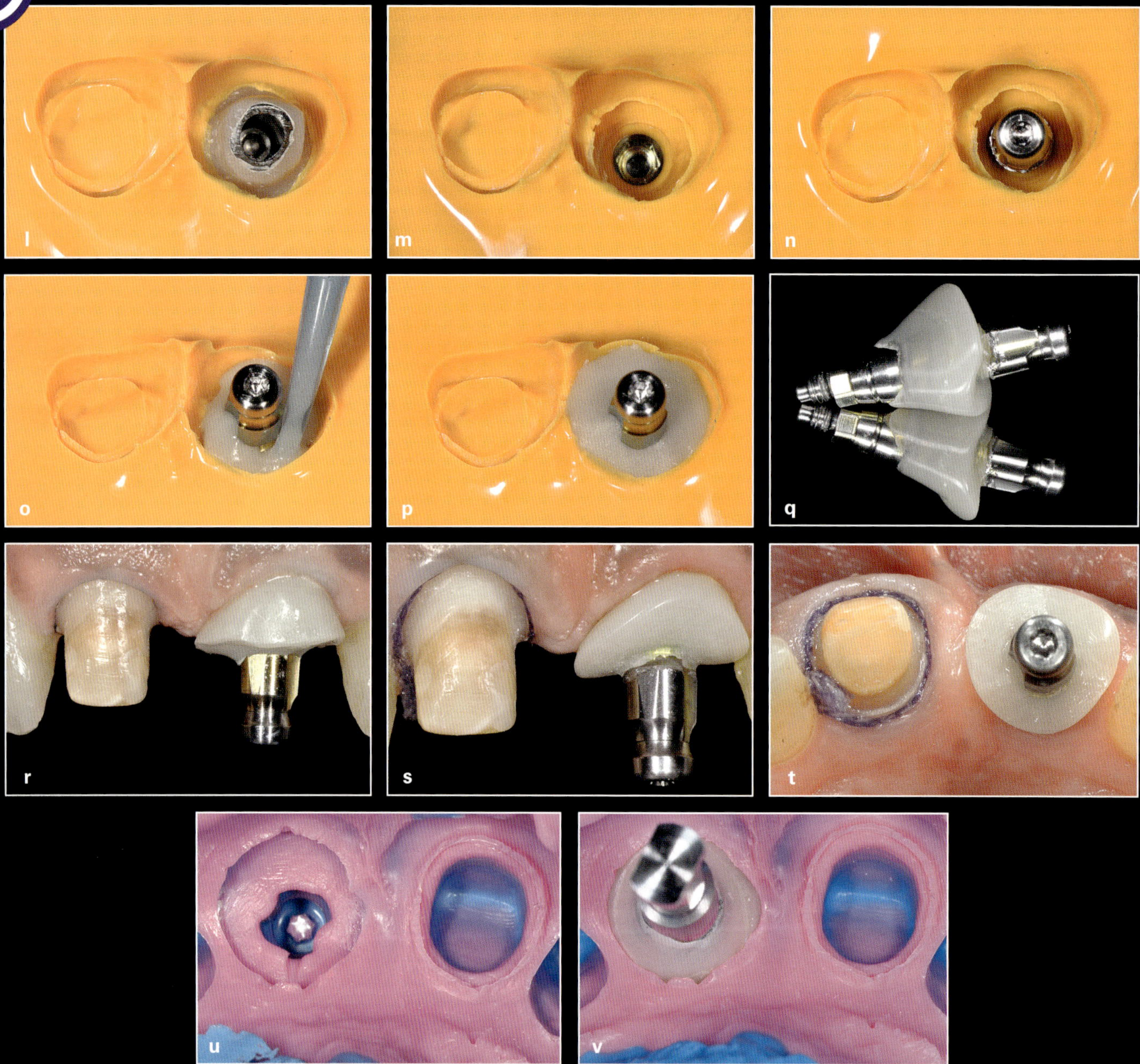

Fig 5-3 *(cont) (l and m)* Once the light-body elastomeric impression material was polymerized, the provisional FDP and the custom anatomical provisional abutment were removed from the analog. *(n)* The impression coping was secured to the implant analog in the medicine cup. Note the space left between the light-body elastomeric impression material and the impression coping. *(o and p)* Autopolymerized acrylic resin (Jet, Lang) was injected into the space between the light-body elastomeric impression material and the impression coping. *(q)* View of the custom impression coping. *(r)* The custom impression coping was tried in the patient's mouth. Note the excess autopolymerized acrylic resin coronal to the free gingival margins. Such excess should be trimmed because it does not support the soft tissue and may compromise a definitive seating of the custom impression coping in the master impression. *(s and t)* Facial and occlusal views of the complete custom impression coping prior to making the master impression. *(u and v)* Views of the master impression (Imprint 4, 3M ESPE) with and without the custom impression coping inserted. Note the cross section of the custom impression coping at the implant site, which is similar to the cross section of the cervical area of the adjacent maxillary central incisor.

Continued from chapter 3

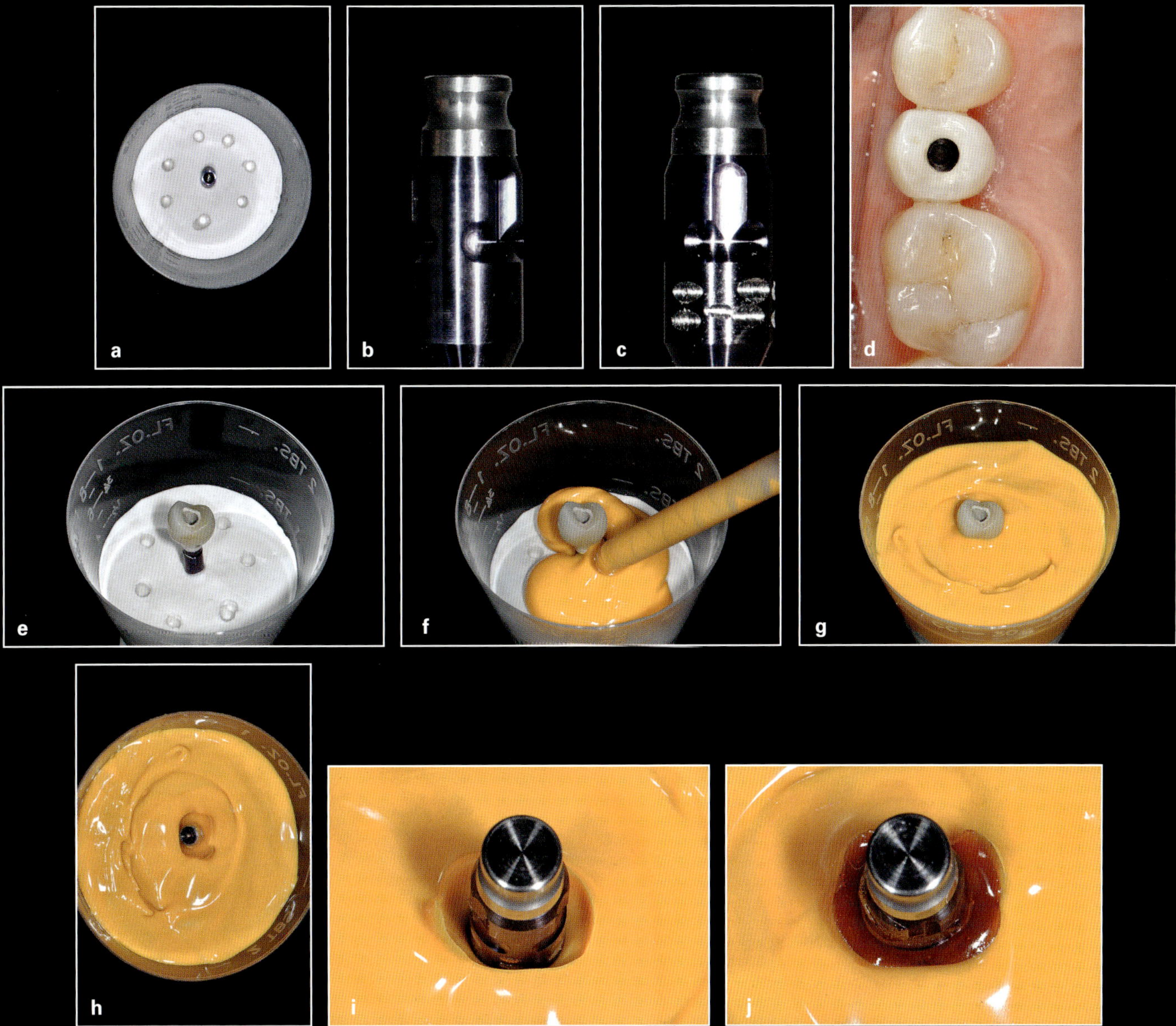

Fig 5-4 *(a)* View of the implant analog (Certain Prevail, Biomet 3i) placed in a medicine cup with the apical two-thirds embedded in dental plaster. *(b and c)* The closed tray impression coping before and after horizontal serrations were made with a high-speed bur to facilitate the retention of the material to be used to modify the impression coping. *(d)* Occlusal view of a screw-retained provisional implant-supported restoration prior to its removal. *(e)* Once removed from the patient's mouth and disinfected, the screw-retained provisional restoration was secured to the implant analog in the medicine cup. *(f and g)* Light-body PVS (Aquasil Ultra) was injected around the provisional restoration to the level of its apical third. *(h)* Once the light-body elastomeric impression material was polymerized, the provisional restoration was removed. Note the cross section of the "socket," which is a copy of the soft tissue emergence profile. *(i)* The impression coping was secured to the implant analog in the medicine cup. Note the space left between the light-body elastomeric impression material and the impression coping. *(j)* Autopolymerized acrylic resin (GC Pattern Resin, GC America) was injected into the space between the light-body elastomeric impression material and the impression coping.

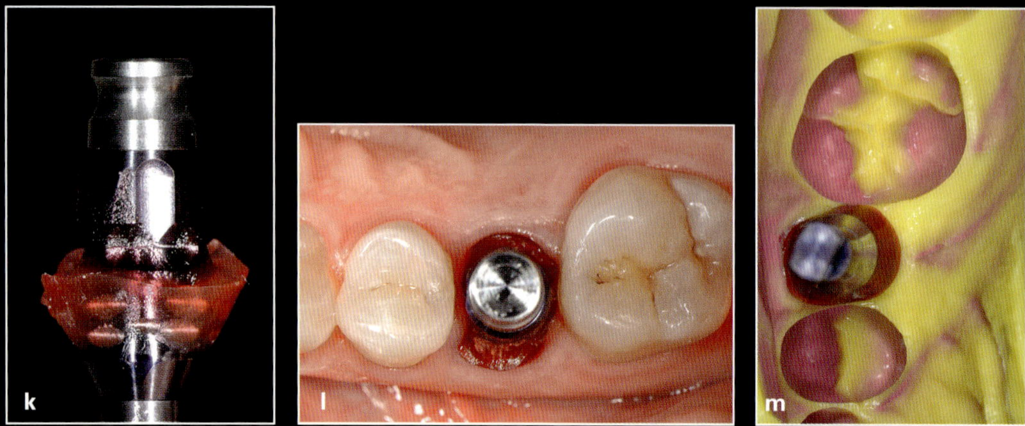

Fig 5-4 *(cont) (k)* View of the custom impression coping. *(l)* Occlusal view of the custom impression coping secured to the implant in the patient's mouth. *(m)* View of the master impression (Imprint 3) with the closed tray custom impression coping inserted.

Ovate Pontics for Tooth-Borne FDPs

Ovate pontic sites are developed surgically and restoratively to facilitate the creation of a cleansable restoration with a pontic that integrates with the soft tissue in an esthetic and healthy manner and simulates the cervical contours of a natural tooth.[56–59] Such a convex pontic with a smooth surface[60,61] exerts slight active pressure on the soft tissue without compromising its blood supply. If patients maintain adequate plaque control with floss and threaders, clinical inflammation of the supporting tissues may not occur.[62,63] The slight pressure created by the ovate pontic may also result in a thin layer of keratinized epithelium covering the pontic site.[62] Time is required for the development of such ovate pontic sites via surgical and/or restorative procedures. The definitive contours of such a pontic site are determined not only by the volume of soft tissue available but also by the intaglio, cervical, and interproximal contours of the provisional restoration, which shapes and supports the pontic site contours.[6,7,59]

Generally, when master impressions are made for an FDP with a pontic, by the time the provisional restoration is removed, the abutment teeth are cleaned, and the tissue is retracted, the soft tissue at the pontic site will have collapsed, and the pseudo papillae created by the provisional ovate pontic will have disappeared due to lack of soft tissue support at the pontic site. Consequently, if no additional measures are taken by the clinician to ensure accurate recording and transfer of the pontic site contours from the patient's mouth to the definitive cast, the dental technician will have to arbitrarily trim the cast at the area of the pontic site, speculating as to the contours of the pontic site on the definitive cast. This will result in an arbitrary design of the intaglio, cervical, and proximal surfaces of the pontic, which may not coincide with the patient's clinical pontic site contours, thereby leading to a pontic designed with contours that differ from those of the pontic of the provisional restoration, which represents the blueprint for the ultimate restorative goal.

Authors have proposed different methods for accurate recording and transfer of clinical ovate pontic sites to definitive casts. Dylina[59] has proposed an ovate pontic circumferential index, which is made via impressing the intaglio surface of the provisional FDP retainers and ovate pontic with PVS impression material[64,65] (Fig 5-5). Such a silicone index is then used by the dental technician as a guide for fabricating the intaglio, cervical, and interproximal contours of the definitive pontic. Chee et al[66] suggested the use of a pickup impression of the provisional restoration and the adjacent teeth in a trayless PVS putty index. Once a master impression is made and the definitive cast is poured, the pontic site on the definitive cast is trimmed, and the working dies are removed. In the next patient visit, the provisional restoration is removed from the patient's mouth and inserted into a trayless putty index with the incisal and facial aspects. A polyether light-body impression material is placed on the exposed intaglio surface of the provisional pontic, and the trayless putty index is seated on the definitive cast, generating a replica of the pontic site.

Others have described the use of the FDP framework or the restoration at the bisque stage for impressing the soft tissue contours at the pontic site using autopolymerized acrylic resin and a light-body silicone[7,67,68] (Fig 5-6). This technique, which uses the FDP framework as a tray to capture the contours of the ovate pontic site and to make a pickup impression of the modified framework ovate pontic to generate a soft tissue cast with a precise pontic site replica, is described here through the illustration of two different

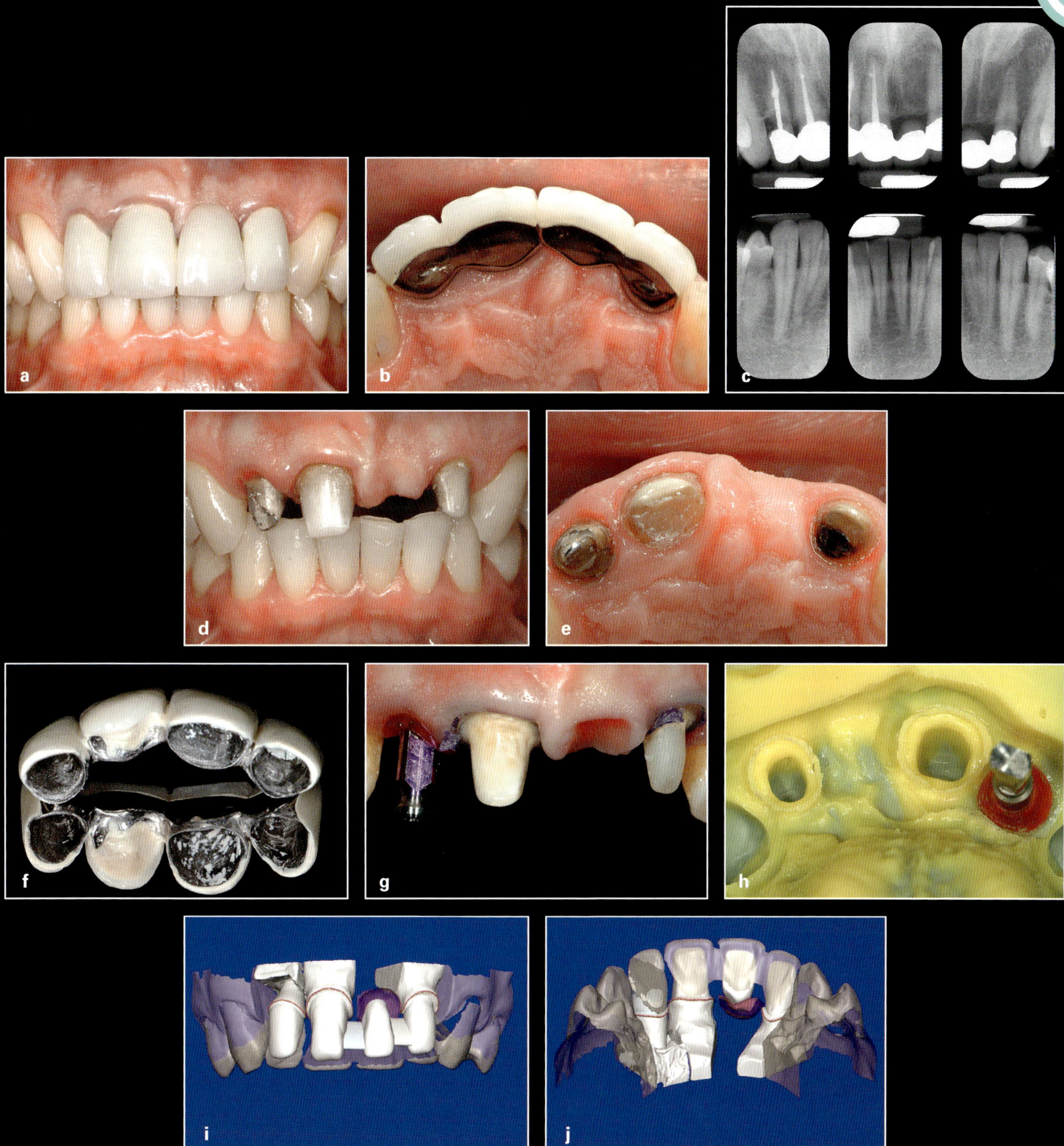

Fig 5-5 *(a and b)* Facial and occlusal views of a failing anterior four-unit FDP. Note the gingival inflammation at the margins of the restoration and the deficient pontic site. *(c)* Periapical radiographs revealed that the maxillary right lateral incisor was not restorable due to secondary caries. *(d and e)* Facial and occlusal views of the anterior maxillary teeth after removal of the failing restoration. Note the horizontal ridge deficiency at the pontic site. *(f)* View of the restoration after its removal. Note the ridge lap design of the pontic. *(g)* Facial view prior to impression making for a three-unit ceramic FDP and an implant-supported crown (NobelReplace NP, Nobel Biocare) to be impressed with a custom impression coping. *(h)* View of the master impression with the custom impression coping inserted in place, transferring the desired soft tissue emergence profile. *(i and j)* Views of the framework and crown coping virtual design on the CAD unit for a ceramic zirconia-based restoration (Lava, 3M ESPE) based on the contours of the provisional restoration.

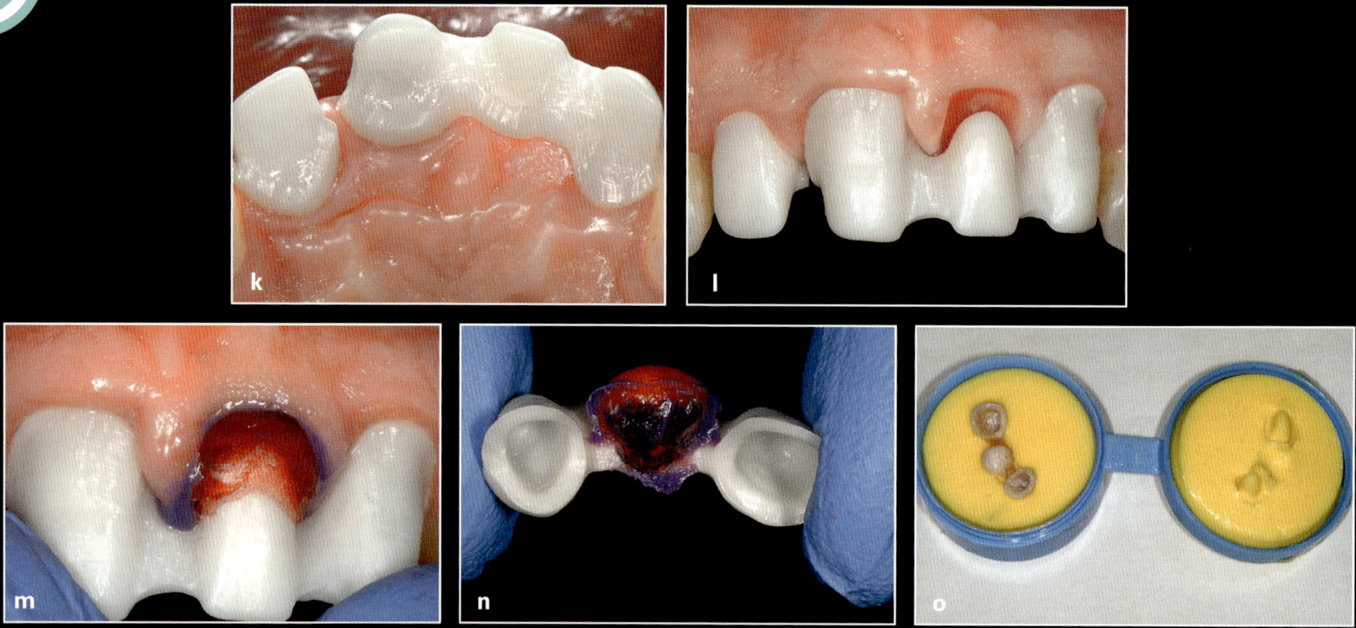

Fig 5-5 *(cont) (k and l)* Occlusal and facial views of the framework try-in for fit assessment and for soft tissue evaluation at the pontic site. Note the space between the pontic and the pontic site and the unique contours of the pontic site, which are similar to the soft tissue contours of the adjacent maxillary central incisor. *(m and n)* The framework was used for impressing the pontic site contours using autopolymerized acrylic resin (GC Pattern Resin) and light-body polyether (Permadyne). *(o)* Because of the unique contours of the pontic site, in addition to the previous procedure, an ovate pontic circumferential silicone index was made using the provisional restoration. It was further used by the dental technician to replicate the intaglio surface of the provisional pontic.

Continued from chapter 4

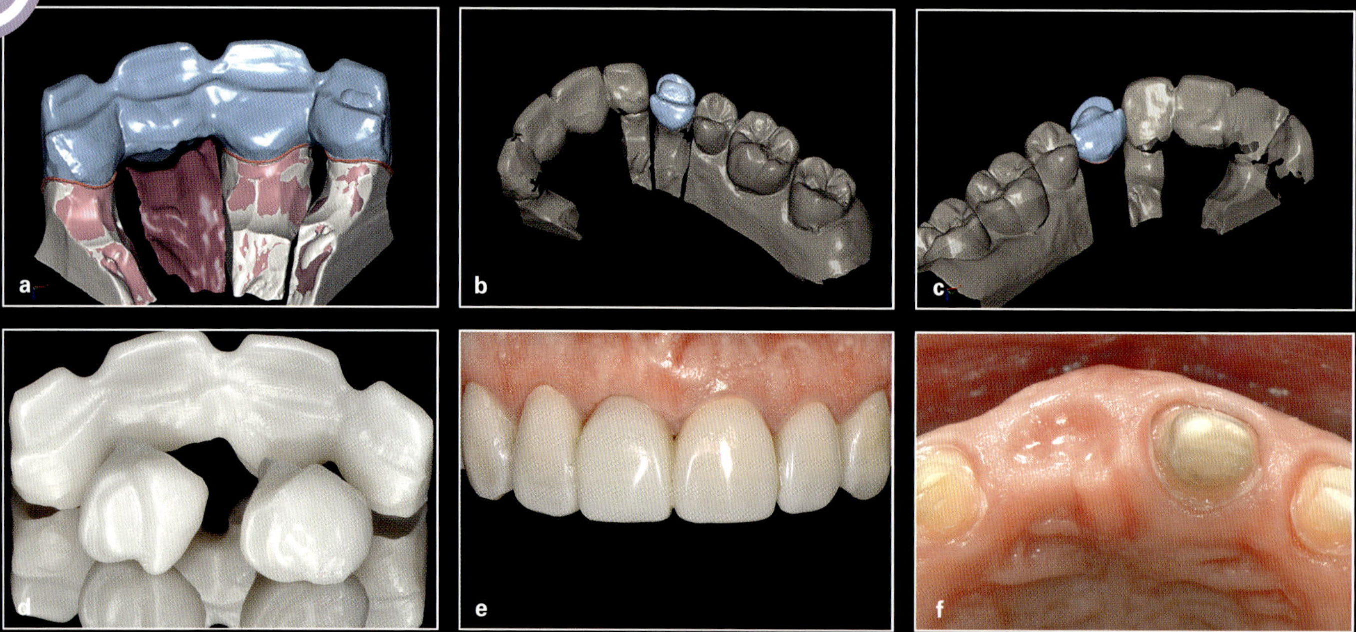

Fig 5-6 *(a)* Palatal view of the virtual design of an anterior four-unit zirconia-based FDP (Lava). Note the extensive palatal struts designed to provide support to the veneering porcelain. Because this type of zirconia is designed for copings and frameworks exclusively, the occlusal contact areas will be made of the veneering porcelain to avoid any concerns of wear of the opposing dentition. *(b and c)* Palatal views of the virtual design of zirconia-based crowns (Lava) for the maxillary canines. Similar design considerations as with the FDP framework have been applied for the crown copings. *(d)* View of the FDP framework and crown copings fabricated based on the virtual designs. *(e)* Facial view of the provisional restoration prior to framework try-in. *(f)* Occlusal view of the pontic site.

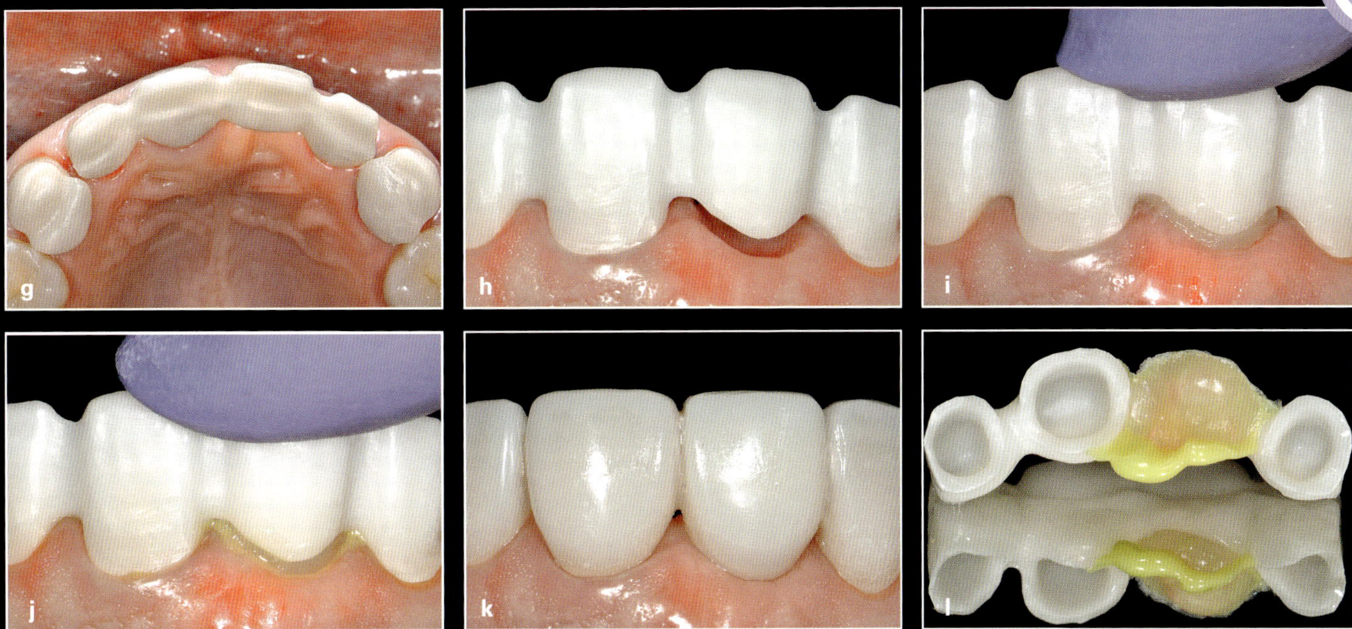

Fig 5-6 *(cont) (g and h)* Occlusal and facial views of the framework try-in for fit assessment and for soft tissue evaluation at the pontic site. Note the space between the pontic and the pontic site. *(i)* Light-polymerized direct composite resin was added to the intaglio surface of the framework pontic and light-polymerized. It was tried in the patient's mouth to record the contours of the pontic. *(j)* The light-polymerized direct composite resin was further refined by adding light-body impression material at the intaglio surface of the pontic and placed in the patient's mouth. *(k and l)* Once set, the framework with the pontic replica was removed and evaluated to ensure similar cervical and interproximal contours to those of the provisional restoration. Once the desired contours were confirmed, the framework was sent to the dental laboratory so that the dental technician could use it as a template for finalizing the cervical, interproximal, and intaglio contours of the definitive pontic.

cases (Figs 5-7 and 5-8). Once the FDP and its framework are designed (see Figs 5-7j to 5-7m and Figs 5-8f to 5-8j) and fabricated (see Figs 5-7n and 5-7o and Figs 5-8k and 5-8l), the patient is seen in the clinic for a framework try-in and recording of the soft tissue contours at the pontic site. The step-by-step procedure is as follows:

1. Remove the provisional FDP and clean the temporary cement from the intaglio surface of the retainers. Clean the abutment teeth with a prophy cup and flour pumice mixed with water.
2. Verify the fit of the FDP framework intraorally in the conventional manner to ensure adequate marginal integrity (see Figs 5-7p and 5-7q). Identify and evaluate the space between the framework pontic and the pontic site. If the restoration is a complete-contour monolithic restoration, assess the interproximal and occlusal contacts as well (see Fig 5-8m). Be advised that during this phase, the soft tissue at the pontic site may collapse due to lack of support (since the provisional restoration has been removed).
3. Remove the framework from the patient's mouth, and reposition and stabilize the provisional restoration (without cement) to regain the previous intaglio, cervical, and interproximal contours of the pontic site (see Fig 5-7r).
4. Paint the intaglio surface of the framework pontic with autopolymerized acrylic resin (PMMA) monomer (GC Pattern Resin). Use a small-diameter brush to pick up PMMA monomer and powder, and add and apply it to the intaglio surface of the framework pontic while creating convex contours (see Figs 5-7s to 5-7v).
5. Remove the provisional restoration from the patient's mouth and immediately seat the framework while applying pressure with the acrylic resin on the pontic site. Use water spray to reduce the exothermic reaction of the acrylic resin. This may cause some tissue blanching because of overcontouring of the framework pontic replica, which may have occurred in the previous step. Wait at least 5 to 10 minutes for the blanching to disappear while spraying the now new framework pontic replica with water to prevent the exothermic reaction from traumatizing the tissue and adjacent abutments. Assess the framework pontic replica contours[7] (see Figs 5-7w and 5-8n).
6. Remove the framework from the patient's mouth, and immediately reposition the provisional restoration in the patient's mouth without cement to ensure that the pontic site is adequately shaped (see Fig 5-7x).

7. Selectively trim the acrylic resin as needed from the framework pontic replica using either an acrylic bur or a sandpaper disk with a low-speed handpiece (see Fig 5-7y). If needed, add acrylic resin in selective areas. Reevaluate the framework pontic replica in the patient's mouth to ensure that its contours are identical to those of the provisional restoration (see Fig 5-7z).
8. Apply polyether or a PVS tray adhesive to the intaglio surface of the framework pontic replica (now made of acrylic resin). Mix the light-body elastomeric impression material (polyether, Permadyne) and apply it to the intaglio surface of the framework pontic replica[7] (see Fig 5-7aa).
9. Remove the provisional restoration from the patient's mouth, seat the framework, and let the light-body impression material set (see Fig 5-7bb). This step will aid in refining the contours of the framework pontic replica and will enhance a precise tridimensional recording of the pontic site. Once the silicone is set, remove the framework from the patient's mouth and reposition the provisional restoration (see Fig 5-7cc).
10. Send the modified framework with the pontic replica to the dental laboratory, which the dental technician will use to modify the definitive cast at the area of the pontic site replica. The pontic site replica on the definitive cast should be carved to create a space between the framework pontic and the pontic site replica on the cast. This space is then filled with a different type of silicone or dental stone, the framework is seated on the cast, and once the silicone is set, the soft tissue contours of the pontic site are copied to the definitive cast, creating a new pontic site replica.
11. An alternative approach is to stabilize the modified framework with a minimal amount of temporary cement or light-body elastomeric impression material in the patient's mouth and then make a pickup impression of the framework (see Fig 5-7dd and Figs 5-8o to 5-8r). The laboratory technician will apply a separating medium to the intaglio of the FDP framework and inject resin into the intaglio of the retainers while pouring silicone at the soft tissue areas. Once it is poured, a new solid soft tissue cast is generated, with a soft tissue simulation silicone material where needed to generate an accurate pontic site replica on the cast (see Fig 5-7ee). Subsequently, the dental technician can design the intaglio, cervical, and interproximal contours of the pontic to mimic the contours generated in the provisional restoration (see Figs 5-8s to 5-8bb).

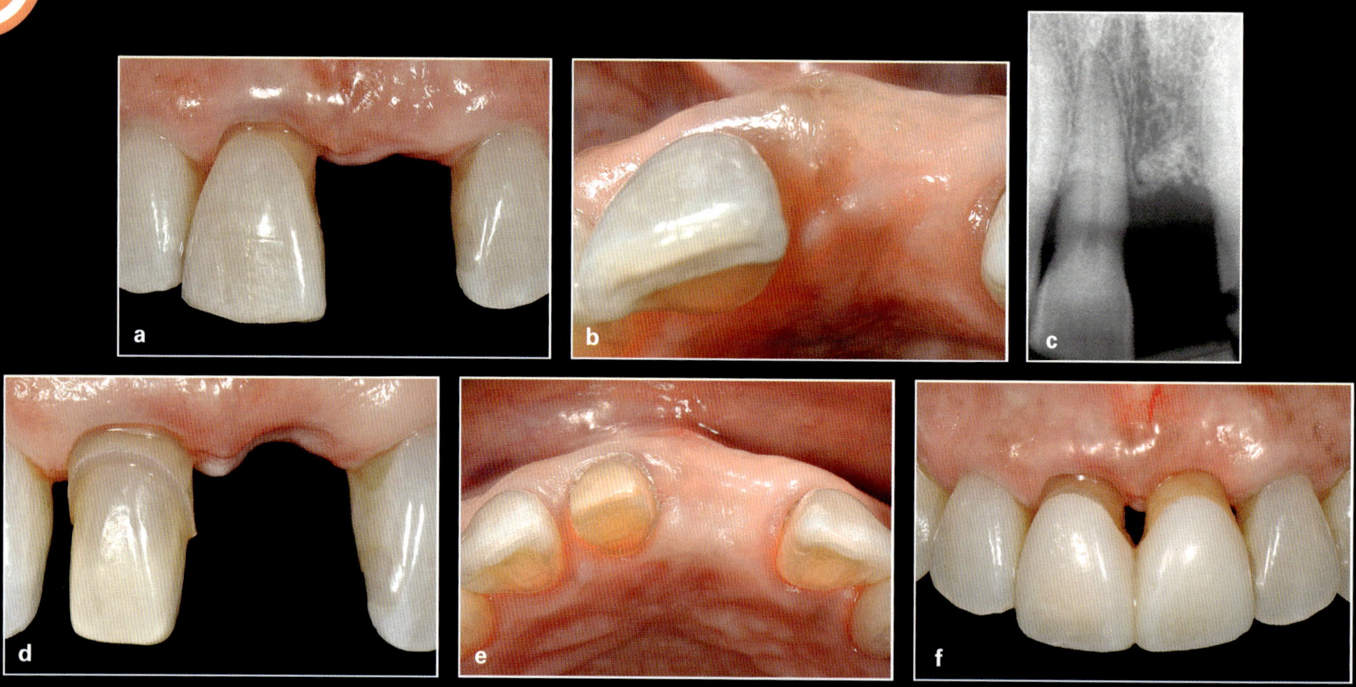

Fig 5-7 *(a and b)* Occlusal and facial views of a patient who lost her maxillary left central incisor. Note the loss of interproximal papillae. *(c)* A periapical radiograph demonstrated moderate horizontal bone loss. It was decided to restore the missing tooth with a cantilever two-unit FDP with the maxillary right central incisor serving as the retainer. *(d and e)* The maxillary right central incisor was prepared in a relatively conservative manner for an FDP retainer, and the finish line was placed supragingivally in enamel. *(f)* A provisional restoration was placed, simulating the shade and the contours of a root of the maxillary right central incisor at the apical portion.

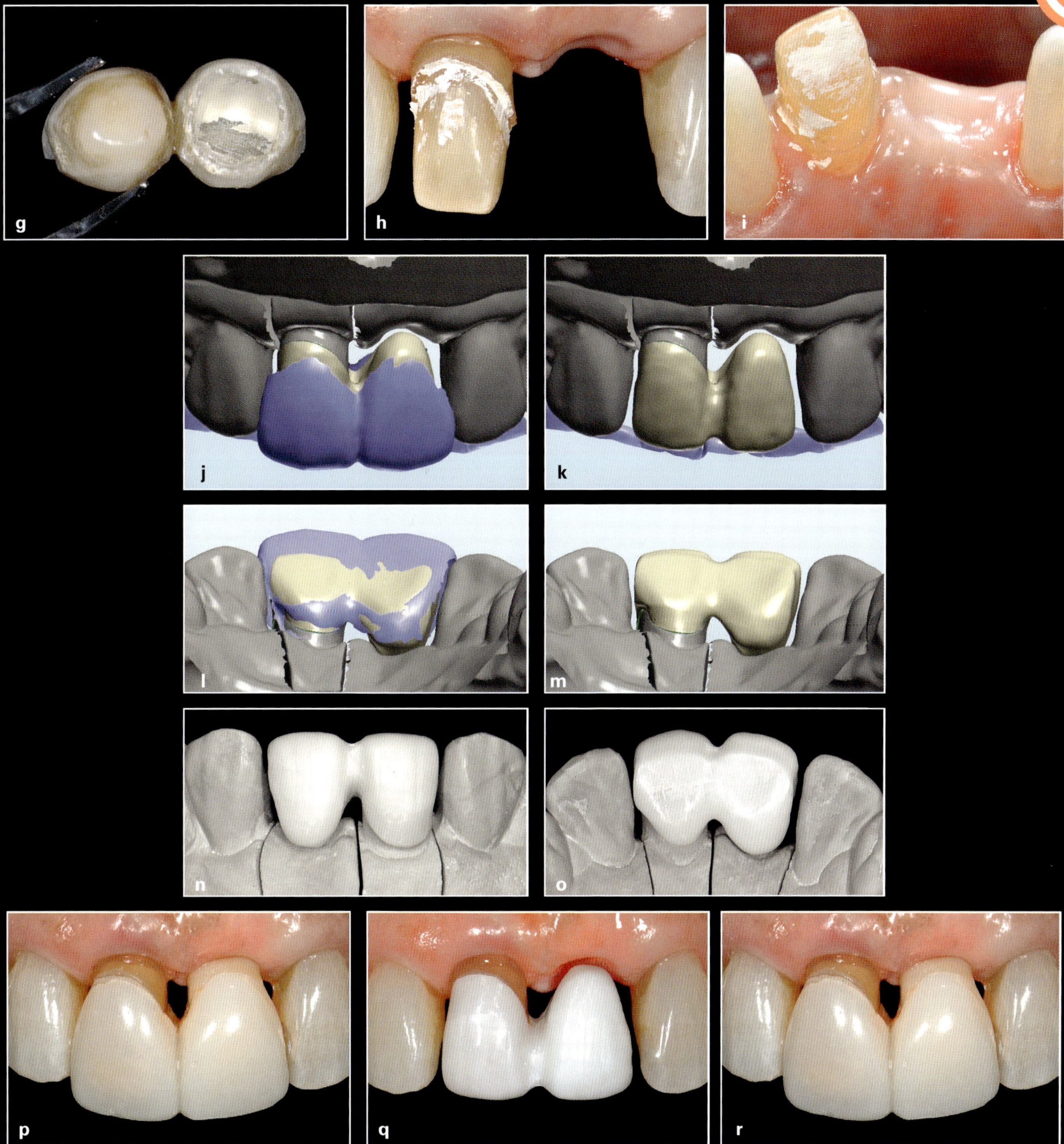

Fig 5-7 *(cont) (g)* Once the provisional restoration was confirmed with the patient from an esthetic perspective, it was removed so that the master impression could be made. The provisional restoration was examined to ensure that there was no temporary cement wash. *(h and i)* Facial and occlusal views demonstrating that some of the temporary cement remained on the prepared tooth surface. *(j and k)* Facial views of the virtual wax-up made based on the contours of the provisional restoration. The design of the framework is verified to ensure adequate support for the veneering porcelain. *(l and m)* Palatal views of the virtual wax-up. The design of the framework is verified to ensure adequate hybrid framework design with the monolithic palatal surface excluding the incisal area, which will be veneered for esthetic purposes. *(n and o)* Facial and palatal views of the definitive zirconia framework (Katana, Kuraray Noritake). *(p and q)* Facial views of the provisional restoration a few months after delivery. Note that the external staining is fading at the cervical aspect *(p)*. The framework try-in demonstrates the space between the framework's ovate pontic and the pontic site *(q)*. *(r)* Once the framework was removed, the provisional restoration was placed intraorally without cement to maintain the soft tissue at the ovate pontic site.

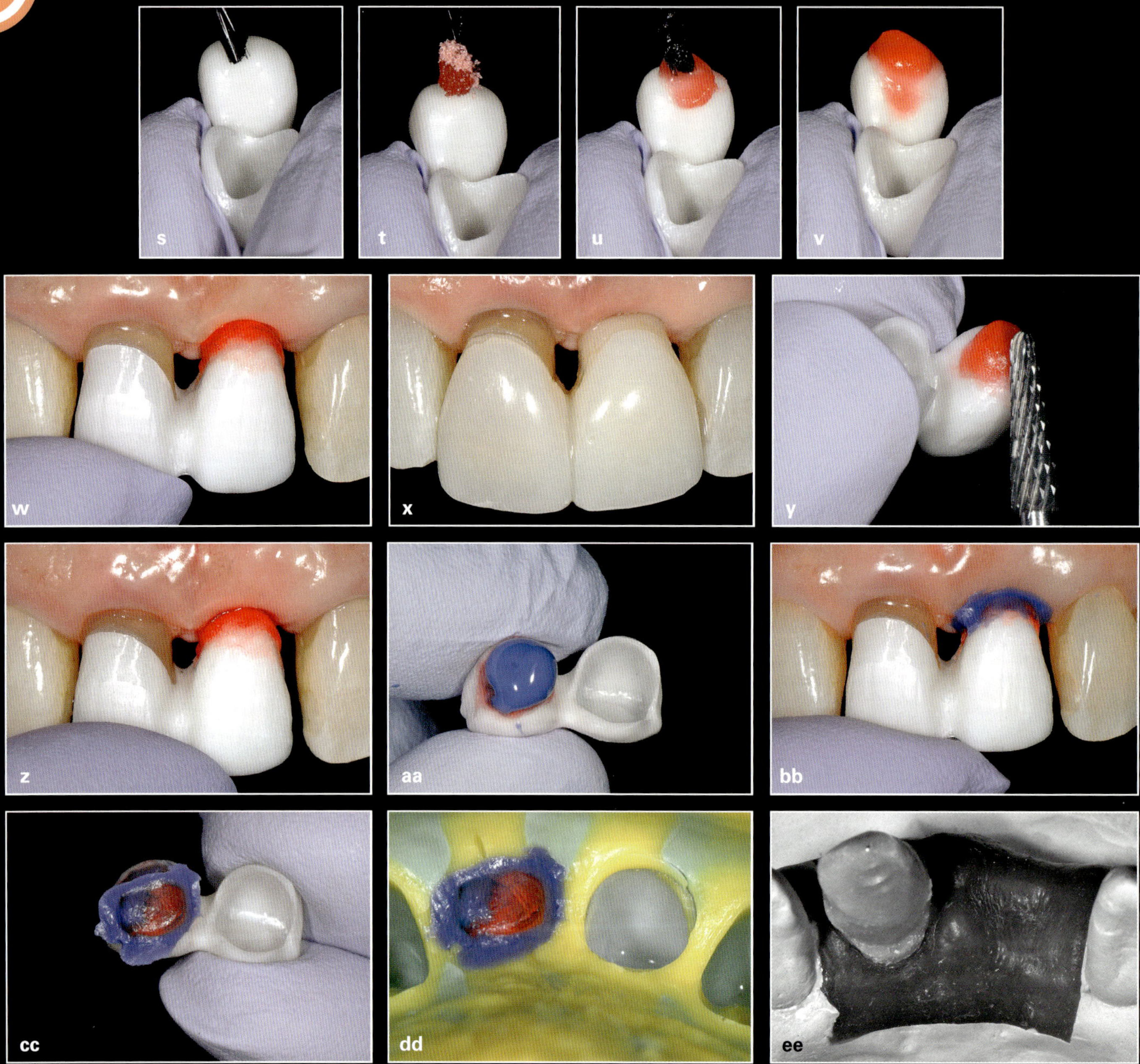

Fig 5-7 *(cont) (s to v)* Autopolymerized acrylic resin (GC Pattern Resin) was used to build up the pontic with a convex contour. *(w)* Once the autopolymerized acrylic resin reached the doughy stage, the provisional restoration was removed, and the framework was seated in the patient's mouth. *(x)* View of the provisional restoration reseated in the patient's mouth immediately after removal of the framework with the modified pontic replica. *(y)* Excess autopolymerized acrylic resin was gently trimmed with an acrylic bur as needed. *(z)* View of the framework tried in again in the patient's mouth with more desired cervical and interproximal contours. *(aa)* View of light-body polyether (Permadyne) applied to the intaglio surface of the pontic. *(bb)* Facial view of the pontic site impressed with the modified pontic replica framework and the light-body polyether. *(cc)* View of the refined ovate pontic replica. *(dd)* View of the pickup impression (Imprint 3), which was made after the FDP framework was stabilized with the modified pontic replica in the patient's mouth. Note the convex contours of the pontic replica. *(ee)* Occlusal view of the stone cast generated from the pickup impression. Note the concave dimple at the pontic site replica.

E
Continued from chapter 4

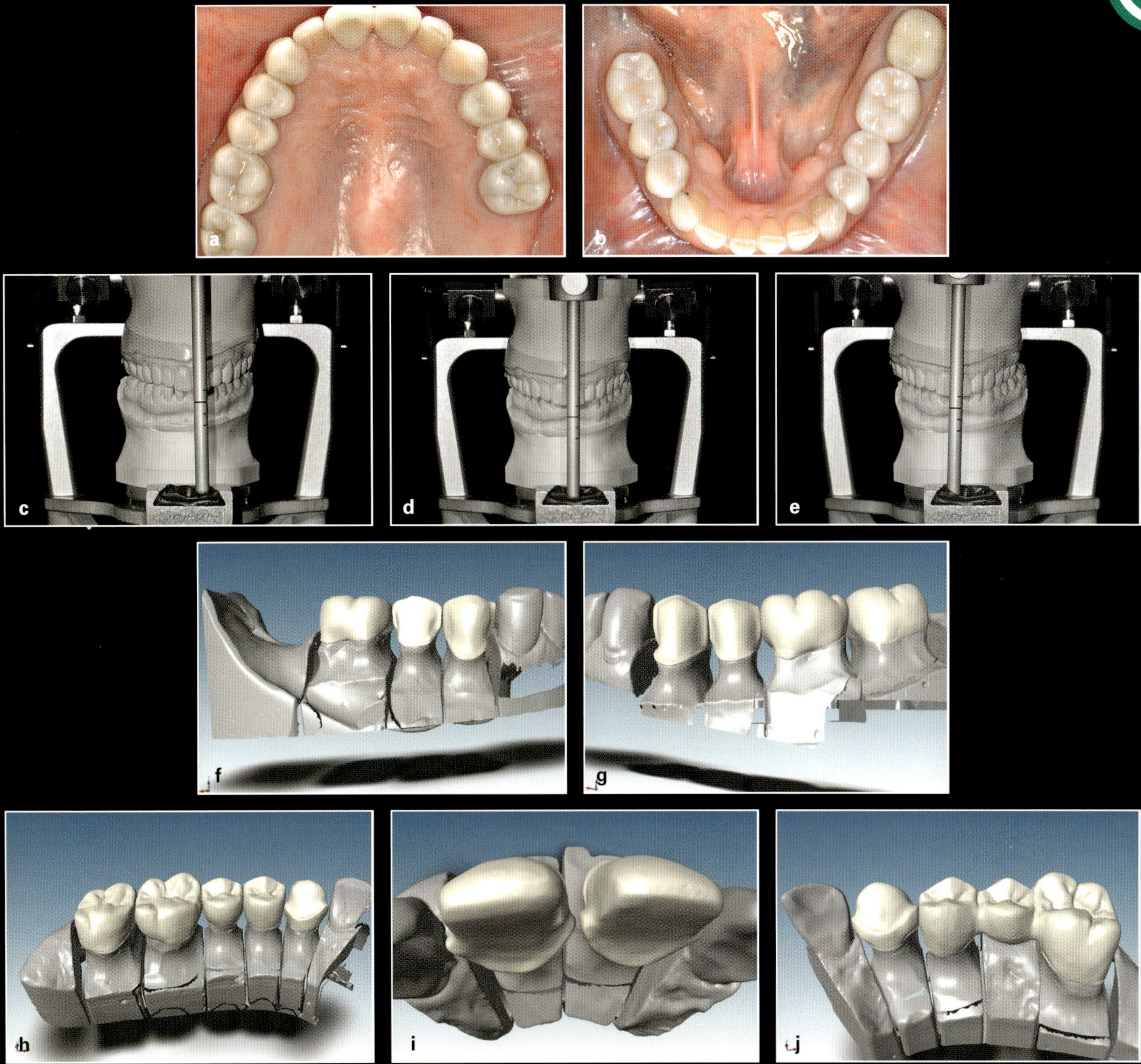

Fig 5-8 *(a and b)* Occlusal views of the maxillary and mandibular provisional restorations. The patient was able to function comfortably for several months with the provisional restorations. *(c to e)* Views of the casts of the maxillary and mandibular provisional restorations mounted on the semi-adjustable articulator. A custom incisal guide table was made while lateral and protrusive excursions were simulated to ensure that the definitive restorations could follow the same functional contours as the provisional restorations. *(f and g)* Views of the virtual design for the mandibular ceramic zirconia-based restorations (Lava Plus, 3M ESPE) based on the provisional restorations. The molars were designed for monolithic zirconia crowns, and the premolars were designed for hybrid zirconia-based crowns. *(h to j)* Views of the virtual design for the maxillary ceramic zirconia-based restorations (Lava Plus) based on the provisional restorations. The molars were designed for monolithic zirconia crowns, the premolars were designed for hybrid zirconia-based crowns, and the central incisors and canines were designed for bilayered zirconia-based crowns.

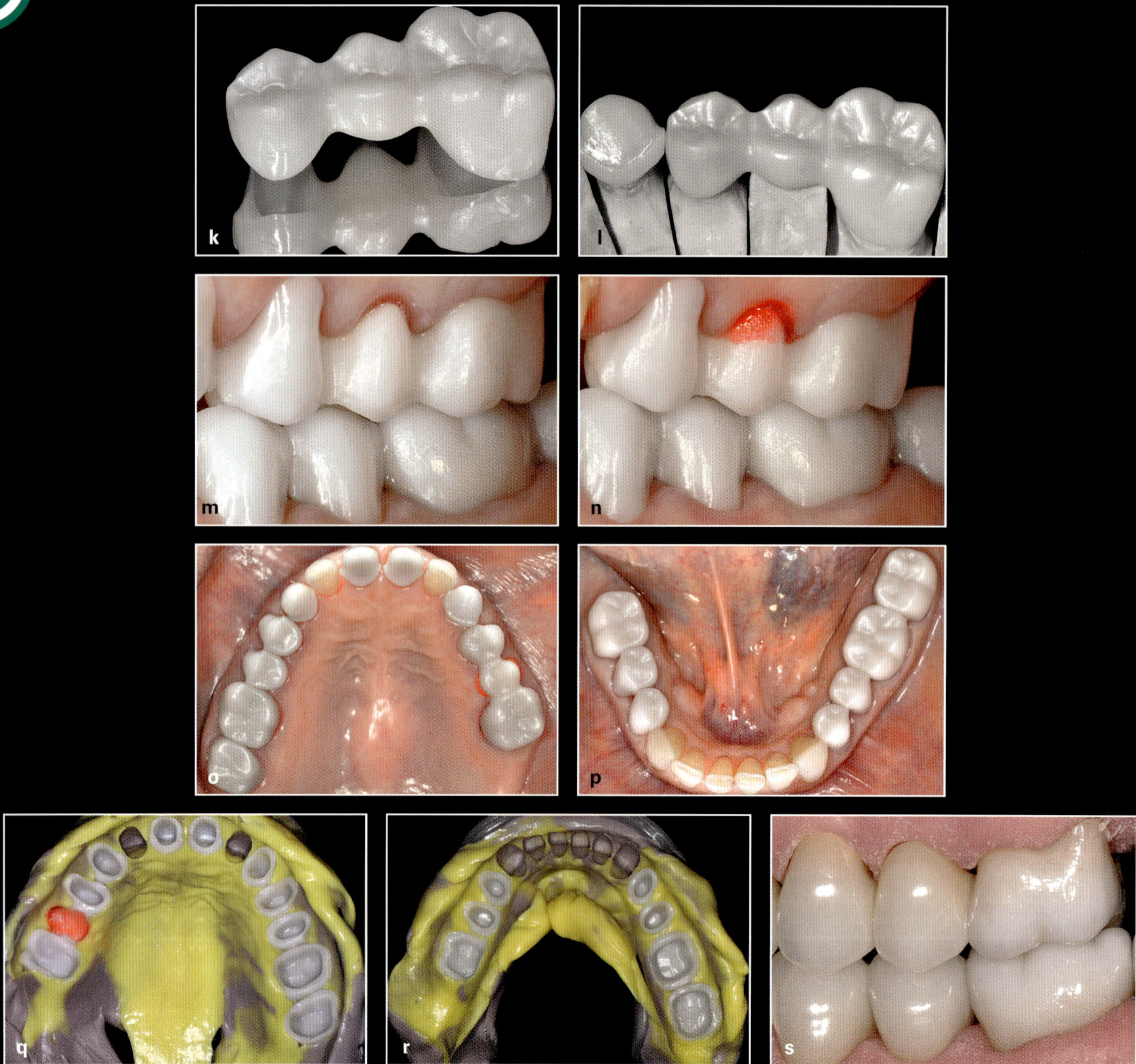

Fig 5-8 *(cont) (k)* View of the milled zirconia FDP framework. Note the relatively short pontic. *(l)* Palatal view of the FDP framework on the definitive cast. Note that there is no space between the pontic and the pontic site on the cast. *(m)* However, during the clinical framework try-in, it was noted that there was a space between the framework pontic and the pontic site. The FDP framework and crown copings were used to evaluate the interproximal and occlusal contacts as well as the internal fit. *(n)* The FDP framework was used for impressing the pontic site contours using autopolymerized acrylic resin (GC Pattern Resin). *(o and p)* Occlusal views of the maxillary and mandibular monolithic restorations, copings, and FDP framework stabilized in the patient's mouth prior to the making of the maxillary and mandibular pickup impressions. *(q and r)* Views of the maxillary and mandibular pickup impressions (Imprint 3) for transferring the natural soft tissue contours around the prepared teeth for crowns and FDP retainers and for the ovate pontic. *(s)* The new casts generated from the pickup impressions, demonstrating adequate soft tissue contours. The pickup impressions enhanced the dental technician's ability to fabricate the restorations with adequate cervical and interproximal contours as well as an adequate intaglio surface for the ovate pontic.

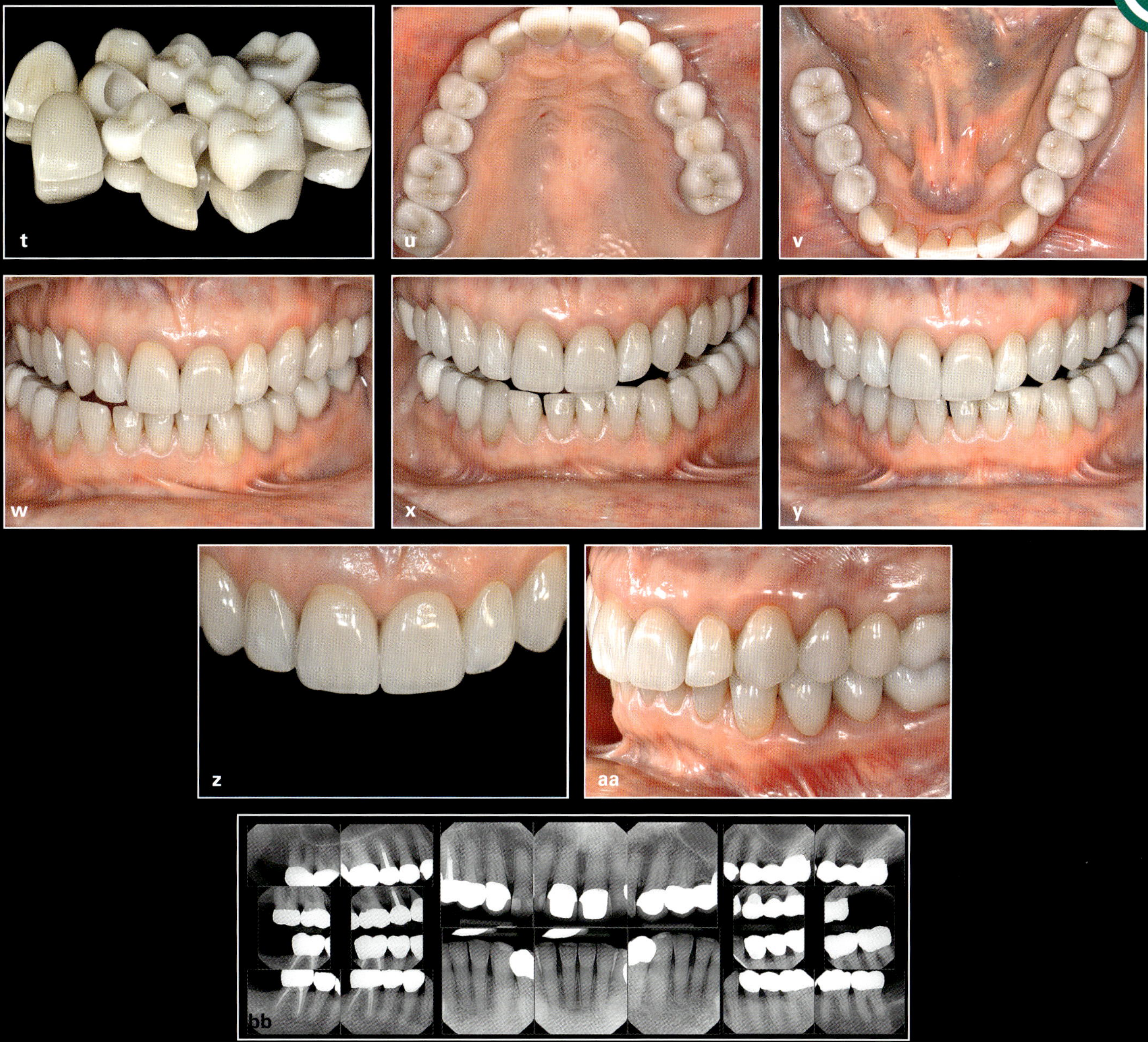

Fig 5-8 *(cont) (t)* View of the three types of ceramic zirconia-based restorations provided to the patient: monolithic for the molars, hybrid for the premolars, and bilayered for the anterior restorations. *(u and v)* Occlusal views of the definitive restorations in the patient's mouth. *(w to y)* Frontal views of the definitive restorations in right and left lateral excursions and in protrusive movement, mimicking the occlusal design achieved with the provisional restorations. *(z)* Frontal view of the anterior maxillary definitive crowns on the central incisors and canines. Note the gingival contours of the restorations and their integration with the soft tissue. *(aa)* Left lateral view of the complete restoration in maximal intercuspal position. Note the blending of the ovate pontic on the maxillary second premolar with the pontic site. *(bb)* Complete-mouth radiographs of the definitive restorations. Note the excellent marginal integrity.

Implant-Supported Ovate Pontics

With implant-supported ovate pontics, clinicians must capture the soft tissue profile around the prospective abutments of the implants for the implant-supported FDP retainers as well as the soft tissue profile around the pontic site at both the cervical and interproximal areas. Few articles have described different techniques for capturing these soft tissue areas. One article described a direct technique of capturing the soft tissue contours intraorally and simultaneously around both the impression copings and pontic site by syringing a low-viscosity dual-polymerized composite resin into the crevice between the transfer coping and the soft tissue at the cervical and interproximal areas to the level of the coronal tip of the papillae.[69] As with implant-supported crowns, the limitation of such direct a technique is that the soft tissue collapses to a certain degree by the time multiple impression copings are secured to the implants intraorally. Other authors described the use of an indirect technique to allow for a more accurate recording and transferring of the soft tissue contours around the implant-supported retainers and ovate pontics (although these techniques may be more time-consuming). One technique is similar to the custom impression coping technique presented for implant-supported crowns with an extension for the pontic using the provisional restoration and a silicone matrix.[70] The other technique captures the soft tissue in two phases. First, the soft tissue contours around the implant abutments are recorded and transferred with the indirect-direct modified impression coping technique as previously described. Subsequently, custom definitive abutments are designed and fabricated, followed by design and fabrication of the framework of the implant-supported FPD. In the second phase, clinicians record and transfer the cervical, interproximal, and intaglio soft tissue contours around the pontic site.[71] The step-by-step procedure for this second phase is as follows:

1. During the patient's FDP framework try-in appointment, remove the implant-supported provisional restoration from the patient's mouth (Fig 5-9a). Evaluate the shape of the ovate pontic site, and fill the space between the free gingival margins and the implant platform with fast-setting PVS or with cotton pellets impregnated with chlorhexidine gluconate to maintain the soft tissue contours.
2. Remove the soft tissue simulation material, which was previously used for the fabrication of the custom implant abutments, from the definitive cast.
3. Syringe/inject any type of light-body elastomeric impression material or a soft tissue simulation material onto the definitive cast at the pontic site area (Fig 5-9b).
4. Immediately secure the provisional implant-supported restoration to the implant analogs on the cast, thus impressing the provisional pontic with light-body elastomeric material and creating a replica of the clinical pontic site on the definitive cast (Fig 5-9c).
5. Once the light-body elastomeric impression material is polymerized, remove the provisional implant-supported FDP from the implant analogs and leave the new pontic site replica as is on the definitive cast (Fig 5-9d).
6. Secure the definitive custom implant abutments to the implant analogs on the definitive cast (Fig 5-9e), and place the FDP framework for evaluation over the elastomer pontic site replica (Fig 5-9f).
7. Paint the intaglio surface of the framework pontic with autopolymerized acrylic resin monomer (GC Pattern Resin) while creating convex contours as previously described in the pontic procedures for tooth-borne FDPs.
8. Seat the FDP framework on the implant abutments, and impress the pontic replica contours with the autopolymerized acrylic resin with the framework pontic, creating an ovate pontic verification replica (Fig 5-9g). Once the material is set, trim the excess autopolymerized acrylic resin with either an acrylic bur or a coarse sandpaper disk (Sof-Lex, 3M ESPE) (Fig 5-9h), and remove the definitive abutments from the definitive cast.
9. To verify the prospective contours of the pontic in the patient's mouth, remove the silicone or cotton pellets from the implant sites, and position the definitive abutments. Follow this with a try-in of the framework to assess the ovate pontic verification replica and the pontic site relationship (Fig 5-9i).
10. Remove the definitive framework and implant abutments from the patient's mouth, and secure the provisional FDP intraorally. Provide detailed instructions to the dental technician for the fabrication of the definitive restoration, with emphasis on layering of porcelain at the intaglio surface of the pontic while using the pontic site replica on the definitive cast as a guide for the definitive cervical, interproximal, and intaglio contours of the definitive pontic.

This technique can be used with slight modifications for transferring soft tissue contours for screw-retained implant-supported FDP pontics (see chapter 7).

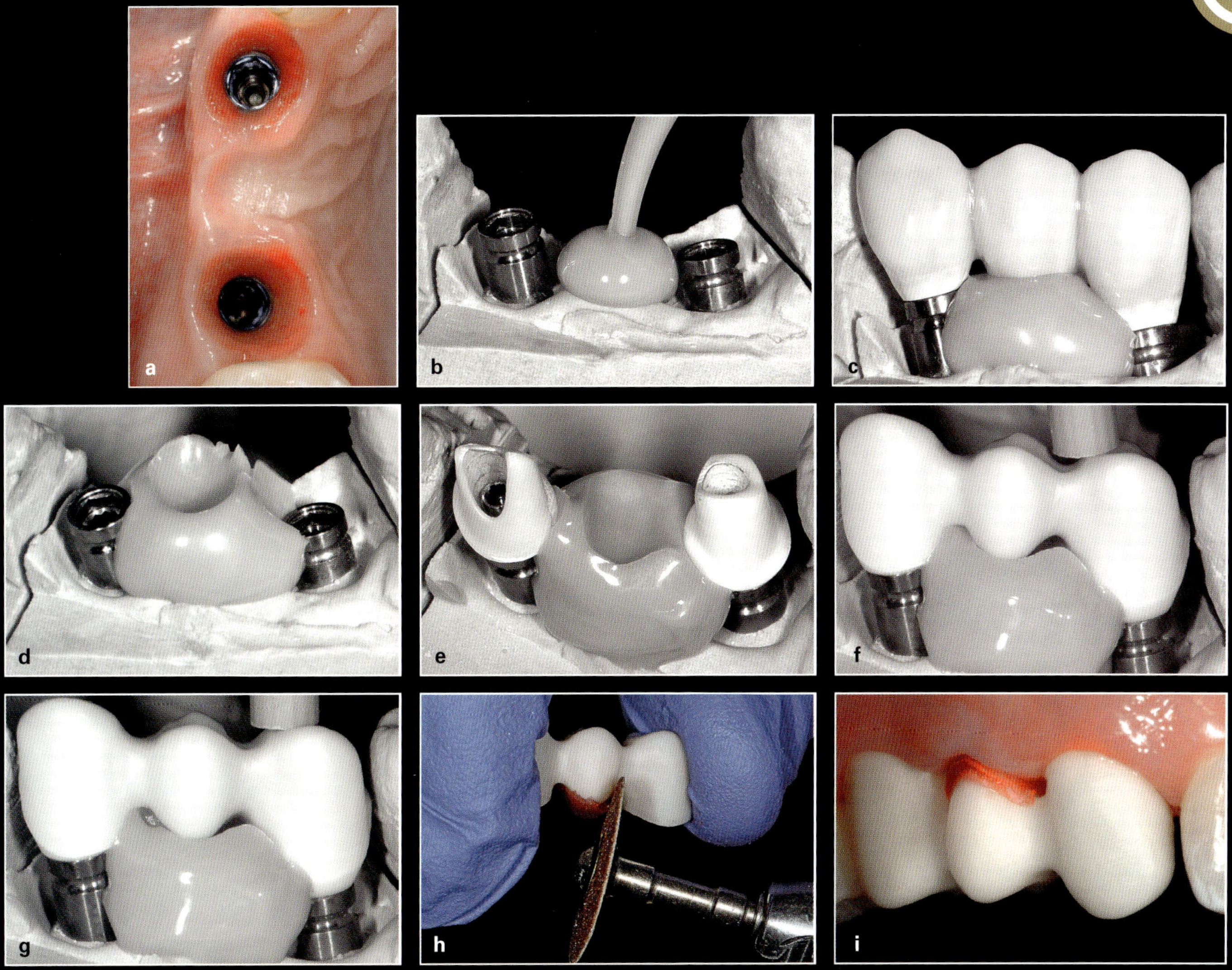

Fig 5-9 *(a)* Occlusal view of the implants (Osseotite Certain, Biomet 3i) and the ovate pontic site at the sites of the maxillary right canine and the first and second premolars designed for a three-unit implant-supported ceramic FDP. *(b)* View of the definitive cast after the soft tissue simulation material was removed and as light-body silicone impression material (Imprint 3) was injected onto the definitive cast at the pontic site replica area. *(c)* The screw-retained provisional restoration was immediately secured to the implant analogs in order to make an impression of the provisional pontic, creating an ovate pontic site replica. *(d)* View of the completely polymerized elastomer pontic site replica after removal of the provisional restoration. *(e)* The definitive zirconia abutments (Atlantis, Astra Tech) secured to the implant analogs. *(f)* View of the zirconia FDP framework (Katana) seated on the abutments. Note the space between the pontic and the pontic site replica. *(g)* The framework was used for impressing the pontic site replica contours using autopolymerized acrylic resin (GC Pattern Resin). *(h)* Excess autopolymerized acrylic resin was removed from the pontic verification replica with a sandpaper disk (Sof-Lex). *(i)* The framework with the pontic verification replica was clinically assessed in the patient's mouth. It was later used by the dental technician as a guide for fabricating the cervical and interproximal contours as well as the intaglio surface of the definitive pontic.

References

1. Shavell HM. Mastering the art of tissue management during provisionalization and biologic final impressions. Int J Periodontics Restorative Dent 1988;8:24–43.
2. Shavell HM. The periodontal-restorative interface in fixed prosthodontics: Tooth preparation, provisionalization, and biologic final impressions. Part I. Pract Periodontics Aesthet Dent 1994;6:33–44.
3. Shavell HM. The periodontal-restorative interface in fixed prosthodontics: Tooth preparation, provisionalization, and biologic final impressions. Part II. Pract Periodontics Aesthet Dent 1994;6:49–60.
4. Kopp FR. Esthetic principles for full crown restorations. Part II: Provisionalization. J Esthet Dent 1993;5:258–264.
5. Bichacho N. Achieving optimal gingival esthetics around restored natural teeth and implants. Rationale, concepts, and techniques. Dent Clin North Am 1998;42:763–780.
6. Jacques LB, Coelho AB, Hollweg H, Conti PC. Tissue sculpturing: An alternative method for improving esthetics of anterior fixed prosthodontics. J Prosthet Dent 1999;81:630–633.
7. Edelhoff D, Spiekermann H, Yildirim M. A review of esthetic pontic design options. Quintessence Int 2002;33:736–746.
8. Kim TH, Cascione D, Knezevic A. Simulated tissue using a unique pontic design: A clinical report. J Prosthet Dent 2009;102:205–210.
9. Kim TH, Cascione D, Knezevic A, Nowzari H. Restoration using gingiva-colored ceramic and a ridge lap pontic with circumferential pressure: A clinical report. J Prosthet Dent 2010;104:71–76.
10. Lewis S, Parel S, Faulkner R. Provisional implant-supported fixed restorations. Int J Oral Maxillofac Implants 1995;10:319–325.
11. Raigrodski AJ, Block MS. Clinical considerations for enhancing the success of implant-supported restorations in the aesthetic zone with delayed implant placement. Pract Proced Aesthet Dent 2002; 14:21–28.
12. Santosa RE. Provisional restoration options in implant dentistry. Aust Dent J 2007;52:234–242.
13. Kan JY, Rungcharassaeng K, Lozada JL, Zimmerman G. Facial gingival tissue stability following immediate placement and provisionalization of maxillary anterior single implants: A 2- to 8-year follow-up. Int J Oral Maxillofac Implants 2011;26:179–187.
14. Chu SJ, Tan JH, Stappert CF, Tarnow DP. Gingival zenith positions and levels of the maxillary anterior dentition. J Esthet Restor Dent 2009;21:113–120.
15. Chu SJ, Tarnow DP, Tan JH, Stappert CF. Papilla proportions in the maxillary anterior dentition. Int J Periodontics Restorative Dent 2009;29:385–393.
16. Hochman MN, Chu SJ, Tarnow DP. Maxillary anterior papilla display during smiling: A clinical study of the interdental smile line. Int J Periodontics Restorative Dent 2012;32:375–383.
17. Hu X, Nahles S, Nelson CA, Lin Y, Nelson K. Analysis of soft tissue display during enjoyment smiling: Part 1—Caucasians. Int J Periodontics Restorative Dent 2013;33:e9–e15.
18. Hu X, Lin Y, Heberer S, Nelson K. Analysis of soft tissue display in Chinese subjects during an enjoyment smile. Quintessence Int 2012;43:105–110.
19. Kapagiannidis D, Kontonasaki E, Bikos P, Koidis P. Teeth and gingival display in the premolar area during smiling in relation to gender and age. J Oral Rehabil 2005;32:830–837.
20. Meijer HJ, Stellingsma K, Meijndert L, Raghoebar GM. A new index for rating aesthetics of implant-supported single crowns and adjacent soft tissues—the Implant Crown Aesthetic Index. Clin Oral Implants Res 2005;16:645–649.
21. Fürhauser R, Florescu D, Benesch T, Haas R, Mailath G, Watzek G. Evaluation of soft tissue around single-tooth implant crowns: The pink esthetic score. Clin Oral Implants Res 2005;16:639–644.
22. Belser UC, Grütter L, Vailati F, Bornstein MM, Weber HP, Buser D. Outcome evaluation of early placed maxillary anterior single-tooth implants using objective esthetic criteria: A cross-sectional, retrospective study in 45 patients with a 2- to 4-year follow-up using pink and white esthetic scores. J Periodontol 2009;80:140–151.
23. Gehrke P, Lobert M, Dhom G. Reproducibility of the pink esthetic score—Rating soft tissue esthetics around single-implant restorations with regard to dental observer specialization. J Esthet Restor Dent 2008;20:375–384.
24. Luo Z, Zeng R, Luo Z, Chen Z. Single implants in the esthetic zone: Analysis of recent peri-implant soft tissue alterations and patient satisfaction. A photographic study. Int J Oral Maxillofac Implants 2011;26:578–586.
25. Bichacho N. Cervical contouring concepts: Enhancing the dentogingival complex. Pract Periodontics Aesthet Dent 1996;8:241–254.
26. Magne P, Magne M, Belser U. The esthetic width in fixed prosthodontics. J Prosthodont 1999;8:106–118.
27. Pameijer JH. Soft tissue master cast for esthetic control in crown and bridge procedures. Esthet Dent 1989;1:47–50.
28. Nayyar A, Moskowitz M, Pollard BL. Improving the emergence profile of dental restorations with accurate reproduction of soft tissue topography. J Esthet Dent 1995;7:26–31.
29. Reich S, Wichmann M, Nkenke E, Proeschel P. Clinical fit of all-ceramic three-unit fixed partial dentures, generated with three different CAD/CAM systems. Eur J Oral Sci 2005;113:174–179.
30. Kohorst P, Brinkmann H, Li J, Borchers L, Stiesch M. Marginal accuracy of four-unit zirconia fixed dental prostheses fabricated using different computer-aided design/computer-aided manufacturing systems. Eur J Oral Sci 2009;117:319–325.
31. Beuer F, Aggstaller H, Edelhoff D, Gernet W, Sorensen J. Marginal and internal fits of fixed dental prostheses zirconia retainers. Dent Mater 2009;25:94–102.
32. Ng J, Ruse D, Wyatt C. A comparison of the marginal fit of crowns fabricated with digital and conventional methods. J Prosthet Dent 2014;112:555–560.
33. Crispin B. Acrylic resin copings: An adjunct to fixed restorative dentistry. J Prosthet Dent 1978;39:632–636.
34. Zuckerman GR. Dies with resin copings for accurate registrations. J Prosthet Dent 1992;67:37–40.
35. Mizrahi B. Modified complete-arch impression technique for facilitating esthetic and biomechanical precision in complete-arch rehabilitation. J Prosthodont 2011;20:474–487.
36. Williamson RT, Breeding LC, Kinderknecht KE. Soft tissue cast aids in establishing interproximal contours for restorations. J Prosthet Dent 1993;69:630–631.
37. Bassiouny MA, Yearwood LL. Establishing the gingival emergence profile of restorations by using a resilient gingival replica. J Prosthet Dent 1996;76:386–389.
38. Tan PL, Ruder GA. Simple(r) soft tissue masque for individual fixed restorations. J Prosthodont 2004;13:192–194.
39. Noh K, Kwon KR, Kim HS, Kim DS, Pae A. Accurate transfer of soft tissue morphology with interim prosthesis to definitive cast. J Prosthet Dent 2014;111:159–162.
40. Su H, Gonzalez-Martin O, Weisgold A, Lee E. Considerations of implant abutment and crown contour: Critical contour and subcritical contour. Int J Periodontics Restorative Dent 2010;30:335–343.
41. Polack MA. Simple method of fabricating an impression coping to reproduce peri-implant gingiva on the master cast. J Prosthet Dent 2002;88:221–223.
42. Spyropoulou PE, Razzoog M, Sierraalta M. Restoring implants in the esthetic zone after sculpting and capturing the periimplant tissues in rest position: A clinical report. J Prosthet Dent 2009;102:345–347.
43. Attard N, Barzilay I. A modified impression technique for accurate registration of peri-implant soft tissues. J Can Dent Assoc 2003; 69:80–83.
44. Elian N, Tabourian G, Jalbout ZN, et al. Accurate transfer of peri-implant soft tissue emergence profile from the provisional crown to the final prosthesis using an emergence profile cast. J Esthet Restor Dent 2007;19:306–314.
45. Chee WW, Cho GC, Ha S. Replicating soft tissue contours on working casts for implant restorations. J Prosthodont 1997;6:218–220.
46. Tsai BY. A method for obtaining peri-implant soft-tissue contours by using screw-retained provisional restorations as impression copings: A clinical report. J Oral Implantol 2011;37:605–609.

47. Breeding LC, Dixon DL. Transfer of gingival contours to a master cast. J Prosthet Dent 1996;75:341–343.
48. Papadopoulos I, Pozidi G, Goussias H, Kourtis S. Transferring the emergence profile from the provisional to the final restoration. J Esthet Restor Dent 2014;26:154–161.
49. Grossmann Y, Pasciuta M, Finger IM. A novel technique using a coded healing abutment for the fabrication of a CAD/CAM titanium abutment for an implant-supported restoration. J Prosthet Dent 2006;95:258–261.
50. Lin WS, Harris BT, Morton D. The use of a scannable impression coping and digital impression technique to fabricate a customized anatomic abutment and zirconia restoration in the esthetic zone. J Prosthet Dent 2013;109:187–191.
51. Lin WS, Harris BT, Morton D. Use of implant-supported interim restorations to transfer periimplant soft tissue profiles to a milled polyurethane definitive cast. J Prosthet Dent 2013;109:333–337.
52. Coelho AB, Miranda JE, Pegoraro LF. Single-tooth implants: A procedure to make a precise, flexible gingival contour on the master cast. J Prosthet Dent 1997;78:109–110.
53. Hinds KT. Custom impression coping for an exact registration of the healed tissue in the esthetic implant restoration. Int J Periodontics Restorative Dent 1997;17:585–591.
54. Buskin R, Salinas TJ. Transferring emergence profile created from the provisional to the definitive restoration. Pract Periodontics Aesthet Dent 1998;10:1171–1179.
55. Barzilay I. Maintenance of gingival contour during prosthodontic procedures: A clinical report. J Prosthet Dent 1999;82:377–378.
56. Dewey KW, Zugsmith R. An experimental study of tissue reactions about porcelain roots. J Dent Res 1933;13:459–472.
57. Abrams L. Augmentation of the deformed residual edentulous ridge for fixed prosthesis. Compend Contin Educ Gen Dent 1980; 1:205–213.
58. Garber DA, Rosenberg ES. The edentulous ridge in fixed prosthodontics. Compend Contin Educ Dent 1981;2:212–223.
59. Dylina TJ. Contour determination for ovate pontics. J Prosthet Dent 1999;82:136–142.
60. Clayton JA, Green E. Roughness of pontic materials and dental plaque. J Prosthet Dent 1970;23:407–411.
61. Tripodakis AP, Constantinides A. Tissue response under hyperpressure from convex pontics. Int J Periodontics Restorative Dent 1990;10:408–414.
62. Zitzmann NU, Marinello CP, Berglundh T. The ovate pontic design: A histologic observation in humans. J Prosthet Dent 2002;88:375–380.
63. Orsini G, Murmura G, Artese L, Piattelli A, Piccirilli M, Caputi S. Tissue healing under provisional restorations with ovate pontics: A pilot human histological study. J Prosthet Dent 2006;96:252–257.
64. Ishibe M, Raigrodski AJ, Mak V. Clinical treatment planning—Case 63: Part I. Seattle Study Club J 2010;15:19–24.
65. Ishibe M, Raigrodski AJ, Mak V. Clinical treatment planning—Case 63: Part II. Seattle Study Club J 2011;15:10–15.
66. Chee WW, Cho GC, Ikoma MM, Arcidiacono A. A technique to replicate soft tissues around fixed restoration pontics on working casts. J Prosthodont 1999;8:44–46.
67. da Fonseca DM, Ankli R, Camara CA. The use of characterized gingival porcelain to restore hard and soft tissue deficiencies. Quintessence Dent Technol 2002;25:117–129.
68. de Vasconcelos DK, Volpato CA, Zani IM, Bottino MA. Impression technique for ovate pontics. J Prosthet Dent 2011;105:59–61.
69. Schoenbaum TR, Han TJ. Direct custom implant impression copings for the preservation of the pontic receptor site architecture. J Prosthet Dent 2012;107:203–206.
70. Ntounis A, Petropoulou A. A technique for managing and accurate registration of periimplant soft tissues. J Prosthet Dent 2010; 104:276–279.
71. Raigrodski AJ, Schwedhelm ER, Chen YW. A simplified technique for recording an implant-supported ovate pontic site in the esthetic zone. J Prosthet Dent 2014;111:154–158.

Abutment Selection for Cement-Retained Implant-Supported Restorations

6

Ariel J. Raigrodski | Jae Seon Kim

In restorative dentistry, an ideal abutment for a tooth-supported complete-coverage restoration is defined as a substructure that properly supports the definitive restoration and adequately interacts with and supports the soft tissue. The location and design of the finish line on the prepared abutment and its junction with the soft tissue are critical for creating an ideal emergence profile and preserving the biologic width. In addition, the abutment color plays a significant role in achieving the desired gingival esthetics, especially in patients with a thin gingival phenotype.[1] The geometric dimensions of the abutment should also allow for adequate ferrule, proper occlusogingival height, and proper total angle of convergence for enhancing the durability of the remaining tooth structure and the prosthesis.[2–7]

In addition to the space occupied by abutments for tooth-supported restorations, abutments for cement-retained implant-supported restorations occupy the space between the free gingival margins and the implant platform and act as a link between the implant and the restoration. Multiple factors must be considered in designing the optimal implant abutment, particularly when esthetics is of primary concern. The biologic, mechanical, and optical properties of the materials used to make the abutment must be comparable to those of natural dentition. Moreover, in terms of design, the implant abutment should be contoured at the cervical area to simulate the cross section of the tooth to be replaced while facilitating and supporting an ideal soft tissue emergence profile.

Generally, stock abutments do not simulate such physiologic form because of their predetermined cylindric contours. The ultimate goal of abutment design is to achieve an adequate interface between the abutment and the margins and cervical and interproximal contours of the definitive restoration while blending both components with the soft tissue functionally and esthetically. Su et al[8] described these interfaces as critical and subcritical contours, both of which affect the soft tissue profile. The critical contour is the area immediately apical to the free gingival margins (with a range of 1 mm), and the subcritical contour refers to the emergence area of the abutment from the implant platform to the critical contour (about 1 mm below the free gingival margins). In addition, the soft tissue color, mainly the value (brightness), may be impacted by the color of the abutment, especially in patients with a thin gingival phenotype.[9–12] Furthermore, different restorative materials may present with different levels of biocompatibility in terms of soft tissue response.[13–19] This chapter discusses these parameters mainly in the context of soft tissue management while emphasizing how the advent of computer-aided design/computer-assisted manufacturing (CAD/CAM) technology facilitates abutment design and abutment material selection for cement-retained implant-supported restorations.

Abutment Classification

Implant abutments can be classified either by design (ie, stock versus custom) or by material and color (ie, metallic versus ceramic).

Classification by design

Stock abutments

Abutment contour and finish line location are extremely critical for achieving an esthetic restorative outcome at the soft tissue–restorative interface. This is where the soft tissue, the subgingival areas and finish line of the abutment and its cervical contours, and the margins and cervical contours of the restoration all converge. Stock abutments are either cylindric or semi-anatomically shaped and are designed by manufacturers based on anatomical averages.[20,21] The diameter at the cervix of any maxillary tooth can vary from 6.5 to 10.0 mm mesiodistally and from 5.0 to 10.0 mm buccolingually.[22] In order to facilitate the positioning of the free gingival margin at the desired location, the implant abutment has to mimic the morphology of the natural root, which selectively varies in dimensions. The cylindric shape of the stock abutment may be limited in providing these kinds of sophisticated contours. These abutments are mainly made of either titanium or zirconia and can be modified in a subtractive manner through preparation.

Stock abutments are popular mainly because of their ease of use and lower cost. However, the disadvantages of stock abutments include the cost of keeping product inventory, higher material cost for metal-ceramic restorations because more metal may be needed to fabricate the definitive restoration, and possible residual excess cement retention due to the limited ability to control the finish line placement of the abutment in relation to the free gingival margins. In addition, preparing a stock zirconia abutment can compromise the physical properties of the zirconia.[23–26] Additional compromises include the inability to ensure the critical minimal thickness of the axial walls of such abutments as well as the inability to ensure the minimum distance between the implant platform and the finish line of the abutment. Therefore, only in limited clinical scenarios in the posterior segments in which the soft tissue is flat and not scalloped can stock abutments be used safely to provide an adequate restorative solution.

Custom abutments

The UCLA abutment was introduced in the early 1980s as the first attempt to create a custom implant abutment. A wax pattern was created on an implant component, invested, and cast.[27,28] With these types of metal abutments, it was also possible to layer feldspathic porcelain apical to the finish line of the abutment subgingivally to mimic root color and fluorescence.[29,30] With the advent of CAD/CAM technology and restorative materials, abutments can be customized with different CAD/CAM systems and fabricated out of titanium, zirconia, and other materials. The following paragraphs describe the rationale for using custom abutments.

Angle correction. Despite the effort involved in treatment planning and the accurate surgical execution of those treatment plans, the implant position may not always be secured in the predetermined position. There is currently a debate among researchers as to whether restoratively driven implant position should always overrule the biologically restricted position in the absence of bone and soft tissue.[31–33] Ultimately, when the endosseous implant gains osseointegration, the restorative dentist must work with the provided implant position to simulate the natural tooth abutment. Custom abutments can provide a wide gamut of angle corrections and subsequently enhance the creation of desired functional and esthetic restorative outcomes.

Soft tissue support. The ideal emergence profile to create a natural-looking restoration can be provided with a custom abutment. Depending on the implant position (apicocoronal, buccolingual, and mesiodistal) as well as the angulation, the emergence profile is shaped using the provisional restoration (Figs 6-1 and 6-2). This will enhance the contours and levels of the facial free gingival margins and the interproximal papillae.[34] In esthetically demanding clinical scenarios in which extra soft tissue refinement is needed, the soft tissue contours are accurately transferred to the dental laboratory (see Figs 6-1f to 6-1h), as previously described in chapter 5. A custom abutment is then designed to meet these expectations and assist with translating the contours achieved with the provisional restoration to the definitive one (see Figs 6-1i to 6-1l and Figs 6-2c and 6-2d).

Control of finish line placement. Custom abutments allow clinicians to control the finish line location while following the scalloping of the soft tissue. Control of the finish line location is critical not only in terms of esthetics but also in terms of preventing residual excess cement retention (Fig 6-3). An implant abutment lacks the tissue attachment (eg, Sharpey's fibers) that is present in natural dentition, so the cement coming out of the margins of the restoration may be driven into the subcritical soft tissue area, resulting in excess cement retention.[35,36] Linkevicius et al[37] evaluated in vitro the amount of residual excess cement that is left around implants and its relation to the apicocoronal placement of the finish line. The study concluded that the amount of residual cement after cleaning increased as the abutment finish line and the restoration margins were located further subgingivally. The greatest amount of cement was left when the finish line of the abutment was placed 2 to 3 mm subgingivally. Control of the finish line location is often limited when stock abutments are used. This may become a critical factor in treatment, especially in areas where access to cleaning is limited such as in interproximal areas and the posterior dentition. Residual excess cement can lead to complications such as inflammatory

Continued from chapter 3

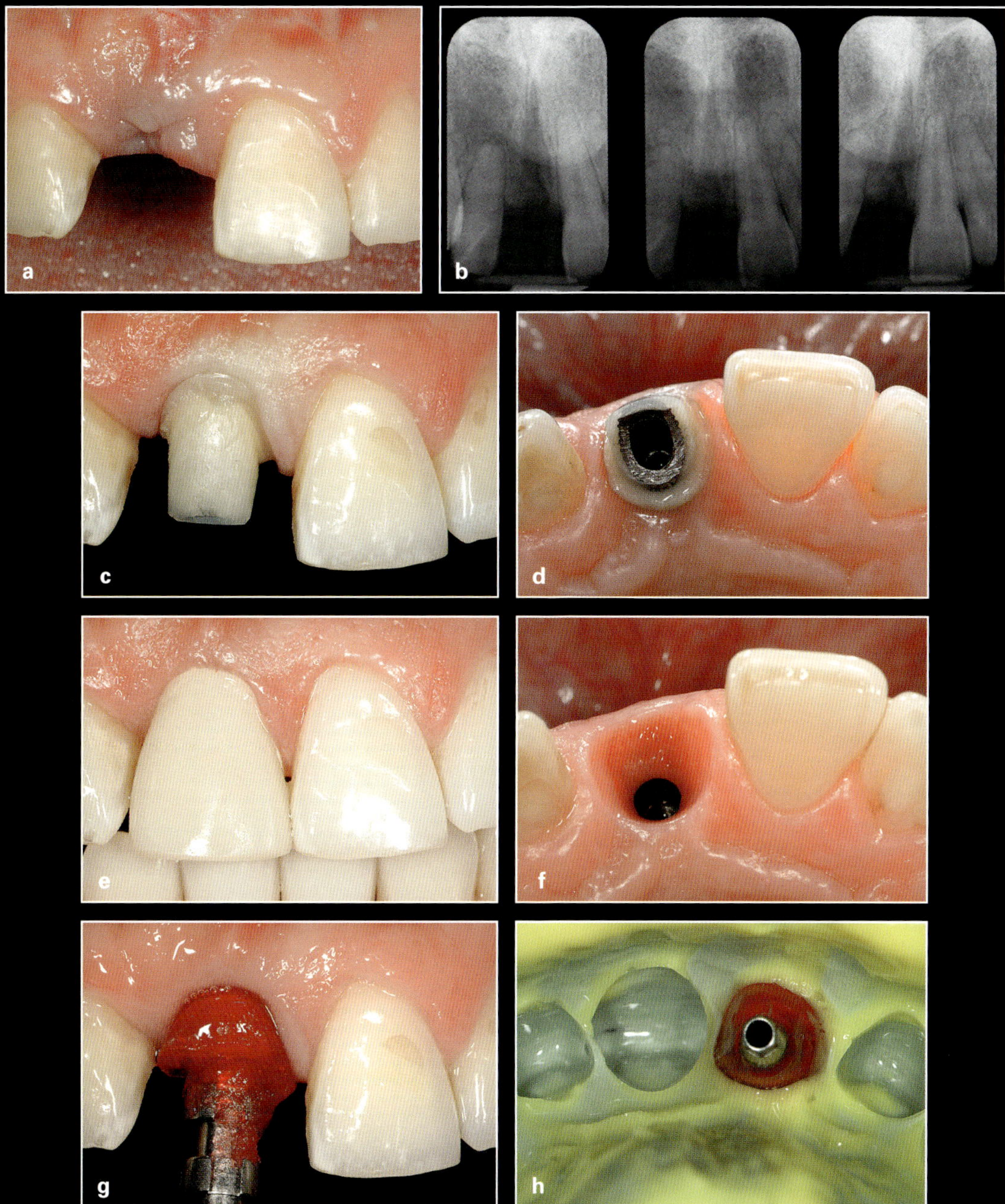

Fig 6-1 *(a)* Facial view of a patient who lost the maxillary right central incisor due to trauma. *(b)* Periapical radiographs of the patient prior to surgical intervention. Guided bone regeneration was performed, and 6 months later, connective tissue grafting was performed at the time of implant placement (Astra Tech Osseospeed 4.0). *(c and d)* Facial and occlusal views of the custom provisional abutment at insertion. Note the soft tissue blanching, which subsided after 10 minutes, and the conservative finish line position, which is slightly below the free gingival margins on the facial and interproximal aspects and supragingival on the palatal aspect. *(e)* Facial view of the provisional restoration a week after delivery. *(f)* Occlusal view of the implant and the soft tissue contours shaped with the provisional restoration. *(g and h)* A custom impression coping was fabricated and used as discussed in chapter 5 to capture the implant position as well as the soft tissue profile, and an open tray master impression was made.

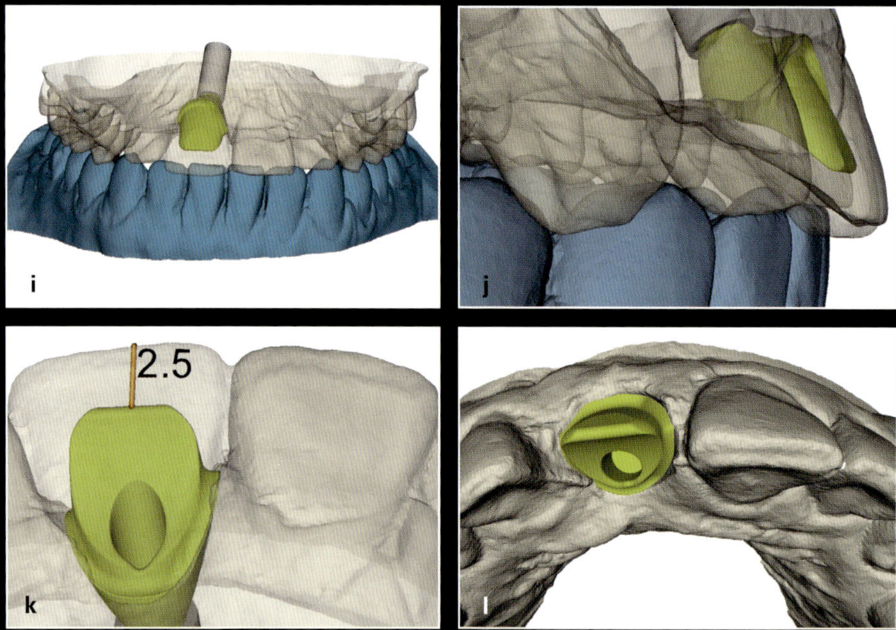

Fig 6-1 *(cont) (i to k)* The definitive cast was scanned with and without a wax-up of the missing tooth based on the contours of the provisional restoration. The scanned images were superimposed to enhance the design of the custom zirconia abutment *(i)*. The CAD design (Atlantis, Astra Tech) allowed for measurements in different areas in relation to the emergence profile, the prospective crown, and the occlusion *(j)*. Rotational and cross-sectional views are available with CAD/CAM systems, which enhance proper abutment design. While reviewing the virtual abutment design, one has to keep in mind the space required for the definitive restoration, whether it is a coping with layered ceramics or a monolithic restoration *(k)*. *(l)* Facial view of the definitive design of the CAD/CAM zirconia custom abutment. While the virtual abutment design is being reviewed, it is critical to assess the subgingival contours and the location of the finish line to ensure the facilitation of residual excess cement removal. The finish line was placed 1 mm below the free gingival margin on the facial aspect (zirconia abutment) and equigingivally on the palatal aspect.

Continued from chapter 5

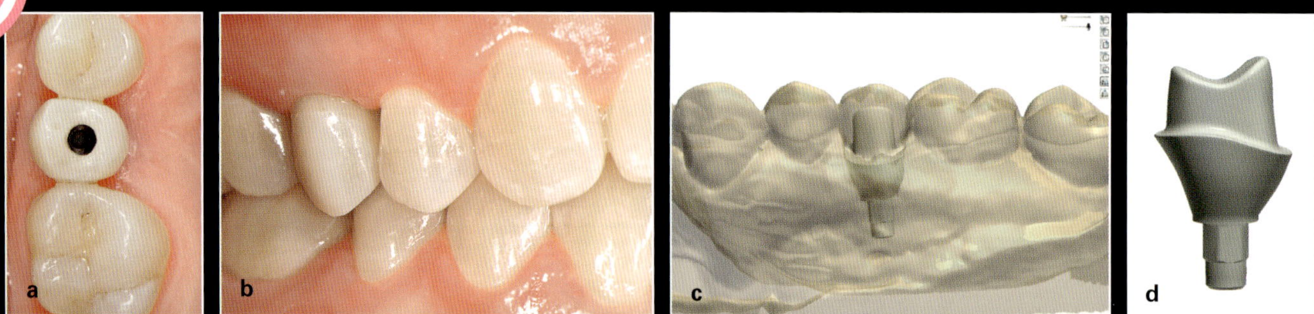

Fig 6-2 *(a and b)* Occlusal and lateral views of the provisional restoration. *(c and d)* The CAD/CAM custom abutment was designed on the CAD unit (3Shape) based on the soft tissue contours and the provisional restoration. The finish line follows the scalloping of the soft tissue. The finish line was placed 1.5 mm below the free gingival margin on the facial aspect (titanium abutment) and equigingivally on the palatal aspect.

G

Continued from chapter 5

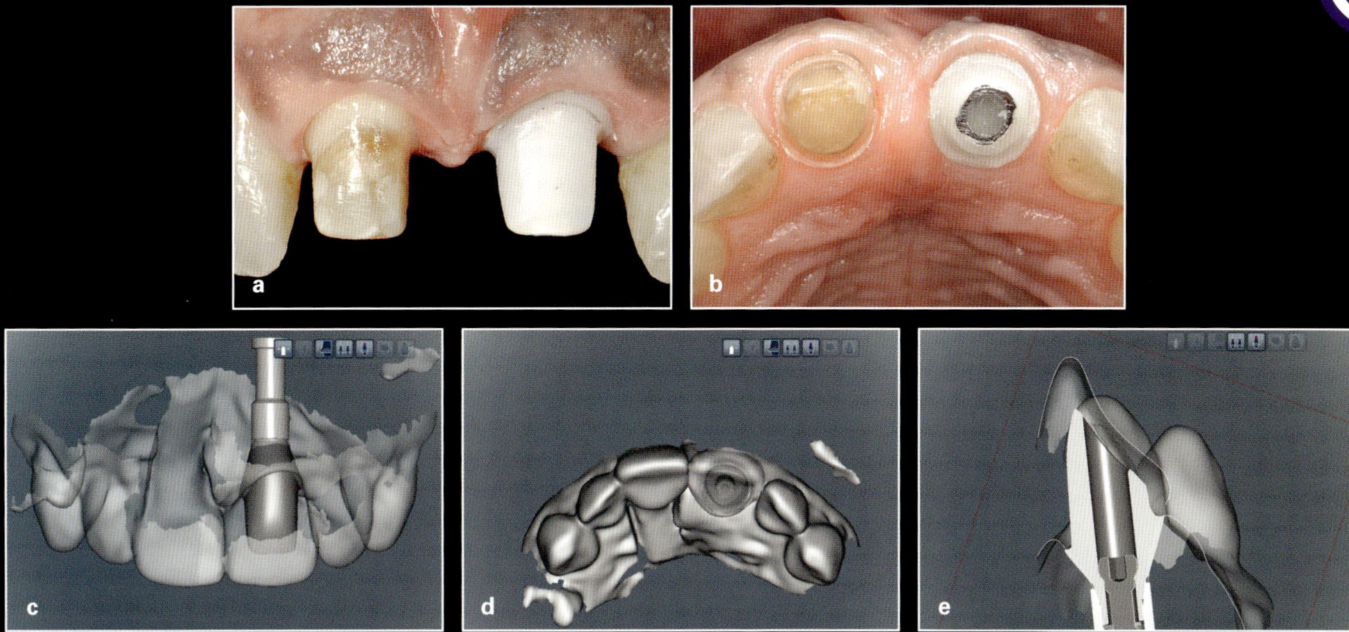

Fig 6-3 *(a and b)* Facial and occlusal views of the provisional custom implant abutment. *(c to e)* The custom titanium abutment was designed on the CAD unit (NobelProcera Optical Scanner, Nobel Biocare) based on the soft tissue contours transferred to the definitive cast as well as the scanned wax-up based on the provisional restoration. The finish line was placed 1.5 mm below the free gingival margins on the facial aspect (titanium abutment) and equigingivally on the palatal aspect *(e)*.

reaction in the periodontium surrounding the implants, and some authors have even linked the excess cement retention to bone loss and loss of osseointegration.[38–40] Whenever restoration margin display has no esthetic liability and adequate axial wall height can be obtained to provide adequate retention and resistance form, designing a supragingival finish line (sometimes even circumferentially) will simplify clinical procedures and long-term maintenance.

Prevention of fracture in ceramic abutments. Zirconia custom abutments made through milling when partially sintered and later through sintering have shown to have fewer microdefects than those made through grinding after the zirconia has been fully sintered.[26] Therefore, the physical properties of zirconia may be compromised whenever the surface is prepared with a bur and may ultimately lead to catastrophic failures in the long term.[23–25]

Financial considerations. Despite the higher cost of custom abutments compared with stock abutments, using a custom abutment can have financial advantages when metal-ceramic implant-supported restorations are fabricated. Because stock abutments are not designed to address the individual clinical restorative space presented by each patient, fabrication of the metal coping/framework for the definitive restoration may require extra metal alloy when these abutments are used. Moreover, additional time may be required by the dental technician to fabricate a coping/framework that properly supports the soft tissue emergence as well the veneering porcelain. Chair time can also be saved with custom abutments because less time is needed for residual excess cement removal, and this saved chair time may make up for the increased cost of the custom abutment.

Classification by material

Metallic abutments

Traditionally in implant dentistry, machined titanium and castable metal abutments were used, but the recent advancement in CAD/CAM technology has led milled titanium abutments to become most prevalent among metallic abutments.[41] Several factors have contributed to the decline in use of high noble alloys for implant abutments. The high price of gold and precious metals, the reduced biocompatibility in terms of soft tissue response compared with titanium,[15] and the lower accuracy due to human error during waxing and casting procedures[42,43] may all be contributing factors. Titanium is mechanically and biologically compatible in the oral environment and has an ample clinical track record.[44–46] However, with titanium abutments, the gray color of the material can reflect through the tissue, especially if the tissue has a thin and/or translucent phenotype.[10,46] Therefore, titanium abutments may be an adequate choice in the posterior segments where esthetic considerations are diminished and functional considerations such as higher occlusal forces and larger chewing surface areas take precedence, or in anterior segments when the patient has a thick soft tissue phenotype (Fig 6-4a). Cast metal or metal-ceramic restorations are mainly used with these types of abutments for restorations in the posterior segments. The restorations on these metallic abutments can be permanently or temporarily cemented, depending on how much retrievability is desired by the clinician for that particular patient.

This does not mean that all metallic abutments cause compromised soft tissue esthetics. A study has shown that gold color blends well with the soft tissue without any shadowing effect.[12] Companies have developed a gold-hue titanium abutment utilizing a titanium nitrate coating technology. This coating is about 3 to 5 microns in thickness (Fig 6-5a). Such abutments still present with excellent biocompatibility in terms of tissue response.[47] Any adjustment of the abutment will remove the nitrate layer and expose the silver/gray titanium color. This may not be a problem for the most part because various restorative materials can effectively block out the gray color once a complete-coverage restoration is cemented to the abutment. However, it becomes a problem if any adjustments have to be made at the finish line or at subgingival areas where the gingival esthetics will be compromised by a gray hue. Thus, as discussed in chapter 5, transfer of the soft tissue profile from the patient's mouth to the definitive cast has to be accurate. Subsequently, the abutment design done via CAD or through fabricating a wax pattern to be scanned later must be impeccable to minimize such adjustments, especially when patients present with the thin soft tissue phenotype. In addition, attempts to color abutments in pink have been unsuccessful in terms of soft tissue color response.[48]

In areas where esthetics is of primary concern and metal abutments are being used, the finish line placement on the buccal aspect should be 1.5 mm below the free gingival margins (Figs 6-4b and 6-4c). Such an approach may reduce the likelihood of any esthetic complications in case of future recession and will not compromise the ability of the clinician to remove residual excess cement. Titanium abutments can also be used in the anterior region when the implant angulation compromises the abutment's axial wall thickness and when the distance from the implant platform to the abutment finish line is limited, depending on the type of implant connection. For titanium abutments, minimal axial wall thickness can be reduced to as little as 0.2 to 0.3 mm. For zirconia abutments, the axial wall thickness should not be reduced to less than 0.5 to 0.7 mm, as any further reduction may facilitate a prospective failure of the abutment.[49,50] Ceramic restorations such as zirconia-based restorations can still be used on titanium abutments either by using a thick zirconia coping (at least 0.6 mm)[51] or by layering various opacious porcelain materials on the zirconia coping of the restoration to effectively block out and mask the titanium abutment[52] (Figs 6-4d to 6-4p and Figs 6-5b to 6-5f).

Implant-supported restorations can be cemented with either temporary or permanent cements. In the past, temporary cements were often used due to frequent screw loosening in external hex machined implants with gold screws. This screw loosening occurred because the external connection of such implants directed the chewing force to the cervical region of the implant.[53] At the time, it was more common to cement the restorations with temporary cement so the abutment and restoration could be retrieved. However, with the increasing popularity of implants with internal connection, various screw head designs, and improved surface treatment on titanium screws, more preload can be achieved, and screw loosening has become less frequent.[54–57] Despite the reduced incidence of screw loosening, however, some clinicians may still prefer to cement the implant restorations with temporary cement for retrievability. With metal abutments and metal-ceramic or cast metal restorations, both types of cements may be considered as viable options. With ceramic restorations cemented on top of metallic abutments, permanent cement is recommended to maximize the physical properties of the restoration and minimize the risk of fractures of the ceramic restorations. Methods to retrieve cement-retained implant restorations have been described in the literature.[58,59]

Ceramic abutments

The advent of CAD/CAM technology has led to the development of various custom abutment fabrication techniques utilizing not only metal alloys but also ceramics. Ceramic implant abutments were introduced in the late 1990s, when alumina preparable abutments emerged on the market.[60,61] Although the optical properties of these alumina abutments were pleasing, the abutments themselves were brittle and extremely susceptible to fracture.[62,63] Currently, the material of choice for ceramic abutments is zirconia, which comes in different designs, colors, and interfaces with the implant platform and with the abutment screw. In several studies, zirconia abutments have demonstrated high clinical success.[64–66] In addition, there were no significant differences between zirconia and metallic abutments in terms of biologic, mechanical, or technical outcomes.[66] Moreover, one study has reported successful use of zirconia abutments even in the posterior segments.[67] However, limitations of these studies such as small sample size and lack of long-term follow-up have to be considered.[68]

Clinicians should remember that the main reason for using zirconia as an abutment material is not its strength or durability but rather the esthetics of the soft tissue and definitive restoration at the soft tissue–restorative interface. Jung et al[10] reported that when more than 2 mm of buccolingual thickness of soft tissue is present, the underlying color of the abutment will not adversely affect the color of the gingiva. However, not all patients have thick soft tissue to mask

Continued from page 131

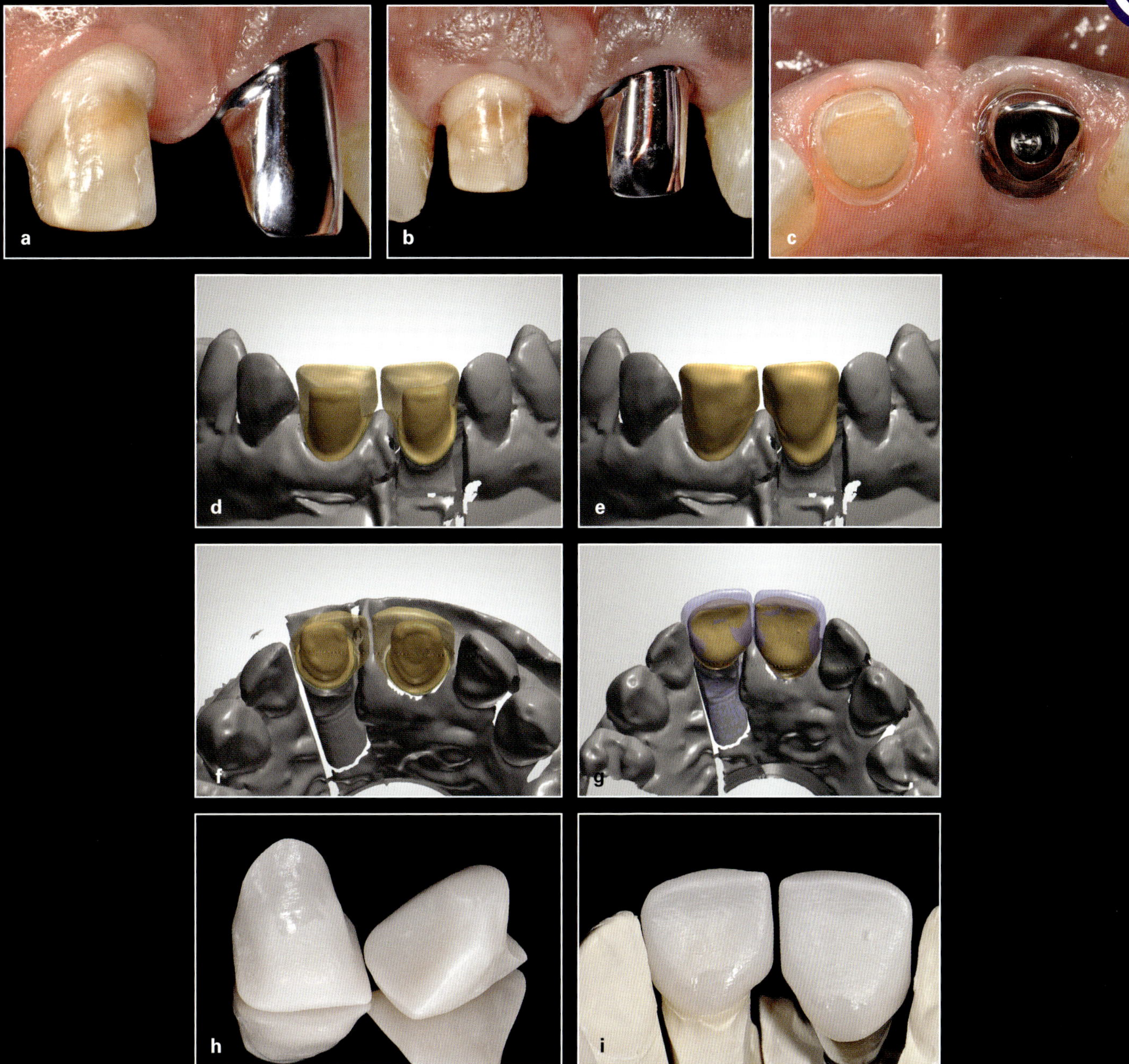

Fig 6-4 *(a)* View of the definitive titanium custom abutment demonstrating that its gray color is not reflected through the tissue due to its thickness. *(b and c)* Facial and occlusal views of the definitive titanium custom abutment with the finish line placed 1.5 mm below the free gingival margins on the facial aspect. Note that the contours of the abutment are similar to a maxillary incisor crown tooth preparation and that the definitive abutment is similar in contours and shape to the provisional custom abutment (see Figs 6-3a and 6-3b). *(d to g)* The copings of the zirconia-based ceramic restorations (Lava Plus, 3M ESPE) were designed on the CAD unit to simulate a coping design similar to a ceramic veneer tooth preparation. This allowed for application of veneering porcelain on the facial and incisal aspects to facilitate the esthetic outcome. The palatal aspect was designed for monolithic zirconia, excluding the palatal incisal aspect, based on the contours of the simulated prospective restorations. *(h and i)* Views of the definitive copings. Note the masking of the titanium abutment to ensure that the value of the restoration was not reduced by the underlying titanium abutment.

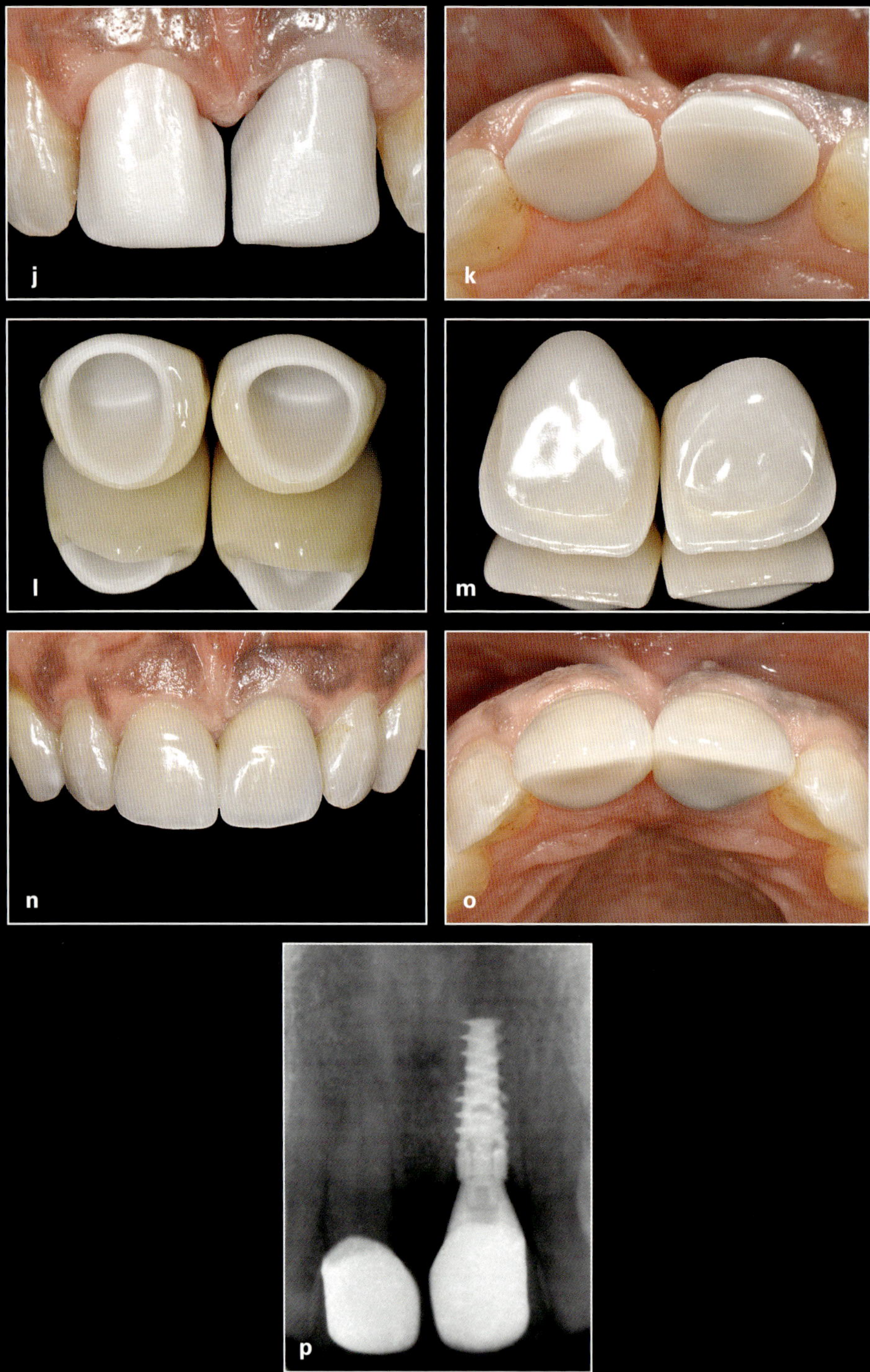

Fig 6-4 *(cont) (j and k)* The hybrid zirconia copings were tried in the patient's mouth. Note that the design of the coping is similar to a ceramic veneer tooth preparation. *(l and m)* Views of the definitive restorations after the application and firing of the veneering porcelain and finishing. Note the zirconia circumferential margins and the palatal monolithic zirconia surfaces. *(n and o)* Facial and occlusal views of the definitive restorations. *(p)* Postoperative radiograph of the definitive restorations.

Continued from page 130

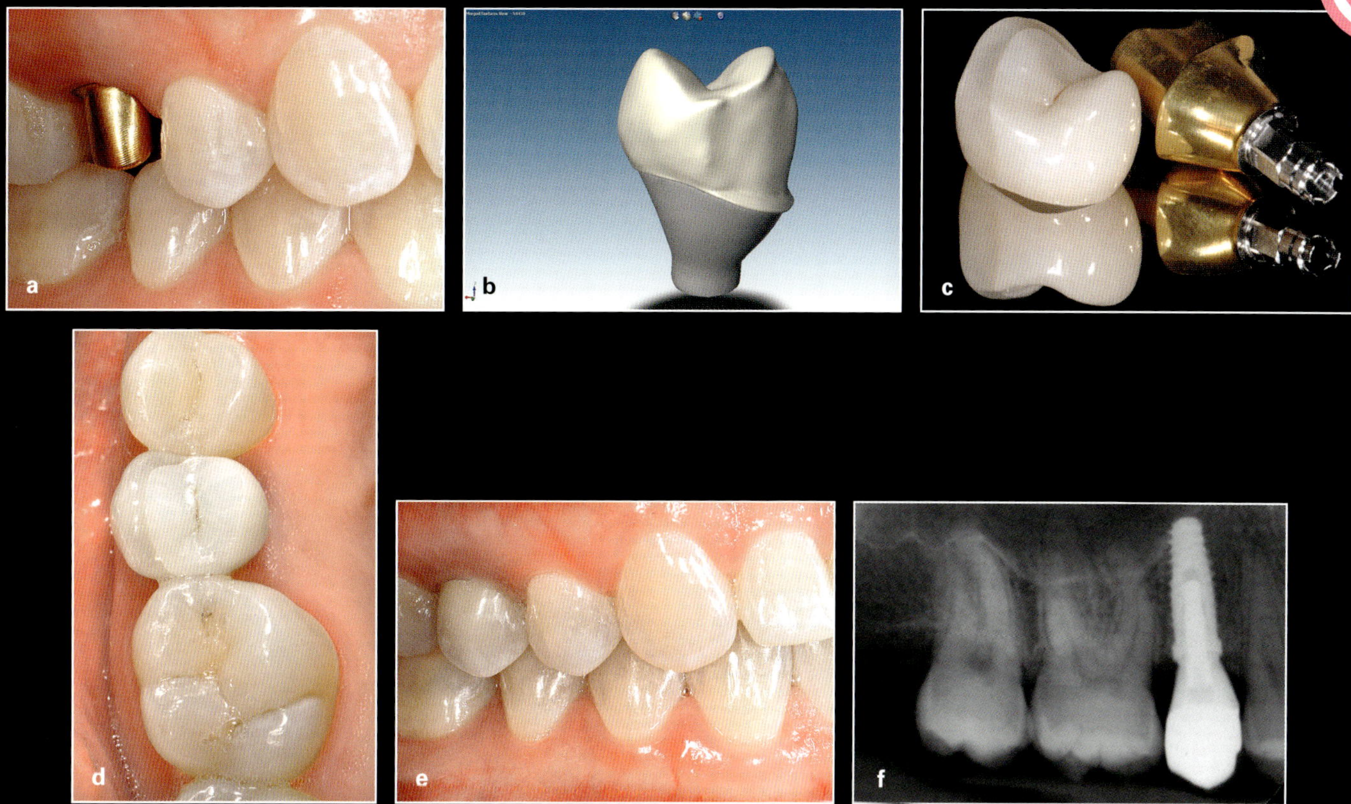

Fig 6-5 *(a)* Buccal view of the CAD/CAM custom titanium abutment (Encode, Biomet 3i). Titanium nitrate coating technology was used to provide the abutment with a gold hue. *(b)* A zirconia coping (Lava Plus) was designed with monolithic surfaces on the occlusal and palatal aspects, while the facial and buccal-occlusal aspects were designed with a virtual cutback to provide space for veneering porcelain. *(c)* View of the definitive zirconia-based crown and the titanium custom abutment. *(d and e)* Occlusal and lateral views of the definitive restoration. *(f)* Postoperative radiograph of the definitive restoration.

the abutment color, and unless soft tissue augmentation procedures are performed successfully, clinicians may need to use tooth-colored abutments such as zirconia in esthetically demanding areas. Multiple studies have shown that zirconia will show the least change of tissue color among all types of abutments.[12,69]

Other material options for tooth-colored abutments, such as lithium disilicate or leucite-reinforced glass-ceramics pressed to metal have shown promising results in in vitro studies.[70,71] However, clinical studies are needed to confirm the use of these materials as predictable options for implant-supported restorations when esthetics is of primary concern.

With tooth-colored abutments such as zirconia, the finish line on the facial and interproximal aspects can be placed more conservatively than on metallic abutments. Supragingival finish line placement on the palatal aspect is recommended whenever possible with whichever abutment material is selected (ceramic or metallic). To avoid esthetic complications in case of future recession and to further facilitate residual excess cement removal, it is recommended to place the finish line 1 mm below the free gingival margins (Fig 6-6). This can be well controlled by measuring the distance between the finish line on a wax pattern (which will later be scanned) and the free gingival margins simulated on a master cast, or via the CAD software during design of the abutment.

Although no study has compared the fracture strength of ceramic restorations permanently cemented versus temporarily cemented to ceramic abutments, it is usually preferred to use permanent cement with ceramic abutments and ceramic restorations. Depending on the type of ceramic (ie, lithium disilicate or zirconia), the maximum fracture strength is reached when the restorations are well bonded to the substructure. If ceramic restorations are cemented temporarily, the maximum fracture strength may not be reached, and micromovements can lead both the abutment and the restoration to fracture.

Continued from page 130

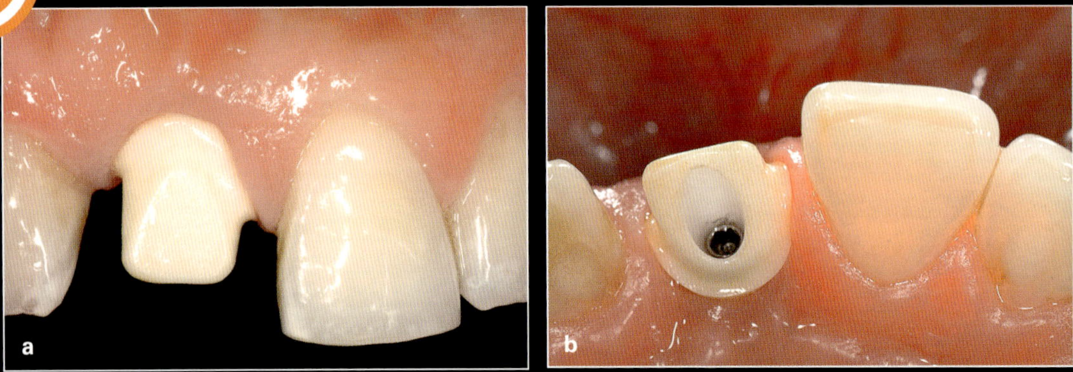

Fig 6-6 *(a and b)* Facial and occlusal views of the CAD/CAM custom zirconia abutment. Note that its supragingival shape is similar to the shape of a tooth preparation for a crown. The finish line of the abutment is placed 1 mm below the gingival margins on the facial aspect and equigingivally and supragingivally on the palatal aspect.

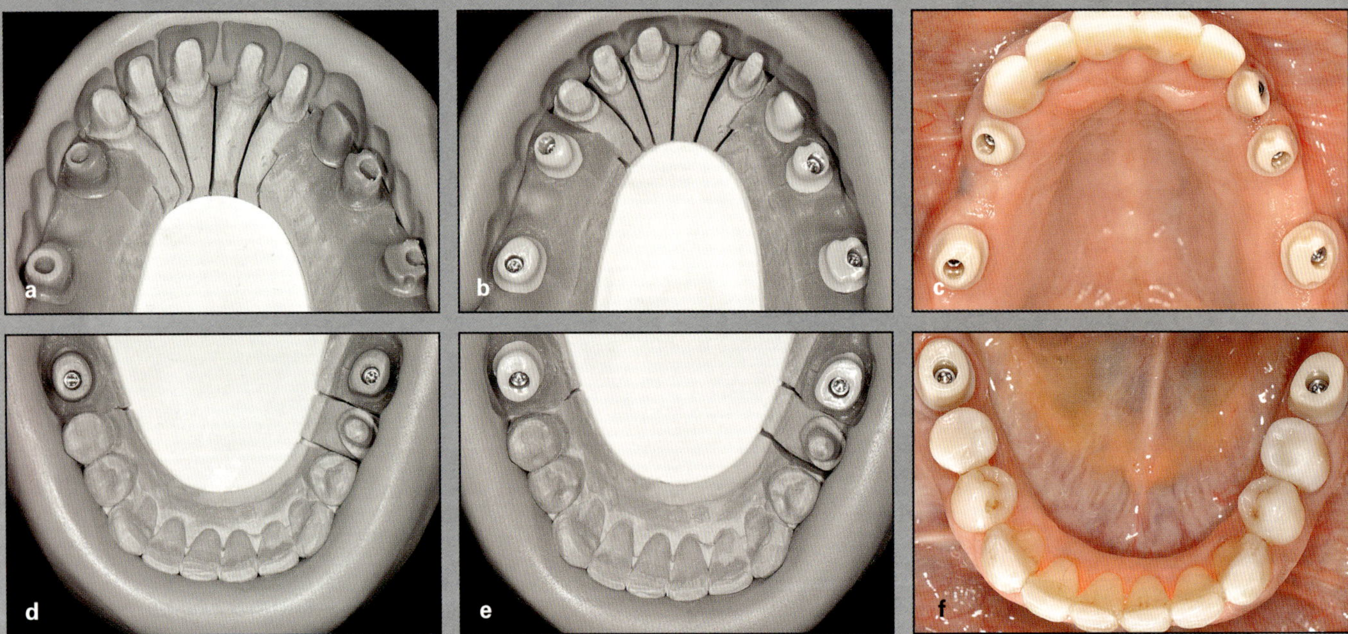

Fig 6-7 *(a and b)* Occlusal views of the maxillary wax patterns made for the custom CAM zirconia abutments (Procera, Nobel Biocare), with a silicone matrix made based on the provisional restorations and the corresponding zirconia abutments on the cast. *(c)* Occlusal view of the maxilla with the zirconia abutments in place. Note the corresponding locations of the finish lines on the cast and in the mouth and the contours of the zirconia abutments, which are similar to the corresponding wax patterns. *(d and e)* Occlusal views of the mandibular wax patterns made for the custom CAM zirconia abutments (Procera), with a silicone matrix made based on the provisional restorations and the corresponding zirconia abutments on the cast. *(f)* Occlusal view of the mandible with the zirconia abutments in place. Note the corresponding locations of the finish lines on the cast and in the mouth and the contours of the zirconia abutments, which are similar to the corresponding wax patterns. (Prosthodontics: Drs Jae Seon Kim, Satoshi Go, and Ariel J. Raigrodski; Periodontics: Dr Stefanie Kretchmar; Orthodontics: Drs Alfonso Navarrete and Adelina Fontes; Abutment design and ceramics: Harald Heindl.)

CAD/CAM Capabilities

CAD/CAM capabilities in designing ideal abutments have shown substantial improvement over the years. However, despite the advanced technology offered by CAD/CAM companies, it is still challenging to fabricate an exact replica of an ideally designed abutment that does not require any adjustment. Clinicians have to critically evaluate and understand the limitations of new technologies and find ways to overcome their shortcomings, which may require waxing up the abutment using traditional techniques and scanning it (Fig 6-7). Clinicians should evaluate the following factors prior to selecting a CAD/CAM system for designing and fabricating custom abutments from titanium or zirconia:

- *Accuracy/precision of fit:* Abutments should precisely and accurately fit on the implant platform. There have been reports of variation in the fit of the abutment to the implant among various CAD/CAM companies.[72,73] This is applied not only to zirconia but to titanium as well. Inaccuracy in fit may compromise not only the abutment but also the implant platform and the surrounding bone and soft tissue by producing titanium particles that can trigger inflammatory responses in the body.[74]
- *Material strength:* Multiple companies provide zirconia abutments for different implant systems, but the physical properties of zirconia from various manufacturers may vary as reported by Flinn et al.[75,76] In addition, a combination of zirconia and metal components can significantly improve the fracture strength of the abutment.
- *Design capabilities:* Abutments can be designed either by manual waxing and then scanning or virtually with the CAD software (Fig 6-8). Enhanced design capabilities, which are constantly evolving, will continue to facilitate the definitive esthetic and functional restorative outcome. Therefore, clinicians and dental technicians should frequently reassess CAD/CAM systems that design and fabricate custom abutments.

Continued from chapter 5

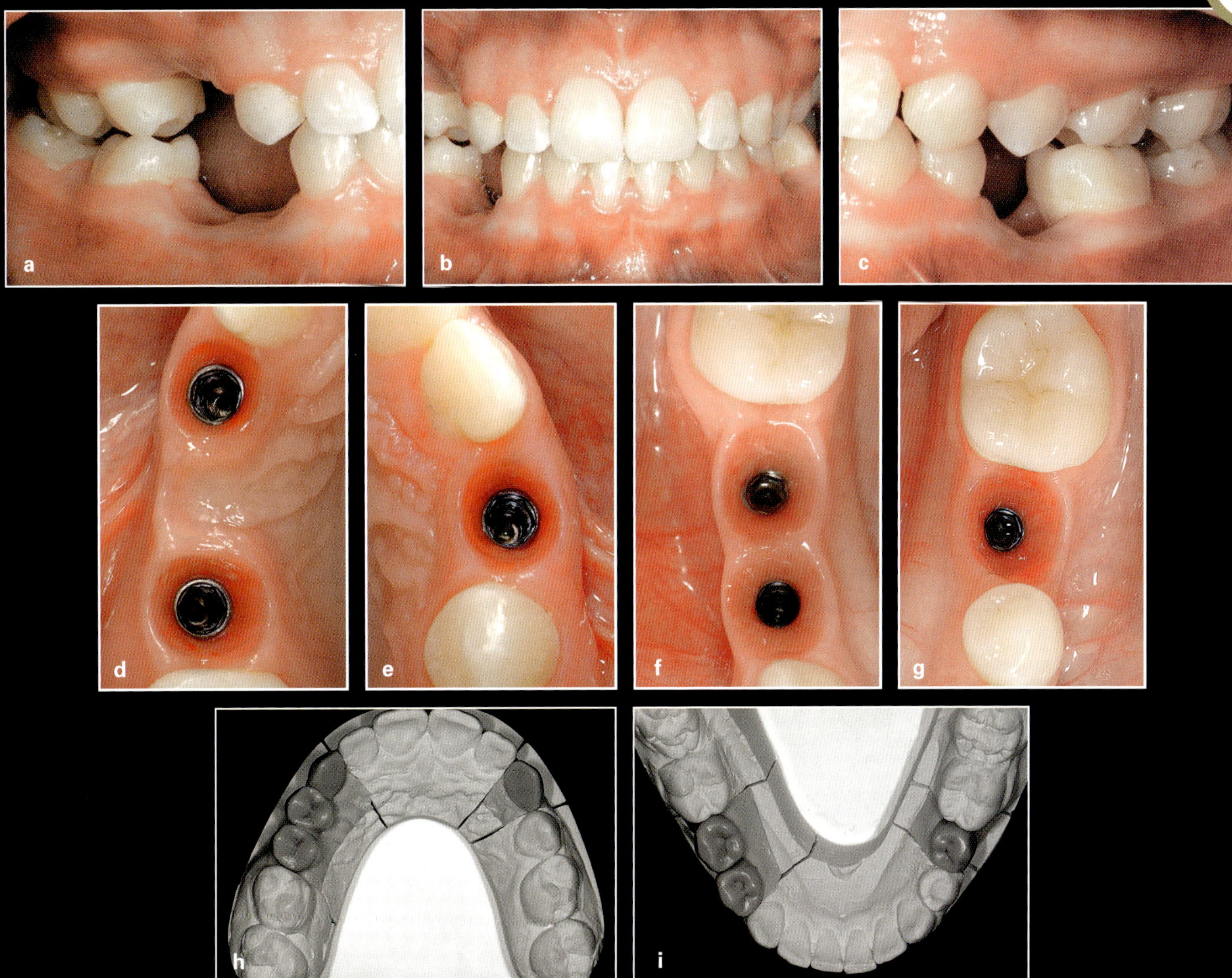

Fig 6-8 *(a to c)* Preoperative frontal and lateral views of a patient with ectodermal dysplasia. The patient underwent orthodontic treatment, bone grafting procedures, and implant placement. *(d to g)* Occlusal views of the implants to be restored with cement-retained implant-supported restorations (Osseotite Certain, Biomet 3i) and the shaped soft tissue prior to master impression making. *(h and i)* A complete-contour wax-up was made on the definitive casts.

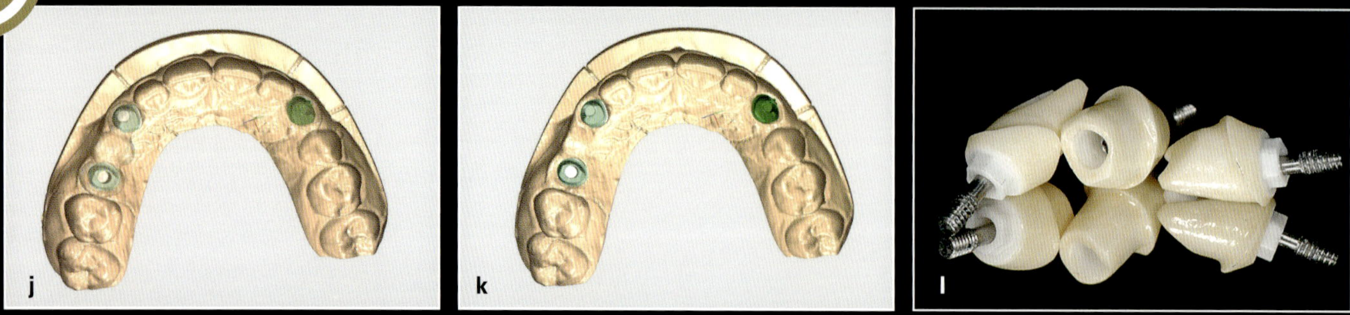

Fig 6-8 *(cont) (j and k)* The definitive maxillary cast was scanned with and without the wax-up to allow for virtual design of CAD/CAM custom zirconia abutments (Atlantis). *(l)* Subsequently, monolithic CAD/CAM zirconia abutments were fabricated.

Implant Platform–Abutment Interface

The type of interface between the implant platform and the abutment plays a significant role in selecting the type of abutment for a cement-retained implant-supported restoration. Zirconia abutments present with different types of implant platform–abutment interfaces. Monolithic zirconia abutments have a zirconia (abutment) to titanium (implant platform) interface and are available for multiple implant systems from multiple manufacturers. However, the first zirconia abutments introduced to the market (ZiReal abutments, 3i Innovations) were designed with a titanium insert bonded to the zirconia abutment body. Brodbeck[77] has advocated the importance of the titanium insert in such abutments for separating the zirconia from the implant platform and therefore preventing any implant platform damage. Currently, custom zirconia abutments with a similar implant platform–abutment interface may be designed and fabricated via CAD/CAM technology (Figs 6-9a to 6-9d). However, one has to critically evaluate how the titanium insert and the zirconia abutment interact with one another and how this may affect the implant platform–abutment interface. Some zirconia abutments (Procera NobelReplace, specifically the trichannel/trilobe platform design, Nobel Biocare) have a titanium component that is friction-fitted to the zirconia component. However, the interface of the abutment with the implant platform is still partially zirconia to titanium, particularly at the circumference of the implant platform. In addition, for such abutments, the screw head is in direct contact with the zirconia wall of the abutment as with monolithic zirconia abutments (Fig 6-10). When the abutment is put under load, the screw head may act as a fulcrum point, which may make the abutment more susceptible to fracture. A study evaluating retrieved fractured zirconia abutments identified friction marks on the abutment screw heads.[49]

Currently, as previously mentioned, many CAD/CAM companies offer zirconia abutments that have a titanium insert. This titanium insert is bonded to the zirconia abutment. Interfacing with the implant platform, it also has a "chimney" that interfaces with the chimney of the abutment. When torqued, the abutment screw head is in contact with that metal chimney (Figs 6-9e to 6-9g). This type of a CAD/CAM zirconia hybrid abutment can have several advantages. First, the fracture resistance of the abutment can be significantly improved due to the titanium insert as reported in several in vitro studies.[63,78–80] Second, damage to the implant platform and to the abutment-implant connection may be prevented. Several studies have shown that after cyclic loading, there is a significant reduction of preload, which may lead to screw loosening.[81,82] Studies[83–85] have also reported that zirconia abutments can cause wear of titanium, and this may potentially damage the abutment-implant connection and/or the implant platform, which may lead to irreversible complications. Third, abutment fracture from the screw head can be prevented. For such CAD/CAM zirconia hybrid abutments, the screw head interfaces with the titanium insert, which extends in one of the systems for at least 3 mm coronally into the abutment (Lava, 3M ESPE) and thus interfaces with the screw.

One concern with such CAD/CAM zirconia hybrid abutments is the bond strength between the titanium insert and the zirconia component of the abutment. However, it has been shown that the use of composite resin cements (with their corresponding bonding agents) in conjunction with controlled air-particle abrasion of the titanium inserts and the zirconia components led to a stable retention between the two components. The bond strength of the investigated luting agents (Panavia 21, Kuraray Noritake; Multilink Automix, Ivoclar Vivadent) exceeded the general limits of fracture resistance of CAD/CAM zirconia hybrid abutments.[86]

Kim et al[78] evaluated maximal load capacity of three different types of zirconia abutments with different implant-

M

Continued from page 138

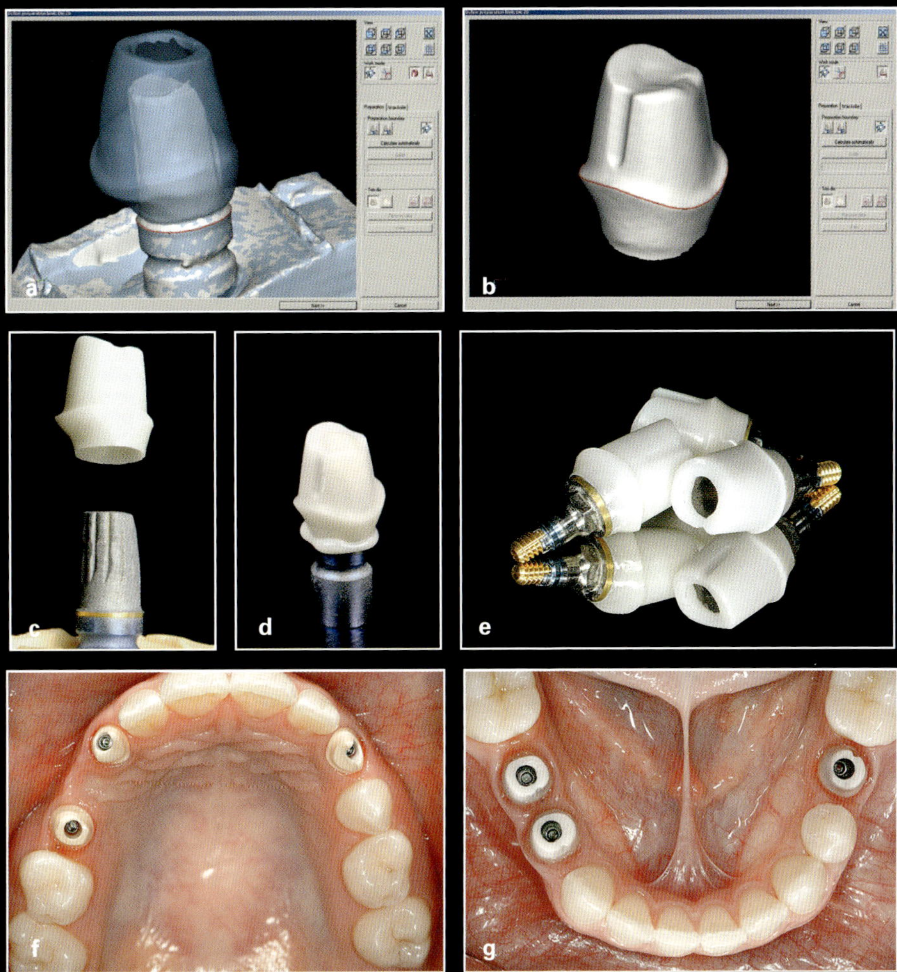

Fig 6-9 *(a and b)* Wax patterns were made and scanned (Lava). The abutment design was then virtually refined on the CAD unit. *(c to e)* The titanium and zirconia components were air-particle abraded at the surfaces to be bonded with 50-µm aluminum-oxide particles at low pressure. They were then silanated and bonded with dual-curing composite resin cement. *(f and g)* Occlusal views of the definitive abutments in the patient's mouth. Note that with the maxillary abutments the screw head is in contact with zirconia, and with the mandibular abutments the screw head is in contact with the metal chimney of the titanium insert.

Fig 6-10 CAD/CAM zirconia abutments (Procera NobelReplace [trichannel/trilobe platform design specifically]) with titanium friction-fitted components. The interface of the abutment with the implant platform is partially zirconia to titanium, particularly at the circumference of the implant platform, and the screw head is in direct contact with the axial walls of the zirconia abutment. (See Fig 6-7 for treating clinicians.)

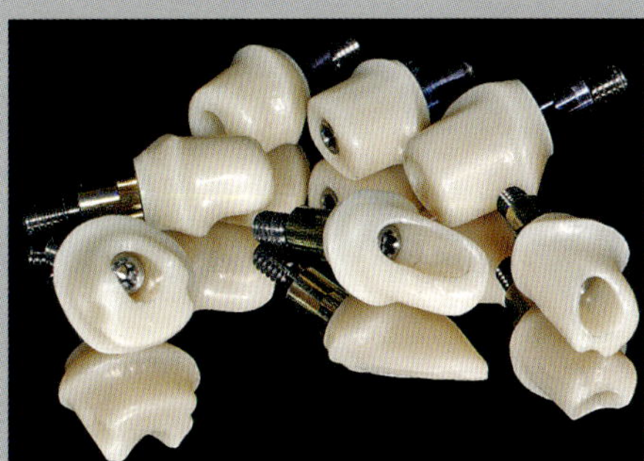

abutment interfaces and also observed the mode of failure and its impact on the implant platform. The three different types of CAD/CAM zirconia abutments used on regular-platform implants (trichannel/trilobe platform design, NobelReplace) were the following: *(1)* monolithic zirconia (Aadva CAD/CAM Zirconia Abutment, GC America), *(2)* zirconia with a friction-fitted titanium component and a zirconia circumference (NobelProcera Abutment Zirconia, Nobel Biocare), and *(3)* zirconia hybrid with a bonded titanium insert in contact with the implant platform and the abutment screw (Lava Zirconia Abutment, 3M ESPE). The screws recommended for the three types of abutment were also different. Monolithic zirconia crowns were bonded on the abutments after thermal cycling, and values of static load to failure were measured. In terms of maximal biting force in the anterior segment, values ranged between 90 and 370 N.[87–89] All groups showed a higher fracture strength. However, the zirconia hybrid group displayed significantly higher values of more than 700 N, as compared to the other two groups, whose values averaged around 500 N. A noteworthy finding was that the mode of failure was different for all groups. Catastrophic failures were seen for groups 1 and 2, whereas partial debonding of the zirconia component of the titanium insert was seen for group 3. The damage pattern of the implant platform was also different among all groups. Group 2 demonstrated more damage to the implant platform than group 1.

Risk Assessment in Abutment Selection

Treatment-planning considerations are critical prior to any treatment rendered. In terms of selecting the abutment material, the functional risk of the patient must be evaluated. The following is a list of functional and mechanical considerations clinicians should weigh while selecting the appropriate abutment material. These considerations may override esthetic concerns. In such clinical scenarios, clinicians may consider avoiding the use of zirconia abutments for implant-supported cement-retained restorations.

- *Abutment-implant connection considerations (flat to flat versus cone to cone):* Metallic abutments may be safer for conical-connection implants, especially if the diameter of the connection becomes critically thin. Seetoh et al[90] demonstrated that the fatigue of zirconia abutments was highly system- and abutment connection–dependent. This study showed consistently high cyclic load to failure for titanium abutments.
- *Parafunction:* Metallic abutments may be safer for patients with parafunctional habits or with high function.
- *Off-axis forces:* Off-axis forces should be minimized as generally recommended for implant-supported restorations and more so for zirconia abutments.
- *Steep guidance in protrusive and lateral excursions:* In some clinical scenarios, off-axis forces cannot be avoided as with anterior teeth. If possible, the occlusion should be addressed as to minimize off-axis forces by shallowing the guidance. If the occlusion cannot be modified restoratively or orthodontically to shallow the guidance, titanium abutments with nitride coating should be considered to facilitate soft tissue esthetics.
- *Narrow-diameter implants in areas of higher occlusal load:* Metallic abutments should be used with narrow-diameter implants where higher occlusal loads are expected. Such is the case for small premolars. The physical properties of zirconia abutments are dramatically reduced when the thickness of the material is significantly reduced. If requirements for esthetics cannot be satisfied with a titanium abutment with nitride coating, zirconia hybrid abutments with a titanium insert may be considered, although scientific evidence is currently lacking to support such a recommendation.
- *Mandibular incisor position:* Because of the narrow dimensions of mandibular anterior teeth, screw-retained restorations are preferred for achieving a robust one-piece abutment-framework complex. Abutments for mandibular incisors are generally small in dimension and have thin axial walls.
- *Consider avoiding zirconia abutments in the canine position:* When an implant-supported restoration is solely guiding the eccentric movements on a canine and the patient displays parafunctional activities, the use of metallic abutments is preferred.

Summary

Custom abutments have several advantages over stock abutments, including angle correction of implants placed in nonphysiologic positions and control of the soft tissue emergence profile and finish line placement. In addition, the mechanical properties for minimally adjusted ceramic abutments are enhanced compared with extensively adjusted stock ceramic abutments. Titanium and zirconia abutments should be selected based on their optical and physical properties as they relate to the functional and optical requirements of clinical scenarios presented by patients and their desires. Future developments in materials and technologies will facilitate the capabilities of clinicians to provide durable, esthetic, and well-designed abutments that can predictably address ample clinical scenarios (Fig 6-11). Current features that must be considered as part of the abutment material selection process are presented in Boxes 6-1 and 6-2.

Continued from page 139

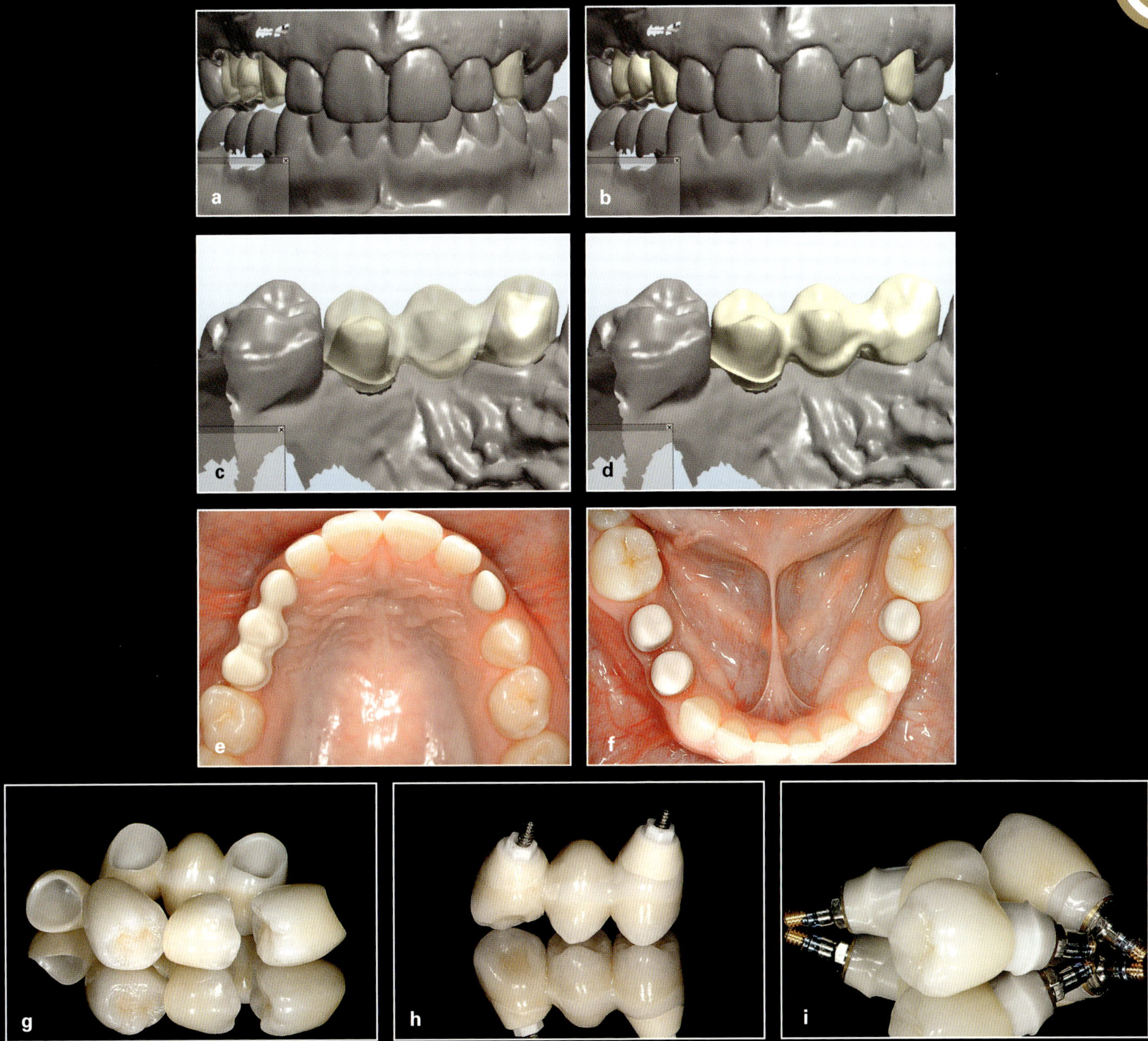

Fig 6-11 *(a and b)* Zirconia-based restorations (Katana, Kuraray Noritake) were virtually designed on the CAD unit. *(c and d)* Views of the maxillary fixed dental prosthesis (FDP) framework designed to ensure adequate support for the veneering porcelain. *(e and f)* Occlusal views of the framework and copings during try-in in the patient's mouth. *(g)* View of the complete zirconia-based restorations. Note the ovate pontic design for the implant-supported FDP. *(h and i)* Views of the maxillary FDP and the mandibular restorations with their corresponding zirconia custom abutments.

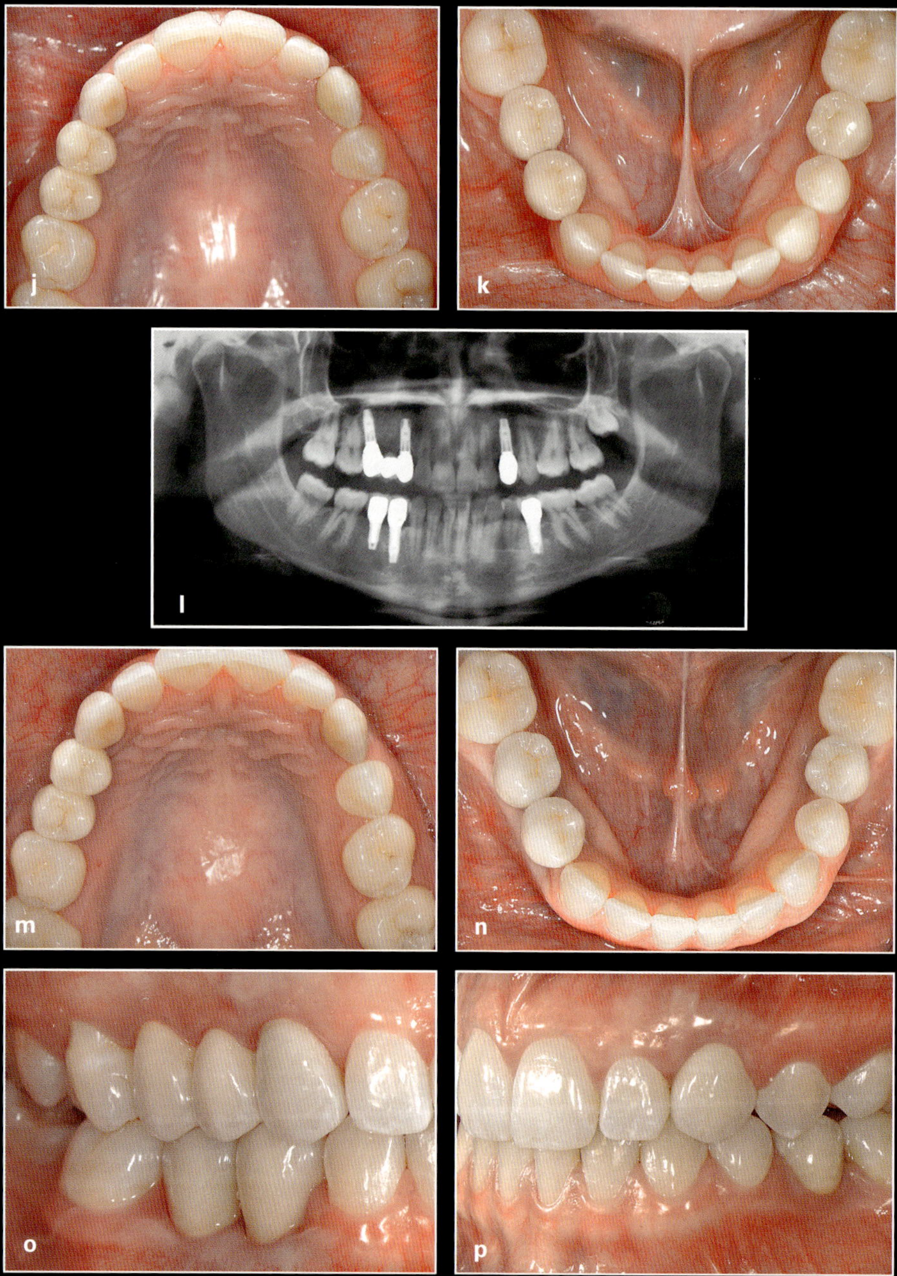

Fig 6-11 *(cont) (j and k)* Occlusal views of the definitive restorations after delivery. *(l)* Panoramic radiograph of the definitive restorations several months after delivery. *(m and n)* Occlusal views of the definitive restorations 6 years after delivery. *(o and p)* Lateral views of the definitive restorations in maximal intercuspal position 6 years after delivery. Note the soft tissue stability and health.

Box 6-1 Features of titanium abutments

- Provide superior physical properties and durability. With ample clinical use, CAD/CAM custom titanium abutments can be predictably used in the posterior segments.
- Present with excellent biocompatibility.
- A minimal axial wall thickness of 0.2 to 0.3 mm is required to retain the durability of the abutment.
- In esthetically demanding clinical scenarios, the finish line should be placed 1.5 mm below the facial free gingival margins.
- To facilitate esthetics at the soft tissue–restorative interface, nitrate-coated titanium abutments can be utilized to mimic yellow-gold color, which displays superior gingival esthetics compared with gray titanium. Therefore, titanium abutments may still be used in the esthetic zone if the soft tissue thickness is adequate (> 2 mm) to block out the yellow-gold color of the abutment.
- Either permanent or temporary cementation can be used for metal-ceramic or cast metal crowns.
- Ceramic restorations such as zirconia-based and high-opacity lithium-disilicate restorations can also be used in conjunction with titanium abutments to effectively block the color of the abutment and provide improved esthetics at the soft tissue–restorative interface. Permanent cementation is recommended for such ceramic restorations.

Conclusion: Titanium abutments should be used in esthetically demanding situations with thick tissue (> 2 mm thick) when implants are malaligned and when mechanical or functional considerations override esthetic ones.

Box 6-2 Features of zirconia abutments

- Highly biocompatible and present with minimal adverse effects on the color of the soft tissue.
- Technique sensitive and susceptible to microstructural degradation and weakening when prepared with a bur. Once the design and the fabrication of the abutment are complete via a CAD/CAM system, adjustments of the abutment in the laboratory and in the clinic should be minimized.
- When a CAD/CAM system is being selected, accuracy and precision of the manufactured abutment, material strength, and accurate designing capabilities are all critical factors, more so with zirconia than with titanium abutments.
- A minimal axial wall thickness of 0.5 to 0.7 mm and adequate height from the implant platform to the finish line of the abutment (depending on the specific implant system used and its implant-abutment connection) must be ensured for durability of the abutment.
- Their use with ceramic restorations facilitates higher translucency over metallic abutments with ceramic restorations, in particular at the subcritical area between the free gingival margins and the implant platform.
- The finish line should be placed 1 mm below the facial free gingival margins on the facial aspect.
- There are different types of abutment-implant and abutment-screw interfaces. Currently, the use of CAD/CAM zirconia abutments with bonded titanium inserts (hybrid zirconia abutments) must be considered to achieve optimal interfaces.
- Permanent cementation for ceramic restorations on zirconia abutments is recommended. Techniques are available to retrieve restorations even when permanently cemented.
- Occlusal and functional risk of the patient should be evaluated, and zirconia abutments should be avoided in patients with high functional risk.

Conclusion: Zirconia abutments may be used in esthetically demanding situations with thin tissue (< 2 mm thick) when implants are adequately positioned and when mechanical or functional risks are relatively low.

References

1. Wang J, Lin J, Seliger A, Gil M, da Silva JD, Ishhikawa-Nagai S. Color effects of gingiva on cervical regions of all-ceramic crowns. J Esthet Restor Dent 2013;25:254–262.
2. Libman WJ, Nicholls JI. Load fatigue of teeth restored with cast posts and cores and complete crowns. Int J Prosthodont 1995;8:155–161.
3. Nicholls JI. The dental ferrule and the endodontically compromised tooth. Quintessence Int 2001;32:171–173.
4. Wiskott HW, Nicholls JI, Belser UC. The relationship between abutment taper and resistance of cemented crowns to dynamic loading. Int J Prosthodont 1996;9:117–139.
5. Isidor F, Brondum K, Ravnholt G. The influence of post length and crown ferrule length on the resistance to cyclic loading of bovine teeth with prefabricated titanium posts. Int J Prosthodont 1999;12:78–82.
6. Goodacre CJ, Campagni WV, Aquilino SA. Tooth preparations for complete crowns: An art form based on scientific principles. J Prosthet Dent 2001;85:363–376.
7. Proussaefs P, Campagni W, Bernal G, Goodacre C, Kim J. The effectiveness of auxiliary features on a tooth preparation with inadequate resistance form. J Prosthet Dent 2004;91:33–41.
8. Su H, Gonzalez-Martin O, Weisgold A, Lee E. Considerations of implant abutment and crown contour: Critical contour and subcritical contour. Int J Periodontics Restorative Dent 2010;30:335–343.
9. Jung RE, Holderegger C, Sailer I, Khraisat A, Suter A, Hämmerle CH. The effect of all-ceramic and porcelain-fused-to-metal restorations on marginal peri-implant soft tissue color: A randomized controlled clinical trial. Int J Periodontics Restorative Dent 2008;28:357–365.
10. Jung RE, Sailer I, Hämmerle CH, Attin T, Schmidlin P. In vitro color changes of soft tissues caused by restorative materials. Int J Periodontics Restorative Dent 2007;27:251–257.
11. Park SE, Da Silva JD, Weber HP, Ishikawa-Nagai S. Optical phenomenon of peri-implant soft tissue. Part I. Spectrophotometric assessment of natural tooth gingiva and peri-implant mucosa. Clin Oral Implants Res 2007;18:569–574.
12. Bressan E, Paniz G, Lops D, Corazza B, Romeo E, Favero G. Influence of abutment material on the gingival color of implant-supported all-ceramic restorations: A prospective multicenter study. Clin Oral Implants Res 2011;22:631–637.
13. Sjogren G, Sletten G, Dahl JE. Cytotoxicity of dental alloys, metals, and ceramics assessed by millipore filter, agar overlay, and MTT tests. J Prosthet Dent 2000;84:229–236.
14. Welander M, Abrahamsson I, Berglundh T. The mucosal barrier at implant abutments of different materials. Clin Oral Implants Res 2008;19:635–641.
15. Abrahamsson I, Berglundh T, Glantz PO, Lindhe J. The mucosal attachment at different abutments. An experimental study in dogs. J Clin Periodontol 1998;25:721–727.
16. Rimondini L, Cerroni L, Carrassi A, Torricelli P. Bacterial colonization of zirconia ceramic surfaces: An in vitro and in vivo study. Int J Oral Maxillofac Implants 2002;17:793–798.
17. Scarano A, Piattelli M, Caputi S, Favero GA, Piattelli A. Bacterial adhesion on commercially pure titanium and zirconium oxide disks: An in vivo human study. J Periodontol 2004;75:292–296.
18. Degidi M, Artese L, Scarano A, Perrotti V, Gehrke P, Piattelli A. Inflammatory infiltrate, microvessel density, nitric oxide synthase expression, vascular endothelial growth factor expression, and proliferative activity in peri-implant soft tissues around titanium and zirconium oxide healing caps. J Periodontol 2006;77:73–80.
19. Raffaelli L, Rossi Iommetti P, Piccioni E, et al. Growth, viability, adhesion potential, and fibronectin expression in fibroblasts cultured on zirconia or feldspatic ceramics in vitro. J Biomed Mater Res A 2008;86:959–968.
20. Daftary F, Bahat O. Prosthetically formulated natural aesthetics in implant prostheses. Pract Periodontics Aesthet Dent 1994;6:75–83.
21. Daftary F. The bio-esthetic abutment system: An evolution in implant prosthetics. Int J Dent Symp 1995;3:10–15.
22. Nelson S, Ash MM Jr. Pulp chambers and canals. In: Wheeler's Dental Anatomy, Physiology and Occlusion, ed 9. St Louis: Saunders, 2009:209–238.
23. Kosmac T, Oblak C, Jevnikar P, Funduk N, Marion L. The effect of surface grinding and sandblasting on flexural strength and reliability of Y-TZP zirconia ceramic. Dent Mater 1999;15:426–433.
24. Luthardt RG, Holzhuter MS, Rudolph H, Herold V, Walter MH. CAD/CAM-machining effects on Y-TZP zirconia. Dent Mater 2004;20:655–662.
25. Iseri U, Ozkurt Z, Yalniz A, Kazazoglu E. Comparison of different grinding procedures on the flexural strength of zirconia. J Prosthet Dent 2012;107:309–315.
26. Jing Z, Ke Z, Yihong L, Zhijian S. Effect of multistep processing technique on the formation of micro-defects and residual stresses in zirconia dental restorations. J Prosthodont 2014;23:206–212.
27. Lewis S, Beumer J 3rd, Hornburg W, Moy P. The "UCLA" abutment. Int J Oral Maxillofac Implants 1988;3:183–189.
28. Lewis SG, Llamas D, Avera S. The UCLA abutment: A four-year review. J Prosthet Dent 1992;67:509–515.
29. Marchack CB, Yamashita T. A procedure for a modified cylindric titanium abutment. J Prosthet Dent 1997;77:546–549.
30. Happe A, Schulte-Mattler V, Fickl S, Naumann M, Zöller JE, Rothamel D. Spectrophotometric assessment of peri-implant mucosa after restoration with zirconia abutments veneered with fluorescent ceramic: A controlled, retrospective clinical study. Clin Oral Implants Res 2013;24(suppl A100):28–33.
31. Garber DA. The esthetic dental implant: Letting restoration be the guide. J Am Dent Assoc 1995;126:319–325.
32. Garber DA, Belser UC. Restoration-driven implant placement with restoration-generated site development. Compend Contin Educ Dent 1995;16:796,800–802,804.
33. Jivraj S, Chee W. Treatment planning of implants in the aesthetic zone. Br Dent J 2006;201:77–89.
34. Parpaiola A, Sbricoli L, Guazzo R, Bressan E, Lops D. Managing the peri-implant mucosa: A clinically reliable method for optimizing soft tissue contours and emergence profile. J Esthet Restor Dent 2013;25:317–323.
35. Weber HP, Cochran DL. The soft tissue response to osseointegrated dental implants. J Prosthet Dent 1998;79:79–89.
36. Listgarten MA, Lang NP, Schroeder HE, Schroeder A. Periodontal tissues and their counterparts around endosseous implants. Clin Oral Implants Res 1991;2:1–19.
37. Linkevicius T, Vindasiute E, Puisys A, Peciuliene V. The influence of margin location on the amount of undetected cement excess after delivery of cement-retained implant restorations. Clin Oral Implants Res 2011;22:1379–1384.
38. Wilson TG Jr. The positive relationship between excess cement and peri-implant disease: A prospective clinical endoscopic study. J Periodontol 2009;80:1388–1392.
39. Korsch M, Obst U, Walther W. Cement-associated peri-implantitis: A retrospective clinical observational study of fixed implant-supported restorations using a methacrylate cement. Clin Oral Implants Res 2014;25:797–802.
40. Linkevicius T, Puisys A, Vindasiute E, Linkeviciene L, Apse P. Does residual cement around implant-supported restorations cause peri-implant disease? A retrospective case analysis. Clin Oral Implants Res 2013;24:1179–1184.
41. Priest G. Virtual-designed and computer-milled implant abutments. J Oral Maxillofac Surg 2005;63:22–32.
42. Kano SC, Binon PP, Bonfante G, Curtis DA. The effect of casting procedures on rotational misfit in castable abutments. Int J Oral Maxillofac Implants 2007;22:575–579.
43. Kano SC, Binon P, Bonfante G, Curtis DA. Effect of casting procedures on screw loosening in UCLA-type abutments. J Prosthodont 2006;15:77–81.

44. Lindhe J, Berglundh T. The interface between the mucosa and the implant. Periodontol 2000 1998;17:47–54.
45. Steflik DE, Corpe RS, Young TR, Buttle K. In vivo evaluation of the biocompatibility of implanted biomaterials: Morphology of the implant-tissue interactions. Implant Dent 1998;7:338–350.
46. Anusavice KJ, Shen C, Rawls HR. Dental implants. In: Phillips' Science of Dental Materials, ed 12. St Louis: Saunders, 2013:499–518.
47. Kim YS, Ko Y, Kye SB, Yang SM. Human gingival fibroblast (HGF-1) attachment and proliferation on several abutment materials with various colors. Int J Oral Maxillofac Implants 2014;29:969–975.
48. Buchi DL, Sailer I, Fehmer V, Hämmerle CH, Thoma DS. All-ceramic single-tooth implant reconstructions using modified zirconia abutments: A prospective randomized controlled clinical trial of the effect of pink veneering ceramic on the esthetic outcomes. Int J Periodontics Restorative Dent 2014;34:29–37.
49. Aboushelib MN, Salameh Z. Zirconia implant abutment fracture: Clinical case reports and precautions for use. Int J Prosthodont 2009;22:616–619.
50. Att W, Yajima ND, Wolkewitz M, Witkowski S, Strub JR. Influence of preparation and wall thickness on the resistance to fracture of zirconia implant abutments. Clin Implant Dent Relat Res 2012;14(suppl 1):e196–e203.
51. Baldissara P, Llukacej A, Ciocca L, Valandro FL, Scotti R. Translucency of zirconia copings made with different CAD/CAM systems. J Prosthet Dent 2010;104:6–12.
52. Yoshida A, Ishhikawa-Nagai S, da Silva J. Opacity control of zirconia restorations. Quintessence Dent Techonol 2010;33:173–185.
53. Binon PP. Implants and components: Entering the new millennium. Int J Oral Maxillofac Implants 2000;15:76–94.
54. Pjetursson BE, Brägger U, Lang NP, Zwahlen M. Comparison of survival and complication rates of tooth-supported fixed dental prostheses (FDPs) and implant-supported FDPs and single crowns (SCs). Clin Oral Implants Res 2007;18(suppl 3):97–113.
55. Pjetursson BE, Tan WC, Tan K, Brägger U, Zwahlen M, Lang NP. A systematic review of the survival and complication rates of resin-bonded bridges after an observation period of at least 5 years. Clin Oral Implants Res 2008;19:131–141.
56. Coppede AR, Faria AC, de Mattos Mda G, Rodrigues RC, Shibli JA, Ribeiro RF. Mechanical comparison of experimental conical-head abutment screws with conventional flat-head abutment screws for external-hex and internal tri-channel implant connections: An in vitro evaluation of loosening torque. Int J Oral Maxillofac Implants 2013;28:e321–e329.
57. Gracis S, Michalakis K, Vigolo P, Vult von Steyern P, Zwahlen M, Sailer I. Internal vs. external connections for abutments/reconstructions: A systematic review. Clin Oral Implants Res 2012;23(suppl 6):202–216.
58. Schwedhelm ER, Raigrodski AJ. A technique for locating implant abutment screws of posterior cement-retained metal-ceramic restorations with ceramic occlusal surfaces. J Prosthet Dent 2006;95:165–167.
59. Tarlow JL. A modified technique to locate the abutment screw access opening of a cemented implant-supported restoration. J Prosthet Dent 2012;108:58–59.
60. Prestipino V, Ingber A. Esthetic high-strength implant abutments. Part I. J Esthet Dent 1993;5:29–36.
61. Prestipino V, Ingber A. Esthetic high-strength implant abutments. Part II. J Esthet Dent 1993;5:63–68.
62. Yildirim M, Fischer H, Marx R, Edelhoff D. In vivo fracture resistance of implant-supported all-ceramic restorations. J Prosthet Dent 2003;90:325–331.
63. Butz F, Heydecke G, Okutan M, Strub JR. Survival rate, fracture strength and failure mode of ceramic implant abutments after chewing simulation. J Oral Rehabil 2005;32:838–843.
64. Glauser R, Sailer I, Wohlwend A, Studer S, Schibli M, Scharer P. Experimental zirconia abutments for implant-supported single-tooth restorations in esthetically demanding regions: 4-year results of a prospective clinical study. Int J Prosthodont 2004;17:285–290.
65. Canullo L. Clinical outcome study of customized zirconia abutments for single-implant restorations. Int J Prosthodont 2007;20:489–493.
66. Zembic A, Sailer I, Jung RE, Hämmerle CH. Randomized-controlled clinical trial of customized zirconia and titanium implant abutments for single-tooth implants in canine and posterior regions: 3-year results. Clin Oral Implants Res 2009;20:802–808.
67. Zembic A, Bosch A, Jung RE, Hämmerle CH, Sailer I. Five-year results of a randomized controlled clinical trial comparing zirconia and titanium abutments supporting single-implant crowns in canine and posterior regions. Clin Oral Implants Res 2013;24:384–390.
68. Chen YW, Sawyer K, Liao SC, Shih HC, Raigrodski AJ. Retrospective dental laboratory survery of zirconia implant abutments [abstract 264]. Presented at the 43rd Annual Meeting of the American Association for Dental Research, Charlotte, North Carolina, 19–22 March 2014.
69. Tan PL, Dunne JT Jr. An esthetic comparison of a metal ceramic crown and cast metal abutment with an all-ceramic crown and zirconia abutment: A clinical report. J Prosthet Dent 2004;91:215–218.
70. Kim S, Kim HI, Brewer JD, Monaco EA Jr. Comparison of fracture resistance of pressable metal ceramic custom implant abutments with CAD/CAM commercially fabricated zirconia implant abutments. J Prosthet Dent 2009;101:226–230.
71. Protopapadaki M, Monaco EA Jr, Kim HI, Davis EL. Comparison of fracture resistance of pressable metal ceramic custom implant abutment with a commercially fabricated CAD/CAM zirconia implant abutment. J Prosthet Dent 2013;110:389–396.
72. de Morais Alves da Cunha T, de Araujo RP, da Rocha PV, Amoedo RM. Comparison of fit accuracy between Procera(R) custom abutments and three implant systems. Clin Implant Dent Relat Res 2012;14:890–895.
73. Garine WN, Funkenbusch PD, Ercoli C, Wodenscheck J, Murphy WC. Measurement of the rotational misfit and implant-abutment gap of all-ceramic abutments. Int J Oral Maxillofac Implants 2007;22:928–938.
74. Mishra PK, Wu W, Rozo C, Hallab NJ, Benevenia J, Gause WC. Micrometer-sized titanium particles can induce potent Th2-type responses through TLR4-independent pathways. J Immunol 2011;187:6491–6498.
75. Flinn BD, deGroot DA, Mancl LA, Raigrodski AJ. Accelerated aging characteristics of three yttria-stabilized tetragonal zirconia polycrystalline dental materials. J Prosthet Dent 2012;108:223–230.
76. Flinn BD, Raigrodski AJ, Singh A, Mancl LA. Effect of hydrothermal degradation on three types of zirconias for dental appplications. J Prosthet Dent 2014;112:1377–1384.
77. Brodbeck U. The ZiReal Post: A new ceramic implant abutment. J Esthet Restor Dent 2003;15:10–23.
78. Kim JS, Raigrodski AJ, Flinn BD, Rubenstein JE, Chung KH, Mancl LA. In vitro assessment of three types of zirconia implant abutments under static load. J Prosthet Dent 2013;109:255–263.
79. Sailer I, Sailer T, Stawarczyk B, Jung RE, Hämmerle CH. In vitro study of the influence of the type of connection on the fracture load of zirconia abutments with internal and external implant-abutment connections. Int J Oral Maxillofac Implants 2009;24:850–858.
80. Stimmelmayr M, Sagerer S, Erdelt K, Beuer F. In vitro fatigue and fracture strength testing of one-piece zirconia implant abutments and zirconia implant abutments connected to titanium cores. Int J Oral Maxillofac Implants 2013;28:488–493.
81. Butignon LE, Basilio Mde A, Pereira Rde P, Arioli Filho JN. Influence of three types of abutments on preload values before and after cyclic loading with structural analysis by scanning electron microscopy. Int J Oral Maxillofac Implants 2013;28:e161–e170.
82. Basilio Mde A, Butignon LE, Arioli Filho J. Effectiveness of screw surface coating on the stability of zirconia abutments after cyclic loading. Int J Oral Maxillofac Implants 2012;27:1061–1067.
83. Stimmelmayr M, Edelhoff D, Guth JF, Erdelt K, Happe A, Beuer F. Wear at the titanium-titanium and the titanium-zirconia implant-abutment interface: A comparative in vitro study. Dent Mater 2012;28:1215–1220.

84. Klotz MW, Taylor TD, Goldberg AJ. Wear at the titanium-zirconia implant-abutment interface: A pilot study. Int J Oral Maxillofac Implants 2011;26:970–975.
85. Nguyen HQ, Tan KB, Nicholls JI. Load fatigue performance of implant-ceramic abutment combinations. Int J Oral Maxillofac Implants 2009;24:636–646.
86. Gehrke P, Alius J, Fischer C, Erdelt KJ, Beuer F. Retentive strength of two-piece CAD/CAM zirconia implant abutments. Clin Implant Dent Relat Res 2014;16:920–925.
87. Paphangkorakit J, Osborn JW. The effect of pressure on a maximum incisal bite force in man. Arch Oral Biol 1997;42:11–17.
88. Helkimo E, Carlsson GE, Helkimo M. Bite force and state of dentition. Acta Odontol Scand 1977;35:297–303.
89. Haraldson T, Carlsson GE, Ingervall B. Functional state, bite force and postural muscle activity in patients with osseointegrated oral implant bridges. Acta Odontol Scand 1979;37:195–206.
90. Seetoh YL, Tan KB, Chua EK, Quek HC, Nicholls JI. Load fatigue performance of conical implant-abutment connections. Int J Oral Maxillofac Implants 2011;26:797–806.

Ceramic Screw-Retained Implant-Supported Restorations

7

Tijana Stijacic | Ariel J. Raigrodski | Robert D. Walter

Historically, the primary rationale for implant therapy was to treat the completely edentulous patient. The early modern era of implant therapy was principally guided by the Brånemark protocol and was dominated by screw-retained restorations. The initial protocol called for the completely edentulous patient to be treated with four to six 3.75-mm, external hex endosseous implants placed in the anterior mandible.[1] Restoration of these dental implants involved multiple parts and prosthetic screws. As implant survival rates increased, clinicians broadened the use of implants to the partially edentulous patient. In addition, there was a transition in the design philosophy to make fixed prostheses simpler in an effort to manage future complications and maintenance issues. One change in design was to introduce cement-retained restorations. The introduction of the UCLA custom abutment in 1988 eliminated the need for a stock transmucosal abutment. Not only did it reduce the number of prosthetic components, but it also provided clinicians with an opportunity to develop an emergence profile, control the finish line placement on the abutment, and restore areas that once were challenged by minimal vertical space.[2] In today's arena of fixed implant-supported restorations, both cement-retained and screw-retained implant-supported restorations are used widely. This chapter discusses treatment considerations for ceramic screw-retained implant-supported restorations, mainly in the context of soft tissue management and long-term maintenance.

Screw-Retained Restorations

Advantages and limitations

The main advantages of screw-retained implant-supported restorations is that they offer reliable retrieval, have decreased space requirements, and may result in healthier tissues because no excess cement cleanup is necessary.[1,3,4] From a long-term maintenance perspective, these restorations offer the advantage of relative ease of accessibility, which may be needed for prosthetic repairs, hygiene, abutment screw tightening or replacement, or removal of a failing implant without causing damage to the prosthesis when multiple implants are restored in a splinted manner.[5]

Conversely, if the implants are improperly positioned, screw-retained restorations can potentially lead to esthetic compromises. Furthermore, wear of composite resin materials used to cover the screw access channel has the potential to result in occlusal instability in the long term.[6] However, with advances in composite resin material formulations, it is hoped that this particular issue will become less of a concern. Another disadvantage is porcelain fracture at the screw access channel due to either unsupported porcelain or limited porcelain thickness.[7] Finally, the anatomy of the maxillary anterior segment may result in a ridge lap design on the cervical aspect of the restoration from the implant platform to the free gingival margins, due to the more palatal implant position and a screw access channel location at the cingulum. This can compromise the patient's access for oral hygiene measures and may even require that the restoration be removed only by the clinician at maintenance appointments.

Indications

The choice between a screw-retained and a cement-retained restoration is not a simple one. It requires careful, comprehensive consideration and case-by-case evaluation. Screw-retained restorations should be considered if the implant position is acceptable from an esthetic standpoint (ie, emergence of the screw access channel at the cingulum of anterior teeth or the central fossa of posterior teeth) as well as a biomechanical standpoint (specifically pertaining to the minimal recommended thickness of the restorative material selected). At the same time, malaligned and less than ideally positioned implants may require use of screw-retained restorations, especially if such an approach does not cause esthetic or biomechanical compromise (Figs 7-1a to 7-1g). This is particularly true in cases where either postdelivery retrieval is absolutely necessary or implant position is such that access for adequate residual excess cement removal and hygiene would be impossible. Such are clinical scenarios involving fixed dental prostheses (FDPs) with a severe horizontal soft and/or hard tissue deficiency that may necessitate utilization of a flange for lip support (Figs 7-1h to 7-1k). Cement use should be avoided in these scenarios because access to the implant abutment and crown surface adjacent to the flange is inherently more difficult. Further, less than ideally positioned implants in the posterior segments that may necessitate a compensatory emergence profile tend to create a similar scenario to that of a cantilevered restoration. In such scenarios, adequate access for residual excess cement removal may prove to be challenging.

With complete-arch restorations involving multiple implants, screw retention is preferred over cement retention because it allows for the possibility to access any of the underlying implants if need be. This is of paramount importance in cases in which one or more implants may present with compromised bone levels at the time of restoration. These implants can be asymptomatic and by all other accounts appear to be osseointegrated. However, it may be difficult to discern whether the bone loss is due to progressive disease or in response to trauma incurred during the surgical procedures of implant placement. Therefore, the ability to remove the restoration and carefully reevaluate the implants at any future point is a clear advantage of screw retention. In addition, implant-supported complete-arch restorations have routinely demonstrated prosthetic technical complications such as fractures of the restorative materials used.[8–10] Therefore, access to these restorations for repairs, adjustments, or replacements as needed is invaluable.

Screw-retained restorations are also indicated for patients with excessive horizontal or vertical ridge deficiencies for whom predictable surgical reconstruction is impossible and who require prosthetic gingival replacement to achieve an acceptable esthetic and functional outcome (Figs 7-1l to 7-1u). This treatment approach allows for gingiva-colored re-

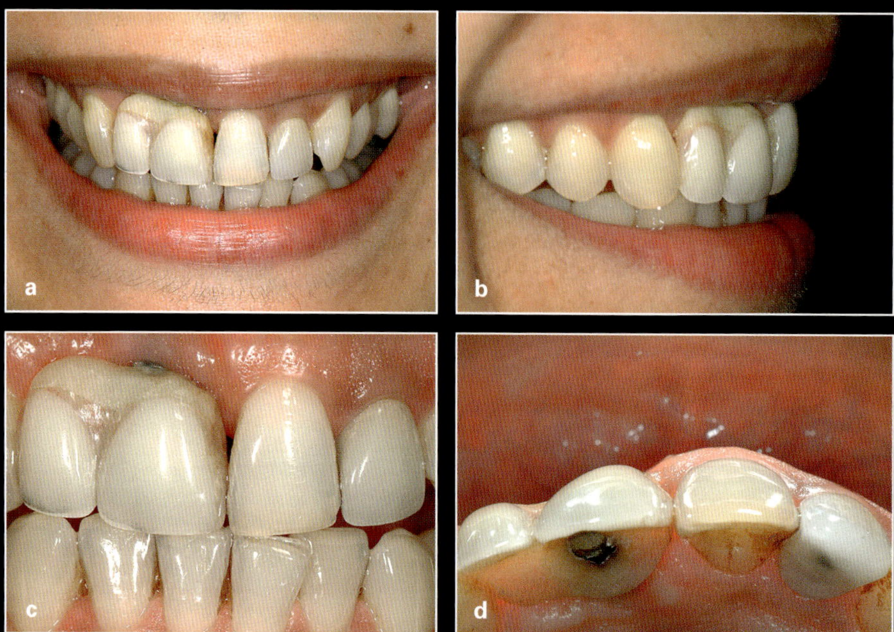

Fig 7-1 *(a and b)* Frontal and lateral smile views of a patient referred with a provisional cantilever implant-supported fixed dental prosthesis (FDP), with a pontic replacing the maxillary right lateral incisor and an implant-supported retainer replacing the maxillary right central incisor. The teeth had been lost due to trauma. Following grafting procedures, an implant (NobelReplace RP 4.3 × 11.5, Nobel Biocare) had been placed and later provisionalized by clinicians in a different state. *(c and d)* Facial view in protrusive contact and occlusal view of the screw-retained provisional restoration. Note the temporary metal abutment showing at the distal aspect of the central incisor implant retainer and the screw access at the distofacial aspect of the implant retainer. Also note the inadequate width-to-length proportions of the implant retainer.

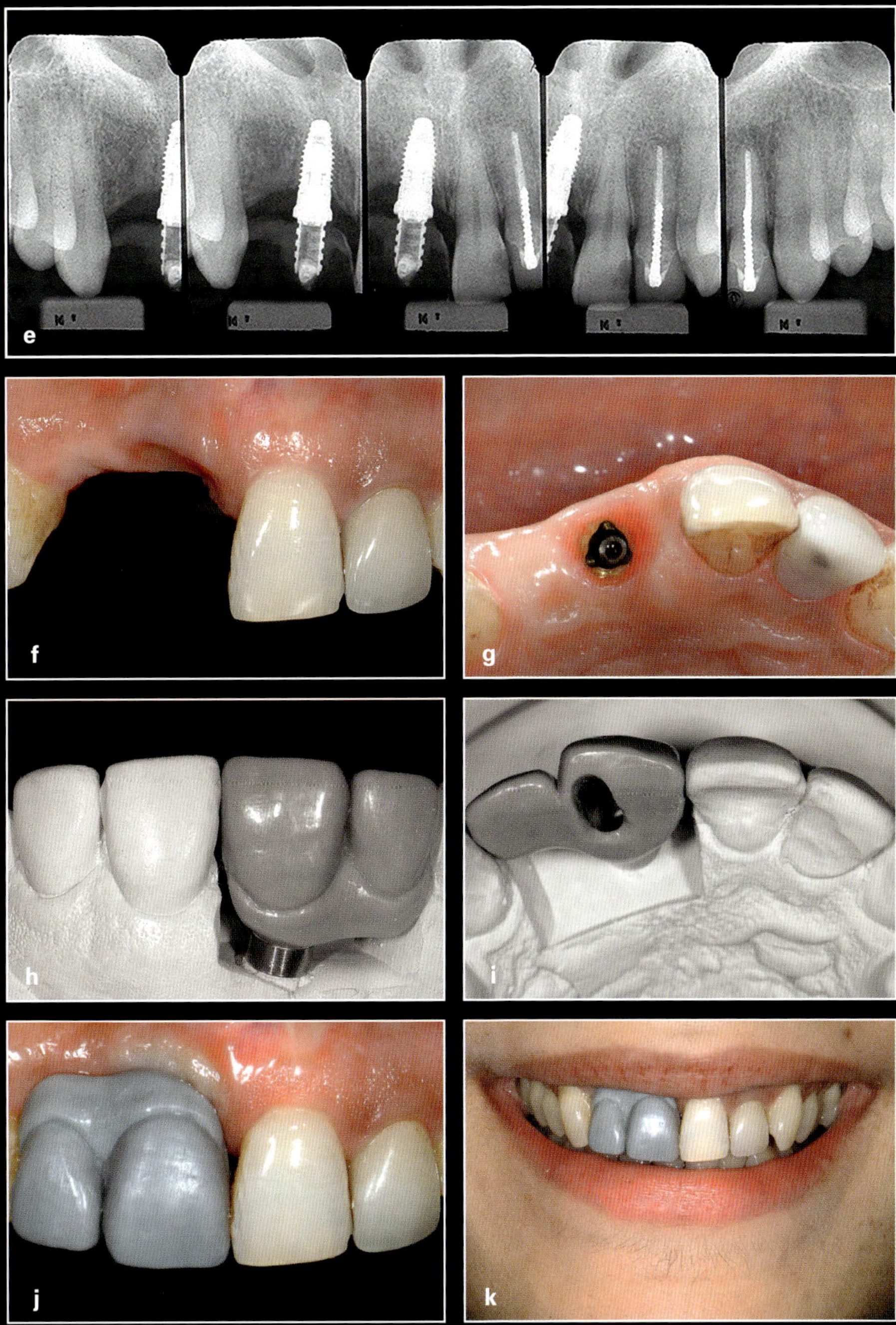

Fig 7-1 *(cont) (e)* Periapical radiographs demonstrated the presence of a provisional screw-retained cantilever FDP with a metal provisional abutment and an implant at the site of the maxillary right central incisor. *(f and g)* The provisional restoration was removed, and a facial view demonstrates a severe vertical residual alveolar ridge defect at the site. An occlusal view demonstrates a severe horizontal residual alveolar ridge defect at the site. The implant was placed too far distally. Because the patient declined additional surgical procedures, at this time it was decided to restore the patient with a screw-retained implant-supported FDP with a gingiva-colored ceramic flange to enhance esthetics and lip support while facilitating long-term maintenance and eliminating the risk of residual excess cement after delivery. *(h and i)* Facial and occlusal views of a complete-contour wax-up on the definitive cast demonstrating slight distobuccal rotation of the prospective retainer of the implant-supported FDP to allow for more thickness of restorative materials at the area of the screw. *(j and k)* The complete-contour wax-up, which included a flange simulation, was tried in the patient's mouth to evaluate the esthetics (including lip support and gingival levels, which will be modified on the central incisor) and phonetics. A major esthetic challenge is blending the restoration with the adjacent tissues at the mesial and distal vertical interfaces, as these interfaces are visible during smiling.

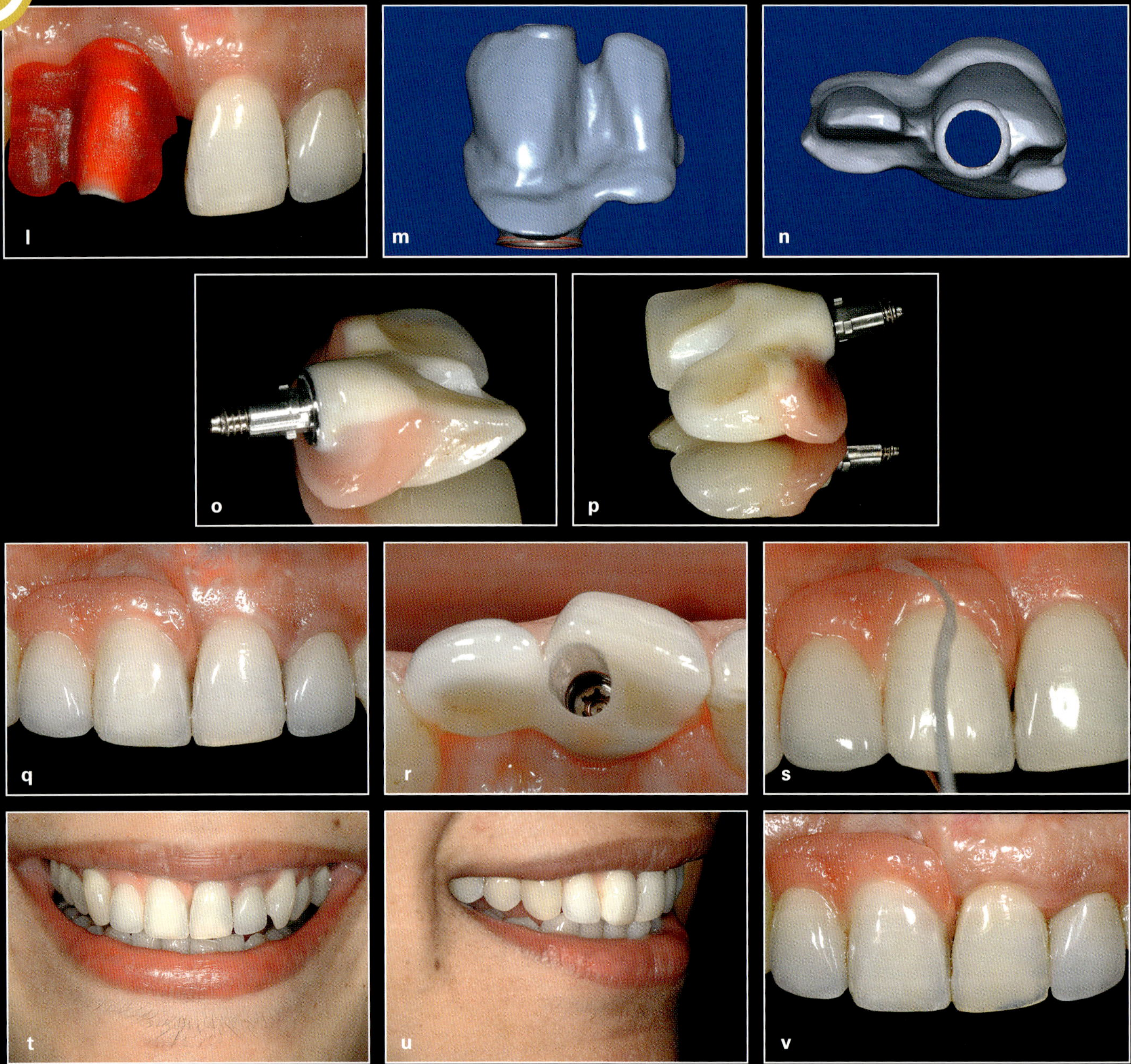

Fig 7-1 *(cont) (l)* A pattern made of an engaging temporary abutment and autopolymerized acrylic resin (GC Pattern Resin, GC America) was used to simulate an abutment-framework complex that included the implant retainer, the pontic, and the flange. *(m and n)* This pattern was scanned for the fabrication of a zirconia-based screw-retained abutment-framework complex with a bonded titanium insert interfacing with the implant and the retention screw (Lava, 3M ESPE). *(o and p)* The FDP abutment-framework complex was layered with zirconia-specific veneering porcelain (Noritake CZR, Kuraray Noritake) to facilitate internal characterization, translucency, and esthetics. Subsequently, the titanium insert was bonded to the zirconia abutment component. *(q and r)* Facial and occlusal views of the definitive restoration demonstrating the distobuccal rotation of the implant FDP retainer to provide adequate thickness to the zirconia abutment-framework complex and veneering porcelain at the distal and incisal areas to facilitate durability. *(s)* Facial view demonstrating the patient's ability to maintain adequate oral hygiene with a threader and floss. *(t and u)* Facial and lateral views of the patient's smile with the definitive restoration in place, demonstrating adequate blending with the adjacent tissues. *(v)* Frontal view at the 5-year recall demonstrating both the high translucency and characterizations at the incisal and interproximal areas as well as at the facial aspect of the restoration.

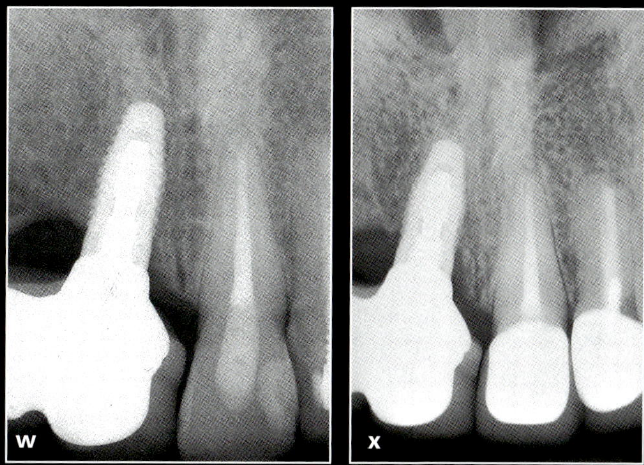

Fig 7-1 *(cont) (w and x)* Postoperative and 5-year recall periapical radiographs.

storative materials, comprised of either ceramic or composite resin, to be applied directly to the framework that carries the teeth, serving as a hard and soft tissue replacement.[11,12] Especially for patients who present with less than ideal hard and/or soft tissue architecture, screw-retained restorations allow for simplified delivery procedures by eliminating the hassle of cement cleanup (Figs 7-1v to 7-1x).

Drawing from principles of conventional fixed prosthodontics, the height of the abutment wall is important for resisting tipping and removal forces. In order to facilitate resistance form for a cemented restoration, the height of the abutment wall must be great enough to interfere with the radial arc pathway of a crown. Therefore, when a crown pivots around a margin, the opposite side of the crown will engage with its adjacent axial wall and hinder the lateral dislodging force. In situations where an implant abutment and crown would not have good retention and resistance form, a screw-retained restoration is a viable treatment alternative. In contrast to natural dentition, dental implants involve more treatment-planning considerations in order to address the biomechanical risks. With tooth loss, a reduced dimension in the residual alveolar ridge often follows. Vertical loss of bone may result in a net increase in the interarch space and consequently elongated replacement teeth. When the crown height becomes too great, biomechanical complications may increase due to increased moment forces on the implant. To address the concern of crown height for single implant restorations, guidelines for the ideal space between the crest of the residual ridge and the occlusal plane were recommended to be between 8 and 12 mm.[13] If a greater interarch space is present, the treatment plan should incorporate a method of implant site development to reduce the vertical space and attempt to minimize the biomechanical risks. In situations where the interarch space is less than the recommended guidelines to allow for an abutment and a crown, a screw-retained restoration offers a reliable solution.

Cement-Retained Restorations

In situations where utilizing a screw-retained restoration would lead to an esthetic compromise (ie, screw access channel on the facial aspect of an anterior restoration) or a functional compromise (ie, screw access channel interferes with cuspal anatomy or unsupported restorative material is left around the screw access channel, making it susceptible to fracture), it may be advisable to consider a cement-retained restoration instead. This does not mean that when implant position is ideal, one cannot use a cement-retained restoration; rather, it becomes a matter of clinician preference. It remains up to the clinician to decide the likelihood of needing to remove the restoration in the future, as that is still the main advantage offered by screw-retained restorations.

Cement-retained implant-supported restorations also may be selected because of the seeming ease of clinical procedures required, especially for clinicians in the early stage of their career and for relatively simple clinical scenarios. Once an abutment is placed, the remaining procedures are very much conventional fixed prosthodontic procedures. Thus, when teeth and implants are simultaneously being restored in the same arch, it may be convenient to use cement-retained restorations from a restorative procedure perspective because the workflow is streamlined for both the clinician and the dental technician.

While the focus of this chapter is ceramic screw-retained restorations, it is important to note that studies have shown no significant difference between cement- and screw-retained restorations for major and minor outcomes with regard to implant survival or crown loss.[14] Major outcomes were defined as those relating to failure of the restoration requiring its replacement. Minor outcomes were defined as those requiring clinician intervention because they threaten the survival of the restoration and/or the implant, such as screw loosening, decementation and subsequent total loss of retention, porcelain fractures that do not necessitate replacement of the restoration, bone loss per month, strain, and marginal gap discrepancies.[14] Likewise, a recent systematic review showed that at 5-year cumulative follow-up, there was no significant difference between screw-retained and cement-retained restorations in terms of biologic complications (soft tissue complications and bone loss greater than 2 mm).[15] Thus, as clinicians continue to use both methods for restoring implants, it remains clear that neither is a form of inferior care.

The following sections of this chapter discuss fundamental principles involved in fabrication of predictable ceramic screw-retained implant-supported restorations, starting with surgical planning and continuing to the definitive restorative material selection. All are considered to play a critical role in the delivery of successful definitive restorations. While the focus remains on multiple-unit implant-supported restorations, discussed concepts can easily be applied to simpler restorations.

Presurgical Planning

Once the decision is made to use a screw-retained restoration, the implant placement should be executed with high accuracy and precision, allowing neither biomechanical nor esthetic challenges to preclude the use of such a restoration. These scenarios emphasize the need for restoratively driven surgical planning and execution when it comes to the implant placement itself.[16] A surgical guide is critical in aiding the execution of such a plan. Guides can be simple (ie, vacuform shells with the buccal or palatal/lingual facings of the planned restorations)[17] or complex (ie, guides with 2-mm drill holes or metal tubes).[18–20] Historically, the problem with surgical guides was the difficulty in correlating a two-dimensional radiograph with the diagnostic casts and wax-up. Advances in three-dimensional (3D) imaging in dentistry (ie, cone beam computed tomography) in combination with the introduction of third-party proprietary implant planning software and associated surgical instrumentation have revolutionized the delivery of care and the predictability of implant placement outcomes. With the use of computer-aided design/computer-assisted manufacturing (CAD/CAM) implant surgical guides, this anatomical relationship can be predictably established and considered prior to surgery[21] (Figs 7-2a to 7-2h). While precision is important with any surgery, it is especially imperative when screw-retained implant-supported restorations are to be restored with multiple splinted units (Figs 7-2i and 7-2j). The authors believe that making a master impression is easiest when all dental implants are as parallel as anatomically possible and all implant platforms are at the same relative depth. This concept allows removal of the impression tray with as minimal interference as possible.

Computer-guided surgery

CAD/CAM implant surgical guides exist in three main categories based on the manner in which they are supported in the mouth during the surgery: tissue borne, bone borne,

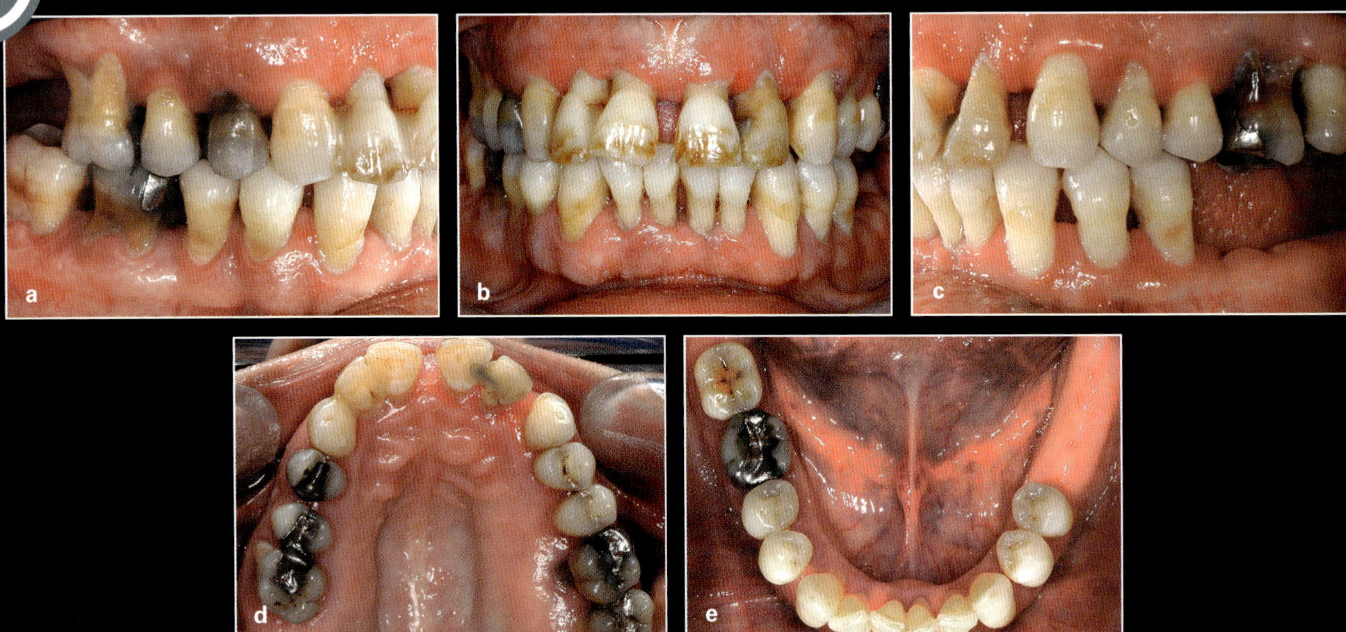

Fig 7-2 *(a to c)* Lateral and facial views in maximal intercuspal position of a patient in his late 50s who presented with severe attachment loss. *(d and e)* Maxillary and mandibular occlusal views demonstrating mild occlusal wear.

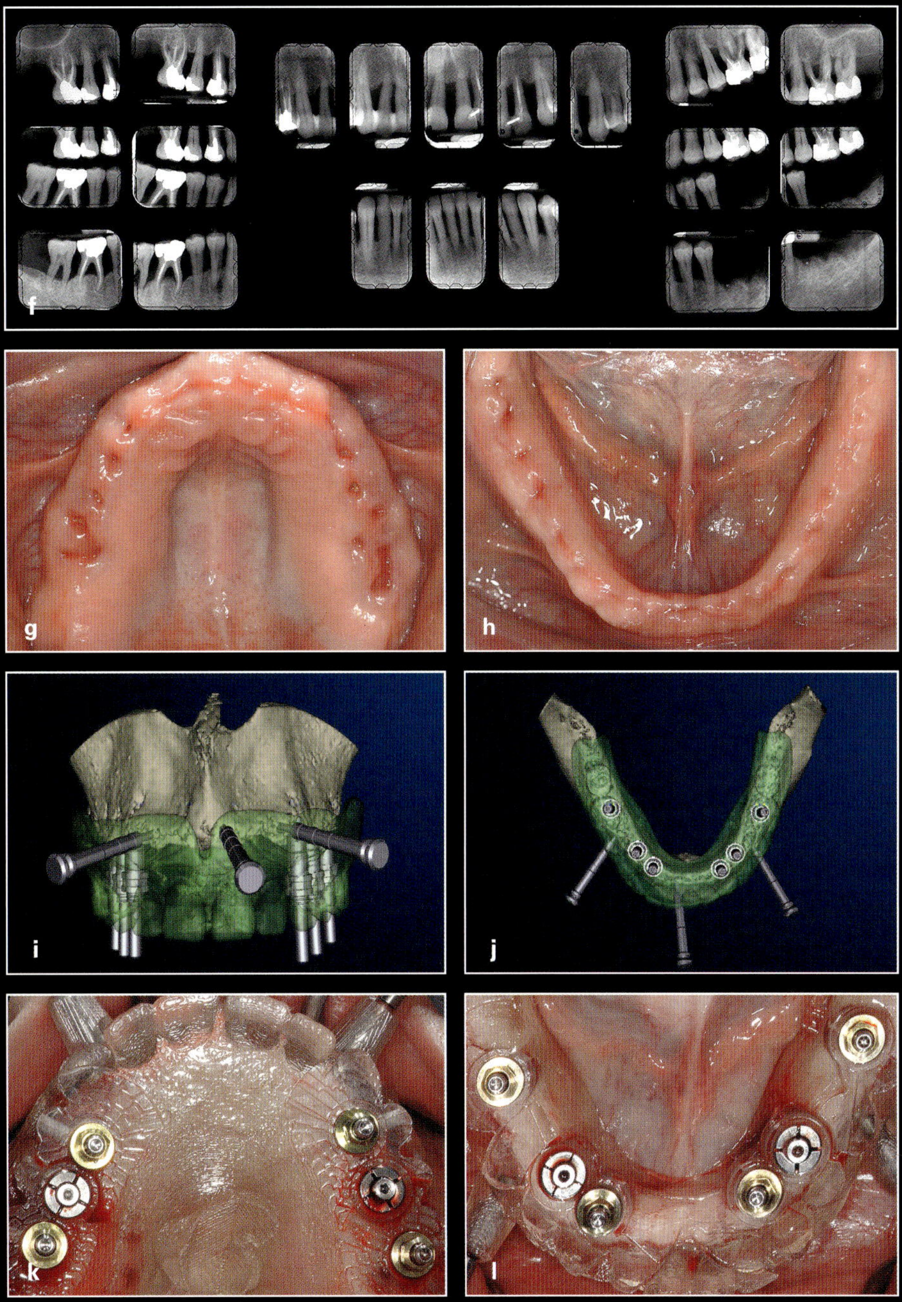

Fig 7-2 *(cont) (f)* Preoperative complete-mouth radiographs demonstrating advanced bone loss. Based on clinical and radiographic findings, the patient was diagnosed with advanced chronic periodontitis. *(g and h)* Occlusal views of the maxillary and mandibular arches a few weeks after complete-mouth extractions and delivery of immediate complete dentures. *(i and j)* Views of the maxillary and mandibular virtual digital treatment plan for implant placement (NobelGuide, Nobel Biocare). Note the designed implant positions for the maxillary complete-arch one-piece screw-retained restoration and the mandibular two posterior and one anterior screw-retained restorations. *(k and l)* Occlusal views of the maxillary and mandibular tissue-borne stereolithographic surgical guides during the implant placement procedure.

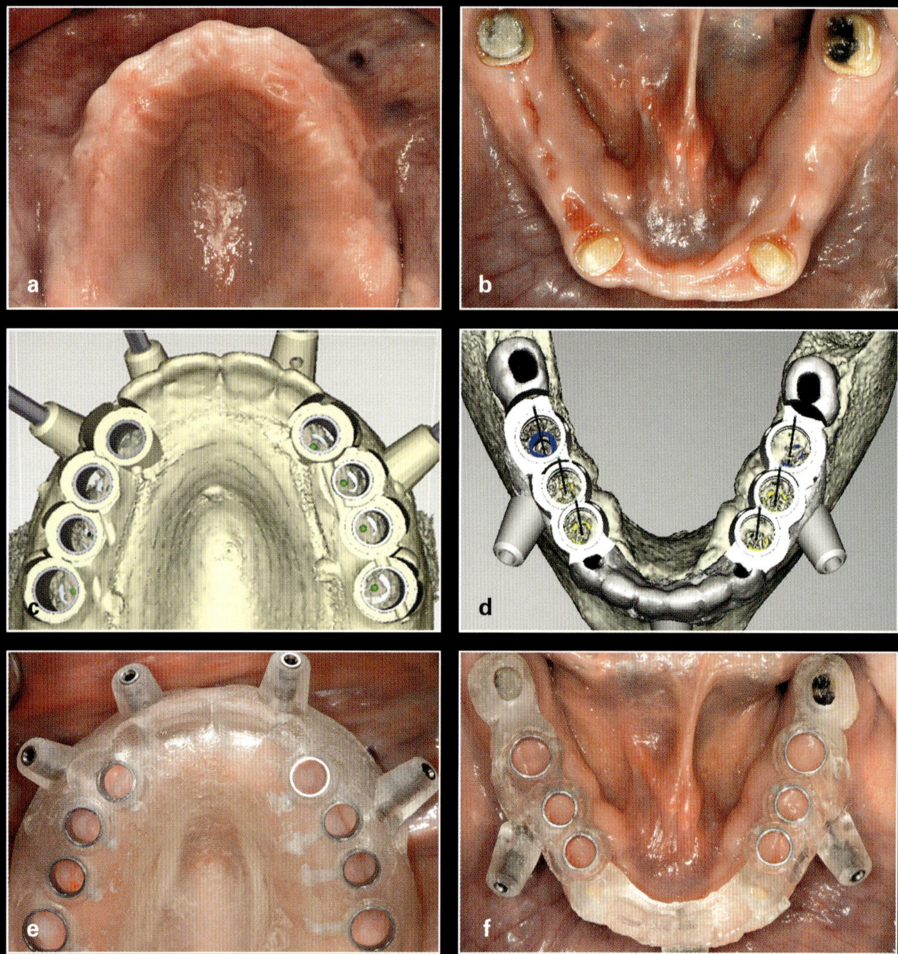

Fig 7-3 *(a and b)* Maxillary and mandibular occlusal views of a patient prior to implant placement for screw-retained implant-supported restorations in the maxillary arch and tooth-borne restorations and screw-retained implant-supported restorations in the mandibular arch. *(c and d)* Views of the maxillary and mandibular virtual digital treatment plan for implant placement (NobelClinicians, Nobel Biocare). *(e and f)* Occlusal views of the maxillary and mandibular tissue-borne stereolithographic surgical guides evaluated intraorally for fit prior to implant placement.

and tooth borne. These computer-aided milled or stereolithographic surgical guides are manufactured based on a virtual digital treatment plan. Such surgical guides are used with implant-specific drilling instrumentation to accurately and precisely place the implants in the same mesiodistal and buccolingual positions, to the same apicocoronal depths, and at the same angulations as planned virtually[21] (Figs 7-2k and 7-2l).

Only a few studies have compared results obtained from conventional guides versus CAD/CAM-generated ones. However, most in vitro[22–24] and clinical[25] studies have demonstrated that CAD/CAM-generated guides result in higher accuracy when it comes to the definitive implant position. Although computer-guided surgery may be more accurate than conventional surgery, an overestimation of its accuracy and underestimation of its error is likely to take place. A threshold for clinically significant error is 2 mm, so this value is routinely employed as the safety margin near vital structures. A clinical study found that mean variations in planned versus placed implant position ranged between 1.0 and 1.6 mm.[26] However, the range for the mean varied from 0 to 6.9 mm.[26] Needless to say, this amount of variation can have serious consequences for patients outside of mean values regarding not only irreversible damage to vital structures but also implant success and potential restorability of the placed implants. In order to facilitate consistent results, correct positioning of the guide is critical[27] (Fig 7-3).

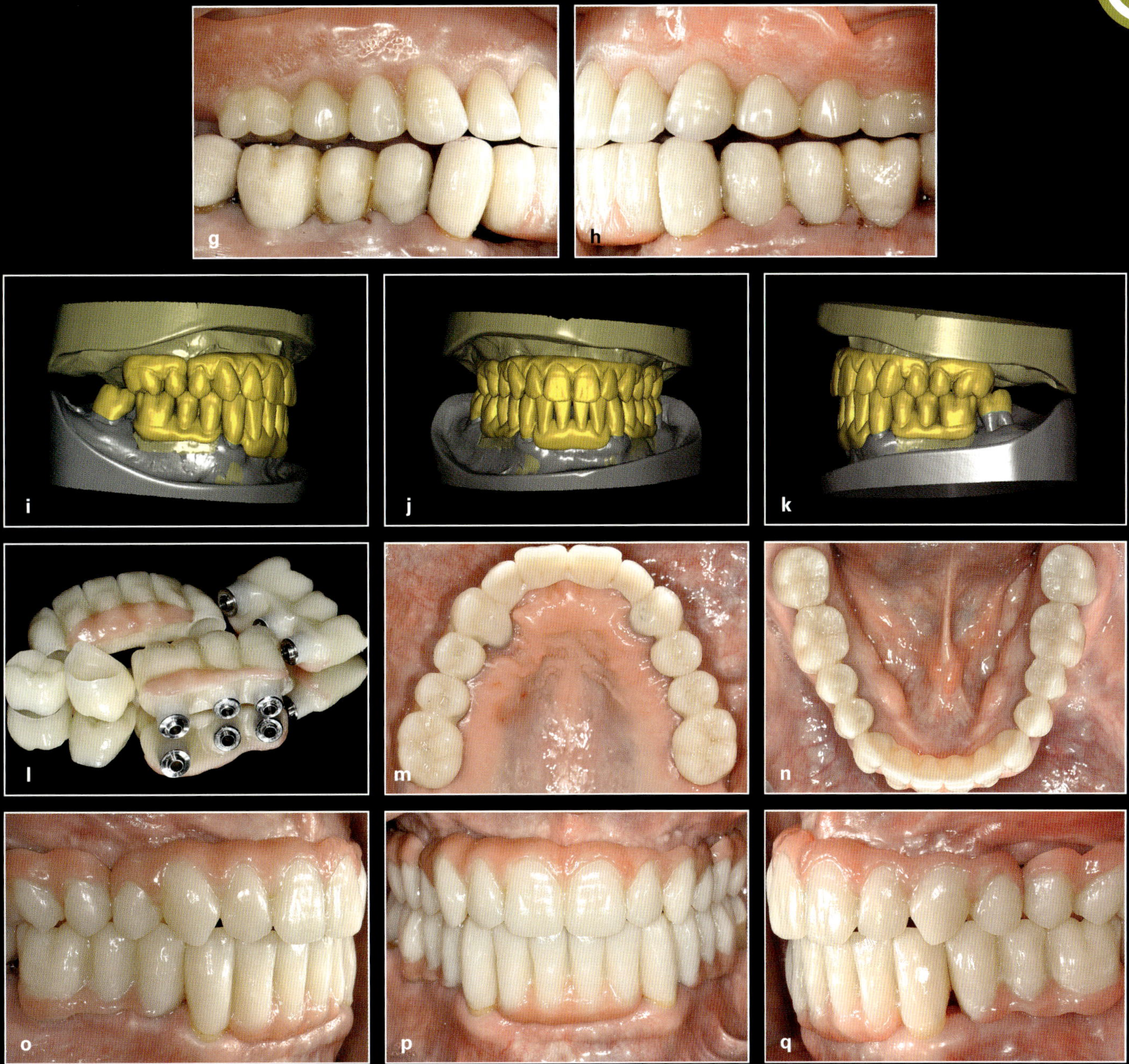

Fig 7-3 *(cont) (g and h)* Lateral views in right and left working movements a few weeks after implant placement (NobelReplace RP and WP, Nobel Biocare) and placement of immediate provisional restorations. Note that the mandibular provisional restorations are not in contact during working movements. *(i to k)* Lateral and frontal views of the virtual design of indirect CAD/CAM screw-retained provisional restorations (Zirkonzahn) designed based on the immediate maxillary denture and the mandibular provisional restorations. *(l)* View of the mandibular indirect provisional restorations milled of acrylic resin block (polymethyl methacrylate [PMMA]) and stained. *(m and n)* Occlusal views of the maxillary and mandibular indirect CAD/CAM provisional restorations in place. *(o to q)* Lateral and frontal views of the indirect CAD/CAM provisional restorations with the gingiva-colored PMMA in centric occlusion, restoring the horizontal and vertical alveolar ridge and soft tissue deficiencies.

Impressions for Screw-Retained Restorations

Concept of fit

In the process of fabricating multiple-unit, splinted, screw-retained implant-supported prostheses, the concept of fit between the restoration and supporting implants is critical. In 1983, Brånemark was the first to define "passive fit." He proposed that it should exist at the 10-µm level to enable bone maturation and remodeling in response to occlusal loads.[28] This concept has long been perceived to be essential to long-term successful osseointegration.[28] In 1985, it was suggested that metal castings with discrepancies greater than 30 µm over more than 10% of the circumference of the abutment interface were unacceptable.[29] This was followed by yet another definition denoting passive fit as the level that did not cause any long-term clinical complications, suggesting that misfits smaller than 150 µm were acceptable.[30] Although these definitions exist and are frequently quoted, they are empirically derived.[31] It is impossible to achieve absolute passive fit clinically,[31–33] and questions remain about the permissible amount of clinical misfit.[34,35] To date, no clinical study has directly pinpointed "inadequate fit" as a direct cause for dental implant complications and failures.[36] Nonetheless, it remains in the best interest of the clinician to aim for a restoration with the least amount of misfit, especially in situations involving multiple-unit splinted implant-supported restorations, as the magnitude of peri-implant strain is affected by the fit of the framework rather than the material from which the framework is fabricated.[37] Therefore, the primary goal of an implant impression is to obtain an accurate definitive cast with an accurate implant analog position, thus improving the likelihood of producing a passively fitting implant-supported restoration.[38,39] Complexity surrounding the attainment of passive fit of the implant prosthesis is directly related to accurate 3D transfer of the implant positions to the working cast.[31,39–41] Factors that can affect the accuracy of an impression and therefore the transfer of implant position include, but are not limited to, impression techniques and materials, splinting of multiple units, implant angulation, and implant apicocoronal depth[38,39,42] (Figs 7-4a to 7-4f).

Impression material

According to a recent review of the literature,[36] polyvinyl siloxane and polyether elastomeric impression materials continue to be the impression materials of choice for implant impressions (Figs 7-4g and 7-4h). Scientific research on combined use of digital impressions with CAD/CAM manufacturing techniques for the fabrication of multiple-unit, splinted implant-supported restorations is still considered to be at a preliminary stage, and more studies are needed to verify their reliability and accuracy prior to their use becoming common practice in the clinical setting.[36] Furthermore, alternative techniques have already been reported in the literature utilizing methods such as photogrammetry[43] to directly obtain the location and orientation of implants. In the future, this could eliminate the need for conventional impression-based methods that tend to incorporate procedural errors and inherent uncontrolled variables.

Impression techniques

Transfer versus pickup

Mode of impression coping transfer has also been investigated. Impression copings can be either picked up as in an open tray technique or transferred as in a closed tray technique, and both methods are accurate. While neither technique has a distinct advantage over the other, the pickup method tends to be favored when several implants are to be impressed.[44–50]

Splinting versus nonsplinting

When managing multiple implants, the issue of splinting versus nonsplinting of the transfer/impression copings at the time of impression-making arises. Much research has been conducted in this area. While some reviews have found more studies to be in favor of splinting,[39] others have failed to find a difference.[36] More recently, no correlation was found between the number of implants being recorded and the utilization of splinting techniques. It appears that in situations in which four to six implants were placed, equal numbers of studies supported and were indifferent to splinting.[36] Therefore, when clinicians consider splinting the transfer copings for making the master impression, perhaps the 3D position of the implants rather than the number of implants to be impressed should be the prime consideration.

Parallel versus angled implant positions

Most studies assessing the implant angulation and impression accuracy utilized only two implants.[36] Only three studies discuss the compounded effect of implant angulation involving three to five implants.[51–53] Presently, more studies are needed to assess the effect of angulation on accuracy of implant impressions in completely edentulous cases involving a greater number of implants. One factor that has been shown to contribute to the inaccuracy of impressions in multiple-unit implant-level impressions is the length of the connection part of the impression coping in implants with an internal connection.[54] Higher forces applied during impression removal in situations involving angled implants are likely to result in strain in the impression material, consequently producing an inaccurate transfer of the 3D implant position to the definitive cast. In instances of implant divergence, where it may be difficult to obtain an accurate impression, it may be more prudent to make use of transmucosal abut-

Continued from page 155

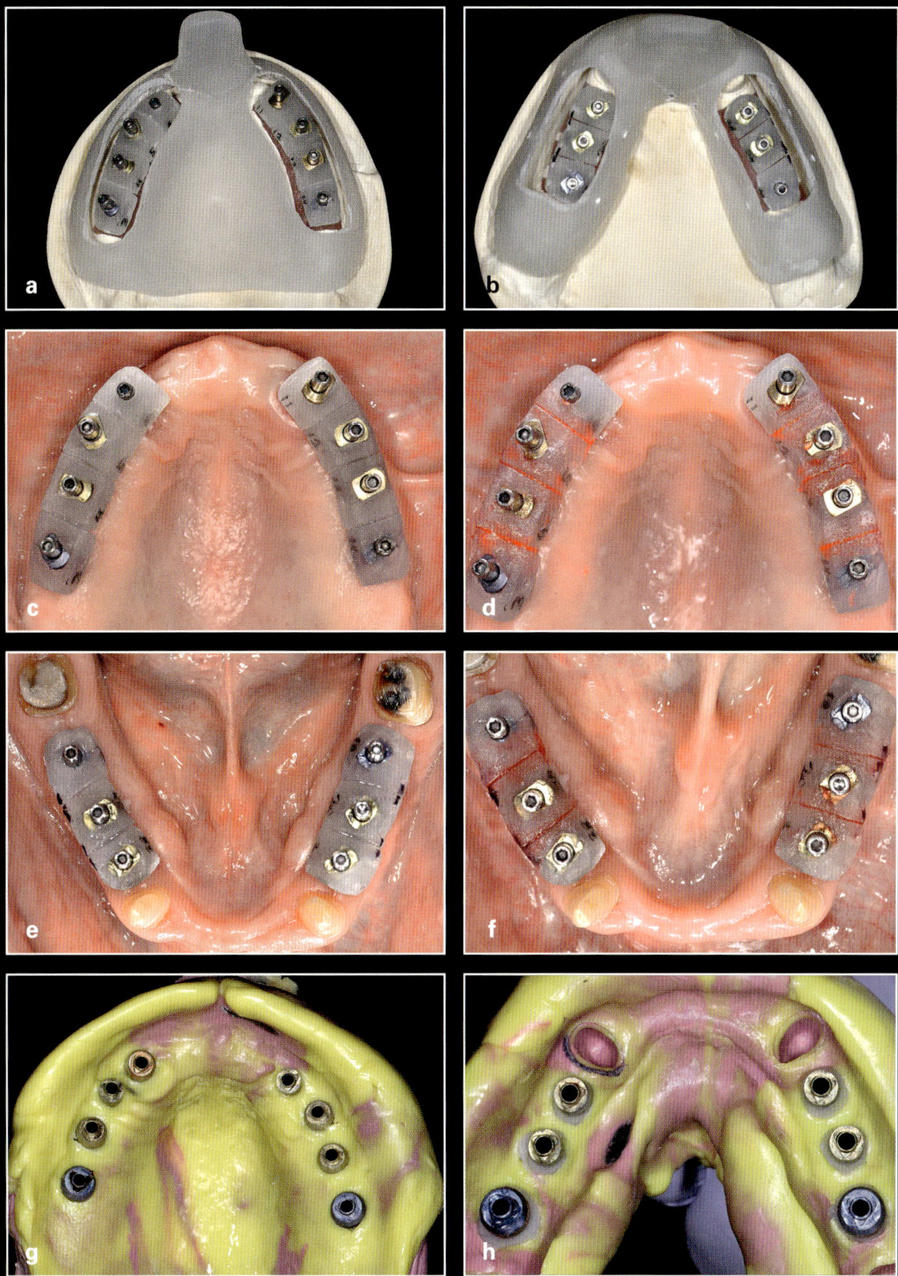

Fig 7-4 *(a and b)* Views of maxillary and mandibular casts generated from closed tray implant impressions. Open tray impression copings were modified with light-polymerized composite resin (Triad, Dentsply) and numbered according to their position. Open impression trays were made for the master impression procedures (Triad). *(c and d)* Occlusal views of the maxillary arch with the open tray impression copings secured to the implant platforms. They were splinted using autopolymerized acrylic resin (GC Pattern Resin). *(e and f)* Occlusal views of the mandibular arch with the open tray impression copings secured to the implant platforms. They were splinted using autopolymerized acrylic resin (GC Pattern Resin). *(g and h)* Views of the maxillary and mandibular master impressions made with heavy-body and light-body impression materials (Imprint 3, 3M ESPE) using the one-step/two-viscosity technique.

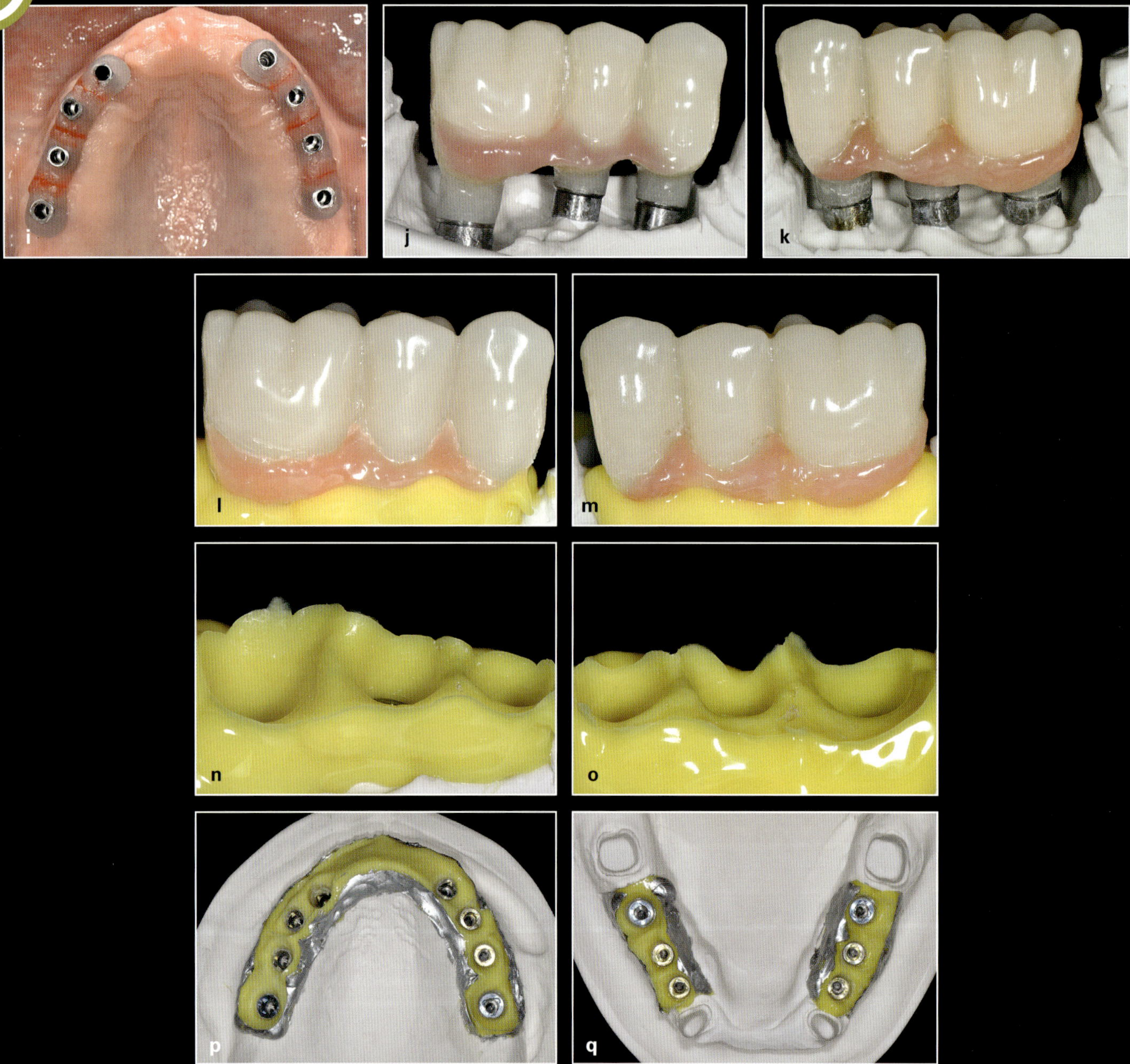

Fig 7-4 *(cont) (i)* Occlusal view of verification jigs used to assess the accuracy of the maxillary definitive cast. Note that the individual components were luted on the cast prior to placement in the patient's mouth. *(j and k)* Lateral views of the mandibular definitive cast with the provisional restoration secured to the implant analogs after the soft tissue simulation material has been removed. *(l and m)* The provisional restoration was removed, and light-body polyvinyl siloxane (PVS) material was syringed around the implant analogs. Subsequently, the provisional restorations were reseated on the implant analogs. The intaglio surfaces of the provisional restorations were impressed and recorded with the PVS material. *(n and o)* Once the PVS material was set, the provisional restorations were removed, revealing the definitive soft tissue contours. *(p and q)* Occlusal views of the maxillary and mandibular definitive casts. The newly recorded soft tissue contours transferred from the patient's mouth were used for the design and fabrication of the definitive restorations.

ments (for angle correction) and fabricate an abutment-level impression. However, abutment-level impressions carry an additional contributing factor for increasing the risk of inaccuracy in terms of fit of the definitive restoration.[55]

Verification of the definitive cast accuracy

Most framework fabrication methods currently in use utilize a definitive cast obtained from a conventional master impression. Typically, the definitive cast is scanned, and the framework is designed to fit the definitive cast. However, in the steps of impression removal from the patient's mouth to the pouring of the impression and setting of the dental stone, inaccuracies can occur. Therefore, several reports[56–58] have suggested the use of a verification jig to improve the accuracy of the definitive cast. Different types of verification jig materials have been evaluated[59] in vitro utilizing readily available auto- or light-polymerizing resin materials (Fig 7-4i). More recently, a study evaluated the difference in the likelihood of achieving passive fit when a framework is fabricated with or without the aid of a verification jig; use of a verification jig was demonstrated to be a valid method to achieve clinically passive fit of the metal frameworks, regardless of the fabrication technique (CAM or lost wax) and the number of implants connected by the framework.[60] In practice, clinical factors can affect the definitive restoration fit by influencing the accuracy of the definitive cast, while technical factors can affect the accuracy of the restoration as it fits on the definitive cast. The step of the verification jig separates clinical from technical factors. If passive fit of the definitive cast is verified, any major errors in the impression can be detected prior to fabricating the definitive framework. This is mainly due to the fact that verification jigs are not typically as rigid as the definitive restoration. However, because passive fit is evaluated in micrometers, verification jigs will only detect gross errors in fit.

Recording and transferring of soft tissue contours

Although the issue of implant apicocoronal position (depth) has been considered, it has been minimally studied,[39] with particular focus on retention of impression copings within the impression material and accurate transfer of 3D implant position. An added challenge with particularly deep implants is the recording of the peri-implant soft tissue profile, which is critical to an accurate portrayal of the emergence profile of the tissue from the platform of the implant through to the free gingival margins, as discussed in chapter 5. This information is crucial in the clinician-technician communication so that the intaglio surface of the restoration can mirror this profile. The soft tissue profile is important not only in highly esthetic regions but also in instances involving multiple-unit splinted implant frameworks or monolithic restorations with multiple pontics spanning the interimplant area (Figs 7-4j to 7-4q). Inadequate allowance for the soft tissue between individual implants can result in the clinician having to adjust the intaglio surfaces of the CAD/CAM framework. This is where framework material properties bear importance, as they are either amenable to clinical adjustment or not. For example, milled titanium frameworks may be adjusted clinically to achieve desired outcomes. Major adjustments, however, which could result in changes of connector dimensions outside manufacturer specifications, are not recommended. Historically, the minimum vertical height of cast alloy metal frameworks was 3 mm.[61] However, the physical properties of milled titanium frameworks are generally better than those of conventional castings because the material is more homogenous. At the time of publication, the only company that published minimal titanium framework dimensions was Biomet 3i (height: 2.5 mm; width: 4.0 mm). This information is not made readily available by other popular manufacturers, who likely have set guidelines. Therefore, while smaller dimensions may be tolerated, these values should be cross-referenced with the particular framework manufacturer. In contrast to milled titanium frameworks, other commonly utilized materials such as zirconia may not be easily manipulated after firing due to their inherent physical properties. Therefore, when using zirconia with a monolithic intaglio surface, it is extremely important to have a detailed treatment plan that includes the definitive design for the restoration so that implant site development and placement can be adequately performed.

Other factors

Other factors that can contribute to impression inaccuracy include, but are not limited to, type of tray used (flexible versus rigid, custom versus stock), reuse of impression copings, and various modifications of impression copings, from adjustments in length to an assortment of surface modifications.[36] When all these factors are considered, it is obvious that an accurate transfer of the 3D implant position and peri-implant soft tissue (and adjacent pontic sites, when relevant) from the patient's mouth to the definitive cast remains a crucial step in the initial development and ultimate long-term success of the implant-supported restoration.

CAD/CAM Technology with Screw-Retained Restorations

While impressions are one source of potential inaccuracy, the method of fabricating definitive prostheses carries its own risk of introducing further inaccuracies. Efforts targeted at improving the adaptation of multiple-unit splinted fixed implant-supported restorations include various technical procedures such as luting and soldering, luting and laser welding, electric discharge machining, and CAD/CAM procedures. The use of CAD/CAM technologies for manufacturing implant superstructures/frameworks has proven to be advantageous in the quality of material processing (lack of porosity), precision of the milled frameworks and superstructures, and passive fit.[62–65] This technology allows the dental technician to design various framework configurations on the computer or via a wax pattern that is subsequently scanned. This results in an anatomical-looking superstructure/framework or a provisional, definitive, or complete-contour restoration that is in harmony with the surrounding dentition and adjacent soft tissue.[66] By eliminating dimensional inaccuracies due to conventional waxing and casting techniques, the precisely fitting multiple-unit framework improves implant longevity and prosthetic success and simplifies the restoration[66,67] (Fig 7-5). While monolithic CAD/CAM zirconia frameworks with zirconia interfaces to implant platforms are available, some CAD/CAM splinted multiple-unit frameworks utilize zirconia frameworks luted to titanium inserts on a verified definitive cast. The latter method provides a titanium-to-titanium contact surface between the framework and the implant platform, rather than zirconia to titanium, and with post–framework/monolithic restoration production, the titanium insert luting may provide an additional step to enhance passive fit.

Continued from page 153

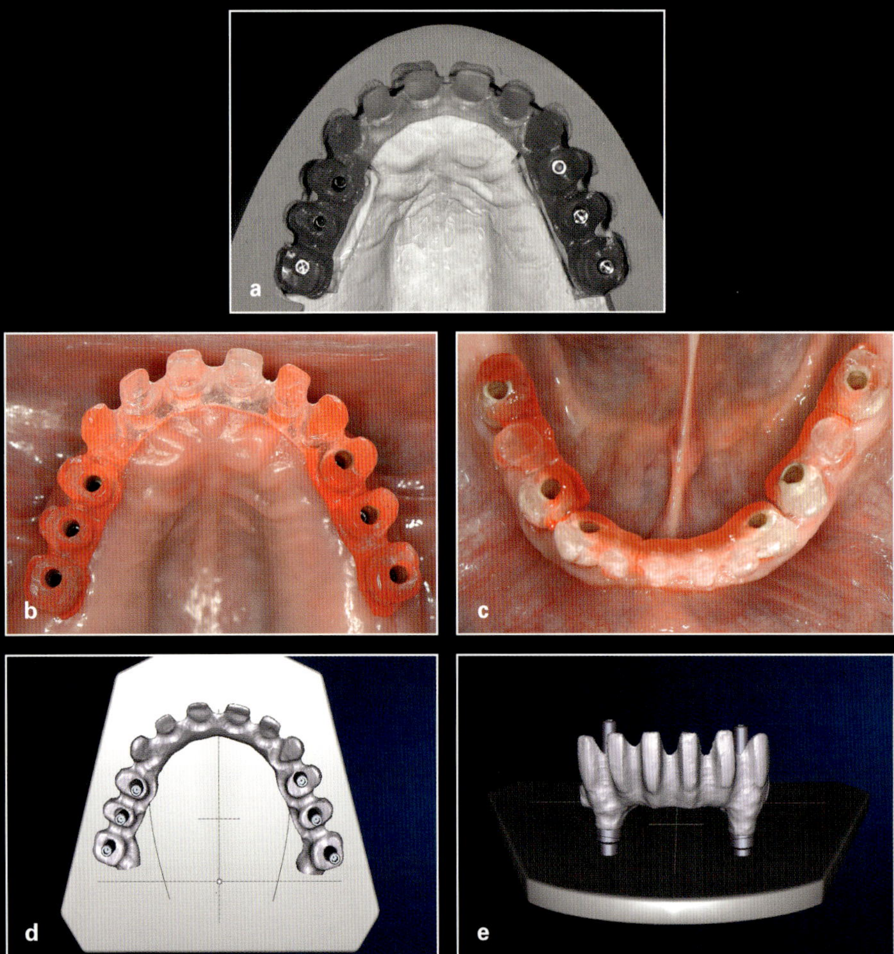

Fig 7-5 *(a)* View of the maxillary definitive cast with the resin pattern (GC Pattern Resin), with the silicone matrix fabricated based on a definitive wax-up. *(b and c)* Occlusal views of the maxillary and mandibular resin patterns, which were also used as verification jigs. Note that the screw access holes are located in favorable positions. *(d and e)* Views of the scanned maxillary and mandibular resin patterns in the CAD unit.

Zirconia

Physical properties

Initially, tetragonal zirconia polycrystals were introduced for biomedical use in orthopedics for total hip replacements.[68] From a microstructural perspective, zirconia is a polycrystalline ceramic without any glassy components. Being polymorphic, zirconia (also known as *zirconium dioxide*) exists in three forms: monoclinic, cubic, and tetragonal. Pure zirconia assumes the monoclinic form at room temperature, which is stable up to 1,170°C. Beyond this temperature, a transformation to the tetragonal phase occurs, which is stable up to 2,370°C, after which point the cubic phase transformation is seen. A transformation from the tetragonal to the monoclinic phase occurs while cooling in a temperature range of about 100°C to 1,170°C. This is associated with a volume expansion of around 3% to 4%, which usually leads to crack precipitation and propagation through pure zirconia.[69]

The addition of stabilizing oxides, such as calcium oxide, magnesium oxide, cerium oxide, and yttrium oxide, to pure zirconia permits generation of multiphase materials known as *partially stabilized zirconia* that possess superior mechanical properties.[70] The physical property of transformation toughening[71] has been shown to stop crack propagation in these materials. The property involves the transformation of the metastable tetragonal phase to the monoclinic phase when tensile stress is applied to the crack tips. The transformation phase is associated with a local volumetric increase of 3% to 5%, which results in generation of localized compressive stresses around the crack tip, thereby squeezing the crack. The metastable tetragonal structure is achieved at room temperature by doping yttrium oxide (3 mol %) with tetragonal zirconia. The ceramic grain size is critical and must be higher than 0.3 μm and less than 0.8 μm.[69,72] With regard to physical properties, in vitro studies have shown flexural strength to range from 900 to 1,200 MPa and fracture toughness to range from 9 to 10 MPa • $m^{1/2}$, while fracture resistance under static load was found to be more than 2,000 N.[70,73] This value, however, does not take into consideration the structural transformations of zirconia's metastable microstructures, which may occur.

This phenomenon was first reported in 1981 as a degradation that occurs at relatively low temperatures (150°C to 450°C) in a gaseous environment and is also referred to as *aging*.[74] Low-temperature degradation was linked to a reaction between water vapor and the yttrium in yttria-stabilized zirconia.[75] The water vapor acted to draw yttrium out to the tetragonal grain surface, where monoclinic nuclei were created. The nuclei grew by further depletion of yttrium until the tetragonal grains transformed completely. The risk of catastrophic degradation arose when the transformed grains were larger than the critical size required to produce microcracks that accommodate expansion and shear strain. This phenomenon was described as a stress-corrosion reaction, resulting in strength reduction.[76] When very thin (0.2-mm) specimens of three different brands of zirconia (Lava, Zirkonzahn, and Zirprime [Kuraray Noritake]) were tested using an accelerated aging model of up to 200 hours (at standard autoclave sterilization conditions), simulating up to at least 200 years in vivo, a significant reduction in mean flexural strength was noted. Nonetheless, the flexural strength of all specimens was greater than 800 MPa, which was still higher than other commercially available ceramic restorative materials.[77] A similar study using the same methodology demonstrated that a newly developed zirconia (ZirTough, Kuraray Noritake) still retained a flexural strength of over 1,200 MPa after up to 200 hours at standard autoclave sterilization conditions.[78]

Mechanisms proposed for the decrease in properties include subcritical crack growth[79,80] and structural changes at the surface or at grain boundaries induced by mechanical energy, moisture, or both. Energy supplied to the material by grinding or polishing will accelerate the transformation influenced by energy and humidity, mainly at the surface of a restoration.[81] Therefore, clinical surface adjustments of monolithic zirconia are not recommended, and every effort should be made to minimize the need for these types of adjustments.

Zirconia as a framework material

With the advent of CAD/CAM technology, clinicians and technicians can now design and mill a one-piece zirconia structure comprising an area simulating an implant abutment (from the implant platform to the free gingival margins) and an area simulating a crown coping or an FDP framework for a screw-retained restoration. Such a structure, termed a *framework* in this chapter, may be more accurately termed an *abutment-framework complex*. An important advantage of zirconia frameworks pertains to the finding that porcelain and glaze firing cycles do not affect the fit of multiple-unit zirconia frameworks.[82] This feature is what allows clinicians to provide patients with complete-arch, multiple-unit, splinted, screw-retained implant-supported restorations layered with corresponding ceramics (Figs 7-6a to 7-6h). However, other studies demonstrating that veneering processes may have a significant influence on the marginal fit of zirconia-based restorations cannot be ignored.[83] It appears that this potential for distortion may arise from the matching of the framework and veneering ceramics used and not only with respect to the coefficient of thermal expansion (CTE). It is speculated that the behavior between zirconia and veneering ceramics may be more complex and warrants further research. More importantly, it should be noted that the preceding conclusions are drawn from studies evaluating tooth-borne frameworks. Implant-supported multiple-unit frameworks tend to contain more bulk, and thus the effect of veneering porcelain firing on potential distortion may be reduced.

Continued from page 160

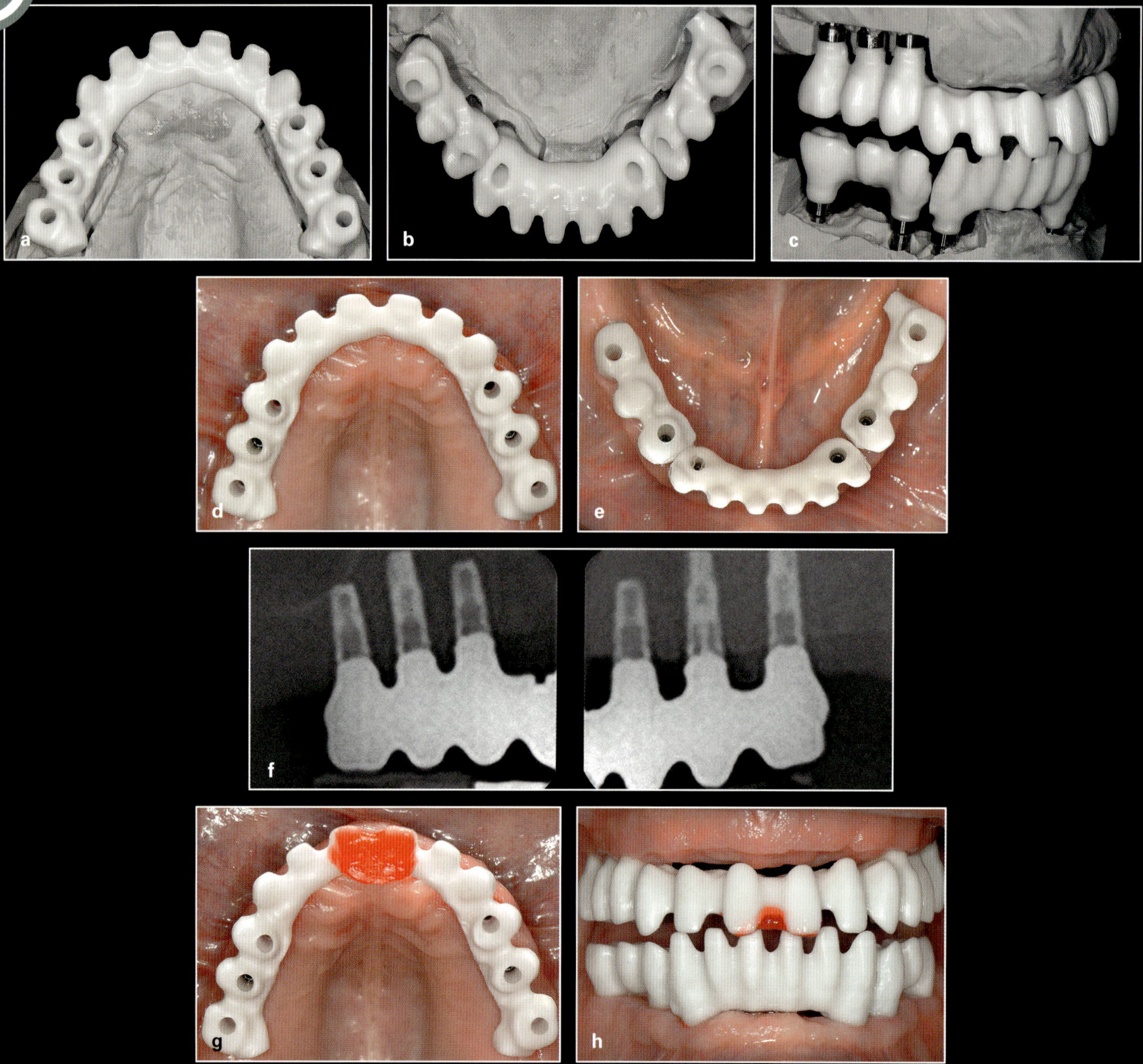

Fig 7-6 *(a and b)* Occlusal views of the maxillary and mandibular abutment-framework complexes on the definitive casts (Procera, Nobel Biocare). *(c)* View of the mounted casts on the semi-adjustable articulator demonstrating fit to the implant analogs. *(d and e)* Occlusal views of the maxillary and mandibular zirconia abutment-framework complexes seated in the patient's mouth. *(f)* Maxillary periapical radiographs demonstrating adequate fit of the complete zirconia abutment-framework complex in conjunction with the one-screw test. Note that the screw is located in the area of the left second premolar. *(g and h)* Views of the zirconia abutment-framework complexes with an anterior custom Lucia jig made of autopolymerized acrylic resin (GC Pattern Resin) at the proposed vertical dimension of occlusion. It was used to reverify the maxillomandibular relationships with a centric relation record.

Biocompatibility

As described in chapters 1 and 6, zirconia presents with superior biocompatibility in terms of soft tissue response. In vitro biocompatibility evaluations of high-purity zirconia showed little mutagenic and carcinogenic tendencies at the local cellular level.[84] Further, in vivo testing of zirconia has shown low to no inflammatory response.[85] Additionally, a clinical study has shown that zirconia allows for significantly less bacterial adhesion than highly biocompatible titanium.[86]

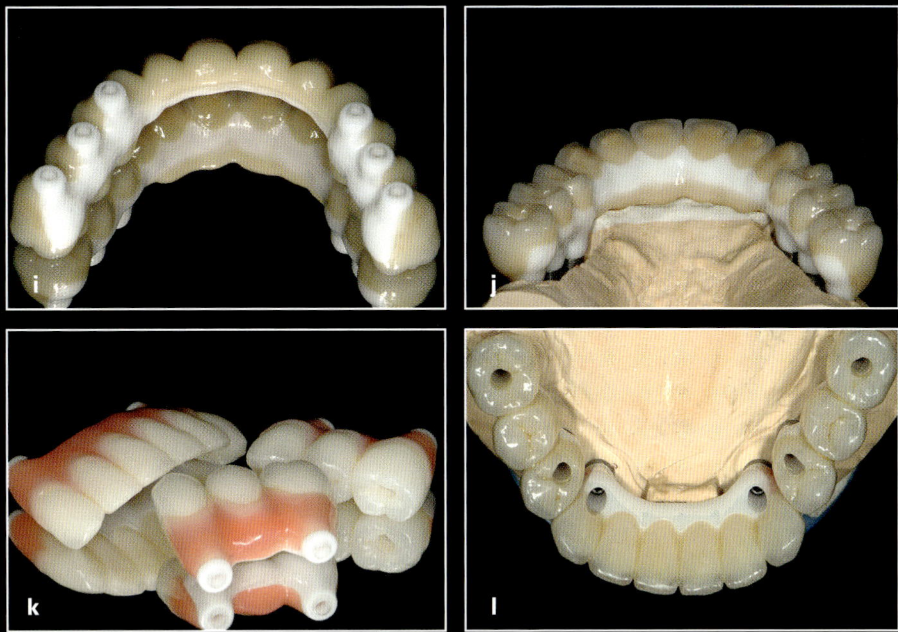

Fig 7-6 *(cont) (i and j)* Views of the intaglio and occlusal surfaces of the definitive complete-arch, zirconia-based, screw-retained restoration layered with the corresponding veneering porcelain (Noritake CZR). Note the non-engaging zirconia circles serving as an index for the restoration's seating onto the implant platforms. Also, note the convex cervical contours of the pontics. *(k and l)* Views of the mandibular zirconia-based restorations layered with indirect composite resin material (Estenia, Kuraray Noritake).

Esthetics

An important part of fabricating esthetic restorations is the management of optical properties and mimicking of natural tooth structure. Dental ceramics have achieved great esthetic qualities for restoring dental implants. The primary advantage of a ceramic restoration is the increase in depth of translucency and light transmission that allows the ceramist and restorative dentist to provide the patient with more natural- and vital-looking restorations.[87] This is not to say that shade matching is easier; however, the added advantage of being able to vary the translucency, shade, and thickness[88,89] of the zirconia substrate as opposed to metal substrates offers a definite advantage. In addition, as discussed in chapter 6, in the context of implant-supported restorations, zirconia does not adversely impair the color of the soft tissue at the emergence area between the implant platform and the free gingival margins, especially when the tissue is thin.[90]

Veneering of zirconia frameworks

In order to achieve maximum esthetic results, much like traditional metal-ceramic restorations, zirconia frameworks are veneered with feldspathic porcelain with matching physical properties. Veneering ceramic materials are primarily composed of glass-ceramics with minor compositional and microstructural differences, depending on the manufacturer. Leucite-reinforced glass-ceramics and nanofluorapatite glass-ceramics are used to veneer zirconia-based restorations[91,92] (Figs 7-6i and 7-6j).

One limitation that has been observed clinically with respect to veneering porcelain is cohesive chipping. In fact, this is regarded as the most common prosthetic complication with zirconia-based restorations.[93–96] Studies evaluating the causal factors of chipping have found that matching the CTEs between the veneering porcelain and the zirconia framework is critical to avoid cracking after firing.[97] Aside from CTE matching, with focus on the veneer-framework interface, tetragonal to monoclinic phase transformation has been observed, which could result in weaker material located at the interface.[98] In terms of framework design, more recent studies have advocated for anatomically designed frameworks, as opposed to arbitrary restoration thickness, in order to support the veneering porcelain.[99–101] In addition, the quality of veneering material should not be discounted, as studies have shown different outcomes depending on the veneering material used and its application technique (layered, pressed, or digitally veneered to the framework/coping).[102–105] Veneering ceramic material with a higher fracture toughness is preferred as well.[92] Methods of combating veneering porcelain chipping have also been found to be re-

Continued from page 158

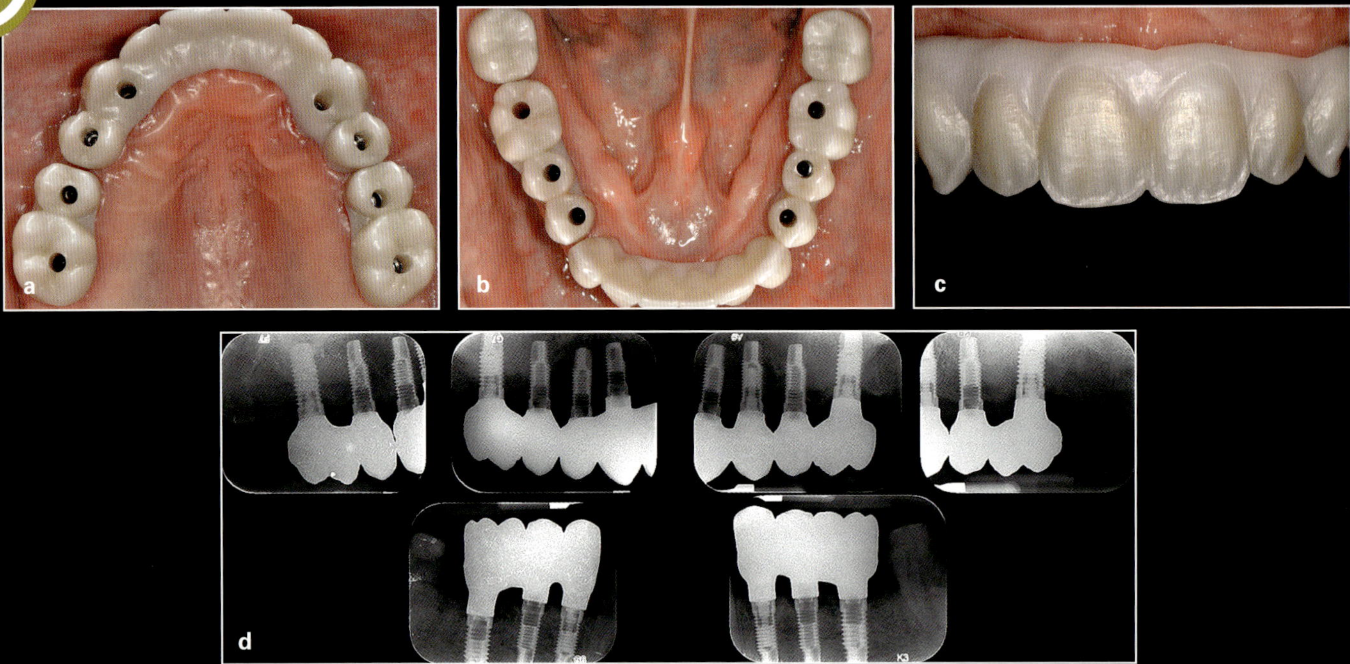

Fig 7-7 *(a and b)* Maxillary and mandibular occlusal views of the unfinished zirconia-based restorations (Prettau, Zirkonzahn), with a monolithic design for the molars and a hybrid design for the rest of the dentition, evaluated for fit as well as occlusion in the patient's mouth. *(c)* Facial view of the unfinished restoration in the maxillary anterior segment with a hybrid design restoration and a zirconia flange. *(d)* The fit of the unfinished restorations was evaluated clinically and radiographically with the one-screw test.

lated to slow cooling and firing regimens during the fabrication of porcelain-fused-to-zirconia restorations.[106] A recent in vitro study demonstrated that failure frequency of veneered zirconia restorations could be reduced by using anatomically designed substructures, a pressed veneering technique, and an adapted cooling protocol.[107]

One way to avoid veneering porcelain chipping with zirconia-based ceramic restorations is to veneer zirconia with lithium disilicate or indirect composite resin.[108] Effects of various veneering materials on stress distribution in implant-supported FDPs have been evaluated. The results revealed that the reduction in stress associated with the use of the composite resin material was 15% compared with feldspathic porcelain[109] (Figs 7-6k and 7-6l). In terms of fracture resistance, no significant difference in the likelihood of failure was found among metal-ceramic restorations and implant-supported restorations veneered with indirect composite resin material.[110] Bonding protocols for zirconia-based restorations are successfully applied to indirect composite resin layering materials. These protocols call for use of 10-methacryloyloxi-decyl-dihydrogen-phosphate (MDP)–containing primers, which have been shown to enhance the bond of composite resin to zirconia.[111]

Monolithic zirconia restorations

The ability to precisely design restorations in the virtual world and to predictably fabricate them in a highly automated fashion has fundamentally influenced clinicians' approaches to implant therapy. Because failures in the form of veneering porcelain chipping in bilayered ceramic restorations are a recognized problem, monolithic zirconia restorations have been developed to overcome such complications. However, the use of monolithic zirconia has not been rigorously investigated for the fabrication of a complete-arch fixed implant-supported restoration. Aside from clinical reports, few longitudinal clinical studies on complete-arch monolithic zirconia have been published in English.[96,112] Nonetheless, short-term results seem to indicate that monolithic zirconia implant-supported restorations may be a viable treatment alternative to metal-ceramic, metal-acrylic, and bilayered zirconia-based restorations.[96] To address esthetic challenges presented by the monolithic design, it was suggested to design such restorations with monolithic surfaces in areas of the restoration where durability and strength (ie, ability to sustain functional and parafunctional forces) are of primary importance as well as in areas where esthetics is a secondary consideration.

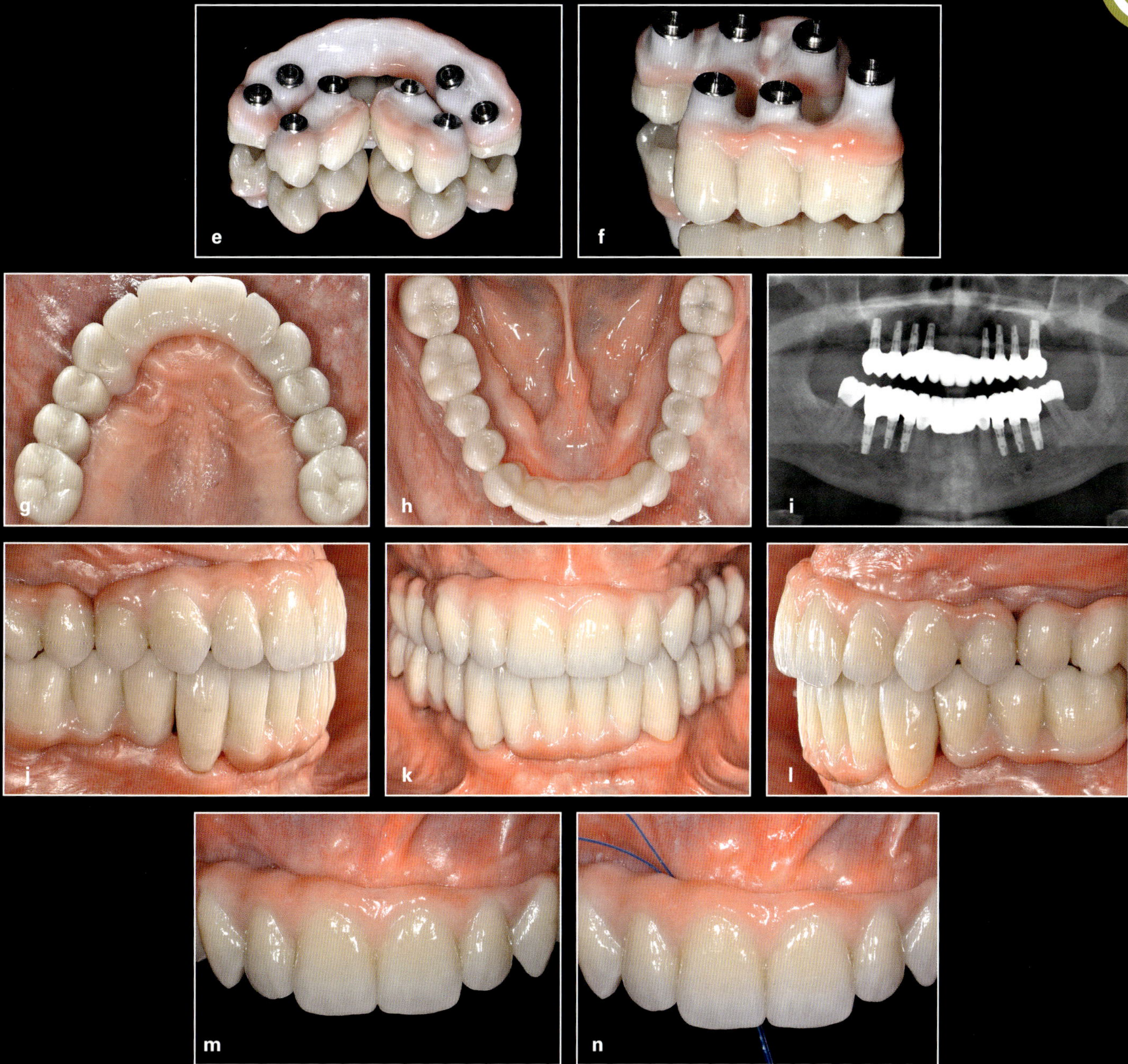

Fig 7-7 *(cont) (e and f)* The intaglio surfaces of the complete zirconia-based, screw-retained implant-supported restorations with the bonded titanium inserts. The critical and subcritical contours of the restorations were designed based on the soft tissue simulation generated from the provisional restorations on the definitive cast. *(g and h)* Occlusal views of the maxillary and mandibular definitive restorations. *(i)* Postoperative panoramic radiograph. *(j to l)* Lateral and frontal views of the definitive restorations with the gingiva-colored stained zirconia in centric occlusion, restoring the horizontal and vertical alveolar ridge and soft tissue deficiencies. *(m)* Frontal view of the maxillary anterior restoration. Note the translucency, surface texture, and characterization achieved with the veneering porcelain layered over the zirconia abutment-framework complex. *(n)* Oral hygiene was successfully maintained at the area of the anterior maxillary flange with a threader and floss.

However, in areas of the restoration where esthetics is of primary concern (such as facial and incisal areas that are visible), the restoration should be virtually designed with a facial and an incisal cutback, also known as a *hybrid design*. Once the cutback is made at the facial and incisal aspects, the area that conceptually resembles a tooth preparation for a veneer restoration will be veneered with the corresponding veneering porcelain by the dental technician to enhance translucency and characterization as well as surface texture[113] (Figs 7-7a to 7-7d).

Similar to other ceramics, anatomically contoured monolithic zirconia restorations have the potential to cause wear of the opposing dentition. The reported hardness of zirconia is in the range of 1,354 to 1,378 Hv, compared with that of zirconia veneering porcelain (481 to 647 Hv), which may potentially correlate to its wear potential.[114,115] Further, the effect of glazed versus polished zirconia and its effect on enamel wear is presently a point of discussion in the literature; some studies show that polished zirconia results in a significantly greater amount of wear,[116] while other studies have shown glazed zirconia to result in greater wear.[117–119] However, different brands of zirconia have been shown to result in different amounts of wear.[120] Nonetheless, multiple in vitro studies have shown that the wear of enamel antagonists is much lower when opposing monolithic zirconia compared with feldspathic porcelain.[117,121–123] Moreover, further research is required on how monolithic zirconia restorations behave in terms of wear against different restorative materials, especially in cases of implant-supported FDPs (Figs 7-7e to 7-7n).

Complete-mouth restorations: Material selection for opposing surfaces

The concept of material selection and pairing in completely restored opposing arches can prove to be critical to the longevity of the restorations, especially in situations involving implants where the damping effect of the periodontal ligament is nonexistent. For complete-mouth implant-supported restorations, one may elect to use ceramic restorations in the maxillary arch because of their superior esthetic properties. An implant framework on the mandibular arch would in turn be restored with resin-based denture teeth or veneered with indirect composite resin material (Figs 7-8a to 7-8g). The purpose of this pairing is to make the mandibular arch more susceptible to wear over time to avoid porcelain chipping. A study evaluating metal-ceramic restorative material behavior demonstrated a higher material reliability when the metal-ceramic restorative material opposed resin-based materials.[124] A more recent in vitro study has demonstrated further validity of the concept of material pairing as shown by the longer life span of a ceramic material when opposing a more resilient resin-based material.[125] This logic allows the clinician to push the mode of prosthetic failure away from a catastrophic failure to a more manageable complication in terms of procedures and cost (Figs 7-8h to 7-8l). Once the mandibular arch sustains enough occlusal wear to justify replacement, the framework can be reveneered. In contrast, if the treatment plan did not have contingency plans for the long-term maintenance phase of the restorative component of the therapy, in the case of severe restorative complication, the restoration would have to be replaced.

Summary

No restorative material or prosthetic design is without limitation. It is clear that restoring missing teeth with screw-retained ceramic prostheses with the available tooth-colored materials and new advanced technologies can deliver both function and esthetics for the dental patient. However, this does not mean that an end point in the development of these types of restoration has been reached. Further material and technologic developments and innovations are necessary in the continuous pursuit of successfully replacing natural dentition.

Continued from page 163

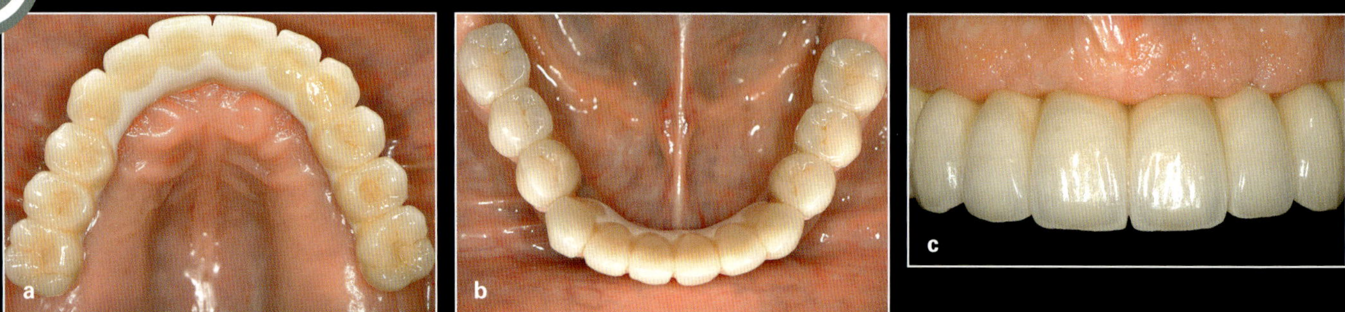

Fig 7-8 *(a and b)* Occlusal views of the maxillary and mandibular complete zirconia-based restorations seated in the patient's mouth. *(c)* Frontal view of the pontics of the maxillary zirconia-based restoration. Note the high chroma root effect used to manage the tooth contours and proportions.

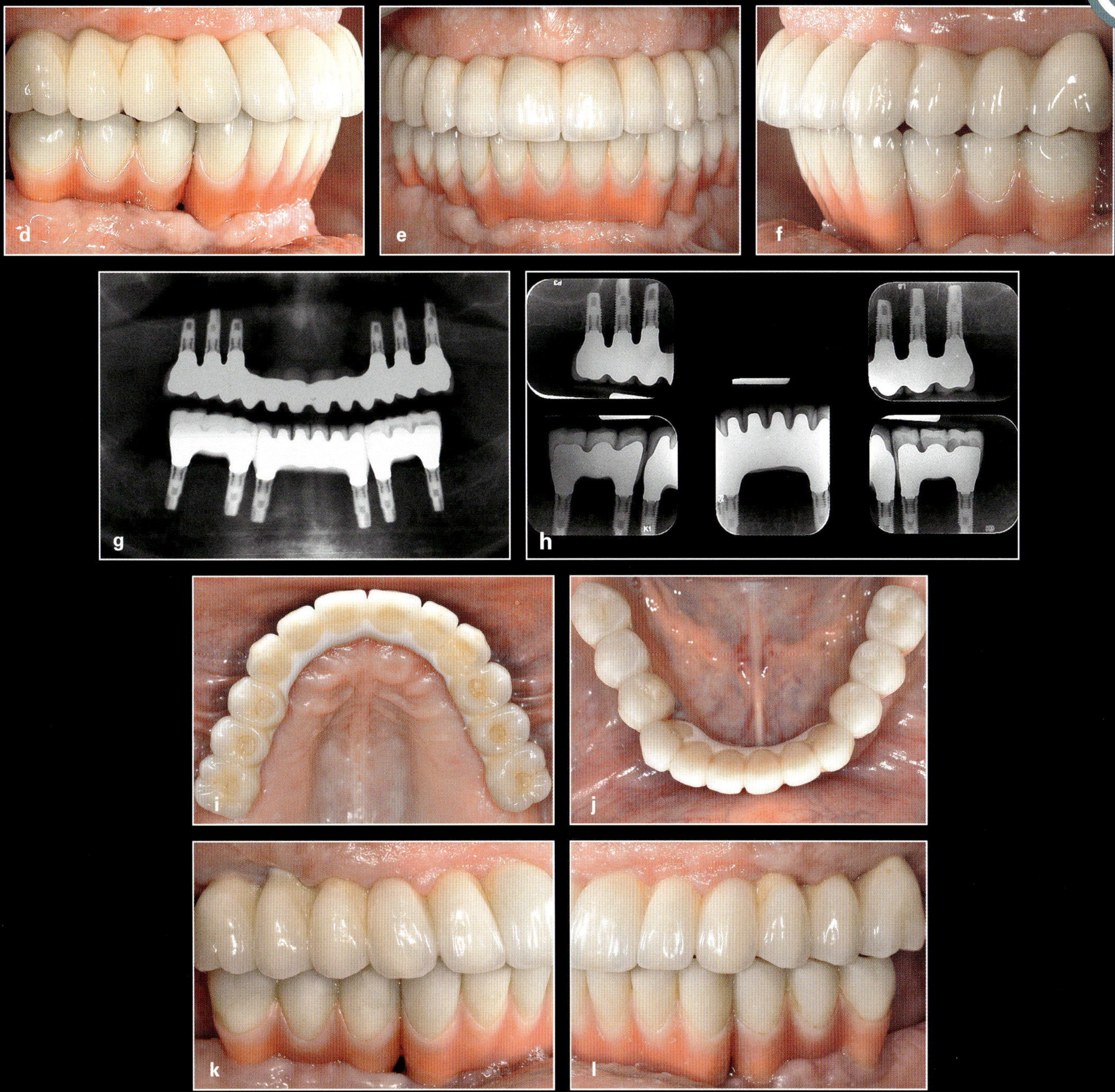

Fig 7-8 *(cont) (d to f)* Frontal and lateral views of the complete restorations in centric occlusion. *(g)* Panoramic radiograph of the patient after delivery of the definitive restoration. *(h)* Periapical radiographs of the patient 5 years after delivery of the restorations. Note the minimal bone remodeling. *(i and j)* Occlusal views of the definitive restoration 5.5 years after delivery. Note the loss of luster of the restoration. In addition, the distolingual cusp of the right mandibular molar that had a cohesive fracture of the veneering composite resin was polished and does not impair the patient's ability to function. *(k and l)* Lateral views of the definitive restoration in centric occlusion 5.5 years after delivery. Note the loss of luster of the composite resin material and the patient's meticulous oral hygiene.

References

1. Adell R, Leckholm U, Rockler B, Brånemark PI. A 15-year study of osseointegrated implants in the treatment of the edentulous jaw. Int J Oral Surg 1981;10:387–416.
2. Lewis S, Beumer J III, Hornburg W, Moy P. The "UCLA" abutment. Int J Oral Maxillofac Implants 1988;3:183–189.
3. Albrektsson T. A multicenter report of osseointegrated oral implants. J Prosthet Dent 1988;60:75–84.
4. Adell R, Eriksson B, Leckholm U, Brånemark PI, Jemt T. A long-term follow-up of osseointegrated implants in the treatment of the treatment totally edentulous jaws. Int J Oral Maxillofac Implants 1990;5:347–359.
5. Nissan J, Narobai D, Gross O, Ghelfan O, Chaushu G. Long-term outcome of cemented versus screw-retained implant-supported partial restorations. Int J Oral Maxillofac Implants 2011;26:1102–1107.
6. Chee W, Felton DA, Johnson PF, Sullivan DY. Cemented versus screw-retained implant prostheses: Which is better? Int J Oral Maxillofac Implants 1999;14:137–141.
7. Hebel KS, Gajjar RC. Cement-retained versus screw-retained implant restorations: Achieving optimal occlusion and esthetics in implant dentistry. J Prosthet Dent 1997;77:28–35.
8. Pjetursson BE, Tan K, Lang NP, Brägger U, Egger M, Zwahlen M. A systematic review of the survival and complication rates of fixed partial dentures (FPDs) after an observation period of at least 5 years. Clin Oral Implants Res 2004;15:625–642.
9. Pjetursson BE, Brägger U, Lang NP, Zwahlen M. Comparison of survival and complication rates of tooth-supported fixed dental prostheses (FDPs) and implant-supported FPDs and single crowns (SCs). Clin Oral Implants Res 2007;18:97–113.
10. Papaspyridakos P, Chen CJ, Chuang SK, Weber HP, Gallucci GO. A systematic review of biologic and technical complications with fixed implant rehabilitations for edentulous patients. Int J Oral Maxillofac Implants 2012;27:102–110.
11. Simon H, Raigrodski AJ. Gingiva-colored ceramics for enhanced esthetics. Quintessence Dent Technol 2002;25:155–172.
12. Coachman C, Salama M, Garber D, Calamita M, Salama H, Cabral G. Prosthetic gingival reconstruction in a fixed partial restoration. Part 1: Introduction to artificial gingiva as an alternative therapy. Int J Periodontics Restorative Dent 2009;29:471–477.
13. Misch CE, Goodacre CJ, Finley JM, et al. Consensus conference panel report: Crown-height space guidelines for implant dentistry. Part 2. Implant Dent 2006;15:113–121.
14. Sherif S, Susarla HK, Kapos T, Munoz D, Chang BM, Wright RF. A systematic review of screw- versus cement-retained implant-supported fixed restorations. J Prosthodont 2014;23:1–9.
15. Jung RE, Zembic A, Pjetursson BE, Zwahlen M, Thoma DS. Systematic review of the survival rate and the incidence of biological, technical, and aesthetic complications of single crowns on implants reported in longitudinal studies with a mean follow-up of 5 years. Clin Oral Implants Res 2012;23(suppl 6):2–21.
16. Garber DA. The esthetic dental implant: Letting restoration be the guide. J Am Dent Assoc 1995;126:319–325.
17. Blustein R, Jackson R, Rotskoff K, Coy RE, Godar D. Use of splint material in the placement of implants. Int J Oral Maxillofac Implants 1986;1:47–49.
18. Engelman MJ, Sorensen JA, Moy P. Optimum placement of osseointegrated implants. J Prosthet Dent 1988;59:467–473.
19. Lee SY, Morgano SM. A diagnostic stent for endosseous implants to improve conventional tomographic radiographs. J Prosthet Dent 1994;71:482–485.
20. Dixon DL, Breeding LC. Surgical guide fabrication for an angled implant. J Prosthet Dent 1996;75:562–565.
21. Orentlicher G, Abboud M. Guided surgery for implant therapy. Oral Maxillofac Surg Clin North Am 2011;23:239–256.
22. Sarment DP, Sukovic P, Clinthorne N. Accuracy of implant placement with a stereolithographic surgical guide. Int J Oral Maxillofac Implants 2003;18:571–577.
23. Nokar S, Moslehifard E, Bahman T, Bayanzadeh M, Nasirpouri F, Nokar A. Accuracy of implant placement using a CAD/CAM surgical guide: An in vitro study. Int J Oral Maxillofac Implants 2011;26:520–526.
24. Park C, Raigrodski AJ, Rosen J, Spiekerman C, London RM. Accuracy of implant placement using precision surgical guides with varying occlusogingival heights: An in vitro study. J Prosthet Dent 2009;101:372–381.
25. Farley NE, Kennedy K, McGlumphy EA, Clelland NL. Split-mouth comparison of the accuracy of computer-generated and conventional surgical guides. Int J Oral Maxillofac Implants 2013;28:563–572.
26. Valente F, Schiroli G, Sbrenna A. Accuracy of computer-aided oral implant surgery: A clinical and radiographic study. Int J Oral Maxillofac Implants 2009;24:234–242.
27. Pettersson A, Kero T, Gillot L, et al. Accuracy of CAD/CAM-guided surgical template implant surgery on human cadavers: Part I. J Prosthet Dent 2010;103:334–342.
28. Brånemark PI. Osseointegration and its experimental background. J Prosthet Dent 1983;50:399–410.
29. Klineberg IJ, Murray GM. Design of superstructures for osseointegrated fixtures. Swed Dent J 1985;28:63–69.
30. Jemt T. Failures and complications in 391 consecutively inserted fixed prostheses supported by Brånemark implant in the edentulous jaw: A study of treatment from the time of prosthesis placement to the first annual checkup. Int J Oral Maxillofac Implants 1991; 6:270–276.
31. Kan JY, Rungcharassaeng K, Bohsali K, Goodacre CJ, Lang BR. Clinical methods for evaluating implant framework fit. J Prosthet Dent 1999;81:7–13.
32. Lee H, Ercoli C, Funkenbusch PD, Feng C. Effect of subgingival depth of implant placement on the dimensional accuracy of the implant impression: An in vitro study. J Prosthet Dent 2008;99:107–113.
33. Papaspyridakos P, Lal K, White GS, Weber HP, Gallucci GO. Effect of splinted and nonsplinted impression techniques on the accuracy of fit of fixed implant prostheses in edentulous patients: A comparative study. Int J Oral Maxillofac Implants 2011;26:1267–1272.
34. Karl M, Graef F, Heckmann S, Taylor T. A methodology to study the effects of prosthesis misfit over time: An in vivo model. Int J Oral Maxillofac Implants 2009;24:689–694.
35. Abduo J, Bennani V, Waddell N, Lyons K, Swain M. Assessing the fit of implant fixed prostheses: A critical review. Int J Oral Maxillofac Implants 2010;25:506–515.
36. Baig MR. Multi-unit implant impression accuracy: A review of the literature. Quintessence Int 2014;45:39–51.
37. Abduo J, Swain M. Influence of vertical misfit of titanium and zirconia frameworks on peri-implant strain. Int J Oral Maxillofac Implants 2012;27:529–536.
38. Chee W, Jivraj S. Impression techniques for implant dentistry. Br Dent J 2006;201:429–432.
39. Lee H, So JS, Hochstedler JL, Ercoli C. The accuracy of implant impressions: A systematic review. J Prosthet Dent 2008;100:285–291.
40. Jemt T, Book K. Prosthesis misfit and marginal bone loss in edentulous implant patients. Int J Oral Maxillofac Implants 1996;11:620–625.
41. Sahin S, Cehreli MC. The significance of passive framework fit in implant prosthodontics: Current status. Implant Dent 2001;10:85–92.
42. Gracis S, Michalakis K, Vigolo P, Vult von Steyern P, Zwahlen M, Sailer I. Internal vs. external connections for abutments/reconstructions: A systematic review. Clin Oral Implants Res 2012;23(suppl 6):202–216.
43. Bergin JM, Rubenstein JE, Mancl LA, Brudvik JS, Raigrodski AJ. An in vitro comparison of photogrammetric and conventional complete arch implant impression techniques. J Prosthet Dent 2013; 110:243–251.
44. Vigolo P, Majzoub Z, Cordioli G. Evaluation of the accuracy of three techniques used for multiple implant abutment impressions. J Prosthet Dent 2003;89:186–192.
45. Vigolo P, Fonzi F, Majzoub Z, Cordioli G. An evaluation of impression techniques for multiple internal connection implant prostheses. J Prosthet Dent 2004;92:470–476.

46. Filho HG, Mazaro JV, Vedovatto E, Assunção WG, dos Santos PH. Accuracy of impression techniques for implants. Part 2: Comparison of splinting techniques. J Prosthodont 2009;18:172–176.
47. Mostafa TM, Elgendy MN, Kashef NA, Halim MM. Evaluation of the precision of three implant transfer impression techniques using two elastomeric impression materials. Int J Prosthodont 2010;23:525–528.
48. Chang WG, Vahidi F, Bae KH, Lim BS. Accuracy of three implant impression techniques with different impression materials and stones. Int J Prosthodont 2012;25:44–47.
49. Ongül D, Gökçen-Röhlig B, Sermet B, Keskin H. A comparative analysis of the accuracy of different direct impression techniques for multiple implants. Aust Dent J 2012;57:184–189.
50. Stimmelmayr M, Erdelt K, Güth JF, Happe A, Beuer F. Evaluation of impression accuracy for a four-implant mandibular model—A digital approach. Clin Oral Investig 2012;16:1137–1142.
51. Carr AB. Comparison of impression techniques for a five-implant mandibular model. Int J Oral Maxillofac Implants 1991;6:448–455.
52. Conrad HJ, Pesun IJ, DeLong R, Hodges JS. Accuracy of two impression techniques with angulated implants. J Prosthet Dent 2007;97:349–356.
53. Jo SH, Kim KI, Seo JM, Song KY, Park JM, Ahn SG. Effect of impression coping and implant angulation on the accuracy of implant impressions: An in vitro study. J Adv Prosthodont 2010;2:128–133.
54. Sorrentino R, Gherlone EF, Calesini G, Zarone F. Effect of implant angulation, connection length, and impression material on the dimensional accuracy of implant impressions: An in vitro comparative study. Clin Implant Dent Relat Res 2010;12(suppl 1):e63–e76.
55. Bartlett DW, Greenwood R, Howe L. The suitability of head-of-implant and conventional abutment impression techniques for implant-retained three unit bridges: An in vitro study. Eur J Prosthodont Restor Dent 2002;10:163–166.
56. McCartney JW, Pearson R. Segmental framework matrix: Master cast verification, corrected cast guide, and analog transfer template for implant-supported prostheses. J Prosthet Dent 1994;71:197–200.
57. Yanase RT, Binon PP, Jemt T, Gulbransen HJ, Parel S. Current issues forum. How do you test a cast framework fit or a full-arch fixed implant-supported prosthesis? Int J Oral Maxillofac Implants 1994; 9:471–474.
58. Hebel KS, Galindo D, Gajjar RC. Implant position record and implant position cast: Minimizing errors, procedures and patient visits in the fabrication of the milled-bar prosthesis. J Prosthet Dent 2000; 83:107–116.
59. De La Cruz JE, Funkenbusch PD, Ercoli C, Moss ME, Graser GN, Tallents RH. Verification jig for implant-supported prostheses: A comparison of standard impressions with verification jigs made of different materials. J Prosthet Dent 2002;88:329–336.
60. Ercoli C, Geminiani A, Feng C, Lee H. The influence of verification jig on framework fit for nonsegmented fixed implant-supported complete denture. Clin Implant Dent Relat Res 2012;14(suppl 1):e188–e195.
61. Taylor TD. Prosthodontic complications associated with implant therapy. Oral Maxillofac Surg Clin North Am 1991;3:979–992.
62. Ortorp A, Jemt T, Bäck T, Jälevik T. Comparisons of precision of fit between cast and CNC-milled titanium implant frameworks for the edentulous mandible. Int J Prosthodont 2003;16:194–200.
63. Al-Fadda SA, Zarb GA, Finer Y. A comparison of the accuracy of fit of 2 methods for fabricating implant-prosthodontic frameworks. Int J Prosthodont 2007;20:125–131.
64. Drago C, Saldarriaga RL, Domagala D, Almasri R. Volumetric determination of the amount of misfit in CAD/CAM and cast implant frameworks: A multicenter laboratory study. Int J Oral Maxillofac Implants 2010;25:920–929.
65. Karl M, Holst S. Strain development of screw-retained implant-supported fixed restorations: Procera implant bridge versus conventionally cast restorations. Int J Prosthodont 2012;25:166–169.
66. Kapos T, Ashy LM, Gallucci GO, Weber HP, Wismeijer D. Computer-aided design and computer-assisted manufacturing in prosthetic implant dentistry. Int J Oral Maxillofac Implants 2009;24:110–117.
67. Apicella D, Veltri M, Chieffi N, Polimeni A, Giovannetti A, Ferrari M. Implant adaptation of stock abutments versus CAD/CAM abutments: A radiographic and scanning electron microscopy study. Ann Stomatol 2010;1:9–13.
68. Piconi C, Burger W, Richter HG, et al. Y-TZP ceramics for artificial joint replacements. Biomaterials 1998;19:1489–1494.
69. Piconi C, Maccauro G. Zirconia as a ceramic biomaterial. Biomaterials 1999;20:1–25.
70. Christel P, Meunier A, Heller M, Torre JP, Peille CN. Mechanical properties and short-term in-vivo evaluation of yttrium-oxide-partially-stabilized zirconia. J Biomed Mater Res 1989;23:45–61.
71. Garvie RC, Hannink RH, Pascoe RT. Ceramic steel? Nature 1975; 258:703–704.
72. Lughi V, Sergo V. Low temperature degradation -aging- of zirconia: A critical review of the relevant aspects in dentistry. Dent Mater 2010;26:807–820.
73. Tinschert J, Natt G, Mautsch W, Augthun M, Spiekermann H. Fracture resistance of lithium disilicate-, alumina-, and zirconia-based three-unit fixed partial dentures: A laboratory study. Int J Prosthodont 2001;14:231–238.
74. Kobayashi K, Kuwajima H, Masaki T. Phase change and mechanical properties of ZrO2-Y2O3 solid electrolyte after aging. Solid State Ionics 1981;3:489–493.
75. Lange FF, Dunlop GL, Davis BI. Degradation during aging of transformation-toughened ZrO2-Y2O3 materials at 250°C. J Am Ceram Soc 1986;69:237–240.
76. Yoshimura M. Phase stability of zirconia. Am Ceram Soc Bull 1988; 67:1950–1955.
77. Flinn BD, deGroot DA, Mancl LA, Raigrodski AJ. Accelerated aging characteristics of three tetragonal zirconia polycrystal dental materials. J Prosthet Dent 2012;108:223–230.
78. Flinn BD, Raigrodski AJ, Singh A, Mancl LA. Effect of hydrothermal degradation on three types of zirconia for dental application. J Prosthet Dent 2014;112:1377–1384.
79. Marx R, Jungwirth F, Walter PO. Threshold intensity factors as lower boundaries for crack propagation in ceramics. Biomed Eng Online 2004;3:41.
80. Taskonak B, Griggs JA, Mecholsky JJ, Yan JH. Analysis of subcritical crack growth in dental ceramics using fracture mechanics and fractography. Dent Mater 2008;24:700–707.
81. Kosmac T, Oblak C, Jevinkar P, Fundunk N, Marion L. Strength and reliability of surface treated Y-TZP dental ceramics. J Biomed Mater Res 2000;53:304–313.
82. Vigolo P, Fonzi F. An in vitro evaluation of fit of zirconium-oxide-based ceramic four-unit fixed partial dentures, generated with three different CAD/CAM systems, before and after porcelain firing cycles and after glaze cycles. J Prosthodont 2008;17:621–626.
83. Kohorst P, Brinkmann H, Dittmer MP, Borchers L, Stiesch M. Influence of the veneering process on the marginal fit of zirconia fixed dental prostheses. J Oral Rehabil 2010;37:283–291.
84. Covacci V, Bruzzese N, Maccauro G, et al. In vitro evaluation of the mutagenic and carcinogenic power of high purity zirconia ceramic. Biomaterials 1999;20:371–376.
85. Warashina H, Sakano S, Kitamura S, et al. Biological reaction to alumina, zirconia, titanium and polyethylene particles implanted onto murine calvaria. Biomaterials 2003;24:3655–3661.
86. Scarano A, Piattelli M, Caputi S, Favero GA, Piattelli A. Bacterial adhesion on commercially pure titanium and zirconium oxide disks: An in vivo human study. J Periodontol 2004;75:292–296.
87. Chiche GJ, Pinault A. Esthetics of Anterior Fixed Prosthodontics. Chicago: Quintessence, 1994:78–94,97–114.
88. Dozic A, Kleverlaan CJ, Meegdes M, van der Zel J, Feilzer AJ. The influence of porcelain layer thickness on the final shade of ceramic restorations. J Prosthet Dent 2003;90:563–570.
89. Baldissara P, Llukacej A, Ciocca L, Valandro FL, Scotti R. Translucency of zirconia copings made with different CAD/CAM systems. J Prosthet Dent 2010;104:6–12.

90. Jung RE, Sailer I, Hämmerle CH, Attin T, Schmidlin P. In vitro color changes of soft tissues caused by restorative materials. Int J Periodontics Restorative Dent 2007;27:251–257.
91. Tang X, Nakamura T, Usami H, Wakabayashi K, Yatani H. Effects of multiple firings on the mechanical properties and microstructure of veneering ceramics for zirconia frameworks. J Dent 2012;40:372–380.
92. Ansong R, Flinn B, Chung KH, Mancl L, Ishibe M, Raigrodski AJ. Fracture toughness of heat-pressed and layered ceramics. J Prosthet Dent 2013;109:234–240.
93. Sax C, Hämmerle CH, Sailer I. 10-year clinical outcomes of fixed dental prostheses with zirconia frameworks. Int J Comput Dent 2011;14:183–202.
94. Raigrodski AJ, Hillstead MB, Meng GK, Chung KH. Survival and complications of zirconia-based fixed dental prostheses: A systematic review. J Prosthet Dent 2012;107:170–177.
95. Papaspyridakos P, Lal K. Computer-assisted design/computer-assisted manufacturing zirconia implant fixed complete prostheses: Clinical results and technical complications up to 4 years of function. Clin Oral Implants Res 2013;24:659–665.
96. Limmer B, Sanders AE, Reside G, Cooper LF. Complications and patient-centered outcomes with an implant-supported monolithic zirconia fixed dental prosthesis: 1-year results. J Prosthodont 2014; 23:267–275.
97. DeHoff PH, Barrett AA, Lee RB, Anusavice KJ. Thermal compatibility of dental ceramic systems using cylindrical and spherical geometries. Dent Mater 2008;24:744–752.
98. Hallmann L, Ulmer P, Wille S, Kern M. Effect of differences in coefficient of thermal expansion of veneer and Y-TZP ceramics on interface phase transformation. J Prosthet Dent 2014;112:591–599.
99. Rosentritt M, Steiger D, Behr M, Handel G, Kolbeck C. Influence of substructure design and spacer settings on the in vitro performance of molar zirconia crowns. J Dent 2009;37:978–983.
100. Mainjot AK, Schajer GS, Vanheusden AJ, Sadoun MJ. Influence of zirconia framework thickness on residual stress profile in veneering ceramic: Measurement by hole-drilling. Dent Mater 2012;28:378–384.
101. Okabayashi S, Nomoto S, Sato T, Miho O. Influence of proximal supportive design of zirconia framework on fracture load of veneering porcelain. Dent Mater J 2013;32:572–577.
102. Al-Dohan HM, Yaman P, Dennison JB, Razzoog ME, Lang BR. Shear strength of core-veneer interface in bi-layered ceramics. J Prosthet Dent 2004;91:349–355.
103. Beuer F, Edelhoff D, Gernet W, Sorensen JA. Three-year clinical prospective evaluation of zirconia-based posterior fixed dental prostheses (FDPs). Clin Oral Investig 2009;13:445–451.
104. Christensen RP, Ploeger BJ. A clinical comparison of zirconia, metal and alumina fixed-prosthesis frameworks veneered with GC Pattern Resin or pressed ceramic: A three-year report. J Am Dent Assoc 2010;141:1317–1329.
105. Ishibe M, Raigrodski AJ, Flinn BD, Chung KH, Spiekerman C, Winter RR. Shear bond strengths of pressed and layered veneering ceramics to high-noble alloy and zirconia cores. J Prosthet Dent 2011;106:29–37.
106. Tan JP, Sederstrom D, Polansky JR, McLaren EA, White SN. The use of slow heating and slow cooling regimens to strengthen porcelain fused to zirconia. J Prosthet Dent 2012;107:163–169.
107. Preis V, Letsch C, Handel G, Behr M, Schneider-Feyrer S, Rosentritt M. Influence of substructure design, veneer application technique, and firing regime on the in vitro performance of molar zirconia crowns. Dent Mater 2013;29:e113–e121.
108. Cho Y, Raigrodski AJ. The rehabilitation of an edentulous mandible with a CAD/CAM zirconia framework and heat-pressed lithium disilicate ceramic crowns: A clinical report. J Prosthet Dent 2014; 111:443–447.
109. Çiftçi Y, Canay S. The effect of veneering materials on stress distribution in implant-supported fixed prosthetic restorations. Int J Oral Maxillofac Implants 2000;15:571–582.
110. Takahashi Y, Hisama K, Sato H, et al. Probability of failure of highly filled indirect resin-veneered implant-supported restorations: An in vitro study. Int J Prosthodont 2002;15:179–182.
111. Komine F, Kobayashi K, Blatz MB, et al. Durability of bond between an indirect composite veneering material and zirconium dioxide ceramics. Acta Odontol Scand 2013;71:457–463.
112. Rojas-Vizcaya F. Full zirconia fixed detachable implant-retained restorations manufactured from monolithic zirconia: Clinical report after two years in service. J Prosthodont 2011;20:570–576.
113. Raigrodski AJ. Managing prosthetic challenges with a CAD/CAM zirconia from bilayered to monolithic. J Cosmet Dent 2014;30:40–52.
114. Pittayachawan P, McDonald A, Young A, Knowles JC. Flexural strength, fatigue life, and stress-induced phase transformation study of Y-TZP dental ceramic. J Biomed Mater Res B Appl Biomater 2009;88:366–377.
115. Shijo Y, Shinya A, Gomi A, Lassila LV, Vallittu PK, Shinya A. Studies on mechanical strength, thermal expansion of layering porcelains to alumina and zirconia ceramic core materials. Dent Mater J 2009;28:352–361.
116. Beuer F, Stimmelmayr M, Gueth JF, Edelhoff D, Naumann M. In vitro performance of full-contour zirconia single crowns. Dent Mater 2012;28:449–456.
117. Janyavula S, Lawson N, Cakir D, Beck P, Ramp LC, Burgess JO. The wear of polished and glazed zirconia against enamel. J Prosthet Dent 2013;109:22–29.
118. Preis V, Weiser F, Handel G, Rosentritt M. Wear performance of monolithic dental ceramics with different surface treatments. Quintessence Int 2013;44:393–405.
119. Stawarczyk B, Özcan M, Schmutz F, Trottmann A, Roos M, Hämmerle CH. Two-body wear of monolithic, veneered and glazed zirconia and their corresponding enamel antagonists. Acta Odontol Scand 2013;71:102–112.
120. Park JM, Park S, Lee K, Yun KD, Lim HP. Antagonist wear of three CAD/CAM anatomic contour zirconia ceramics. J Prosthet Dent 2014;111:20–29.
121. Jung YS, Lee JW, Choi YJ, Ahn JS, Shin SW, Huh JB. A study on the in-vitro wear of the natural tooth structure by opposing zirconia or dental porcelain. J Adv Prosthodont 2010;2:111–115.
122. Kim MJ, Oh SH, Kim JH, et al. Wear evaluation of the human enamel opposing different Y-TZP dental ceramics and other porcelains. J Dent 2012;40:979–988.
123. Rosentritt M, Preis V, Behr M, Hahnel S, Handel G, Kolbeck C. Two-body wear of dental porcelain and substructure oxide ceramics. Clin Oral Investig 2012;16:935–943.
124. Anderson MR, Chung KH, Flinn BD, Raigrodski AJ. An in vitro study of the effect of different restorative materials on the reliability of a veneering porcelain. J Prosthet Dent 2013;110:521–528.
125. Stijacic T, Chung KH, Flinn BD, Raigrodski AJ. Effect of tooth-colored restorative materials on reliability of heat-pressed lithium disilicate [epub ahead of print 17 December 2014]. J Prosthodont 2014 doi:10.1111/jopr.12243.

8

Delivery Procedures

Ariel J. Raigrodski | Matthew R. Anderson

The various techniques used to deliver fixed restorations can have a direct impact on the surrounding soft tissues. However, sometimes little consideration may be given to the dentogingival complex around the restorative site during delivery procedures. The soft tissues surrounding a restorative site should not be discounted as an inconvenience to work around or as an aspect of the patient's oral environment that can be manipulated without risks or consequences.[1] As discussed in previous chapters, once clinicians understand the central role a healthy dentogingival complex plays in the esthetic outcome and long-term prognosis of a restoration, they can appreciate how the interplay of restorative steps and procedures leading up to delivery of the restoration can influence the success of a given therapy.

The key to not only maintaining soft tissue health but also enhancing the definitive esthetic outcome of restorations at the soft tissue–restorative interface is understanding the interplay among three considerations: *(1)* tooth and abutment finish line, *(2)* restorative margins, and *(3)* soft tissue quality, quantity, and health.[2] To maintain a harmonious and healthy relationship between any definitive restorations and the surrounding soft tissues, it is important to follow the principles and steps outlined in this chapter during the delivery of any type of indirect restoration. Such a relationship will help facilitate long-term success and, more importantly, patient acceptance of the treatment rendered.

Ceramic Veneers

Ceramic veneers are a conservative and highly esthetic restorative mode of treatment with long-term success that is heavily substantiated within the literature.[3–5] It has been demonstrated that when ceramic veneers are adequately placed, favorable clinical soft tissue response is expected.[5] The success and survival of any ceramic veneer and its esthetic outcome hinge on a meticulous delivery protocol that ensures effective adhesive cementation. A strong and lasting bond between the tooth surface and the ceramic veneer—via a dental adhesive and composite resin cement—is essential for the longevity of the restoration.[5–8] Adequate isolation that prevents contamination of the bonding site by oral fluids is paramount to achieving good adhesion. Contaminants from oral and bodily fluids, such as saliva, crevicular fluid, and blood, can decrease the adhesion and bond strength among the tooth substrate, the dental adhesive and composite resin cement used for delivery, and the ceramic veneer.[5,9] Consequently, this can contribute to the formation of discolored margins, poor marginal integrity, secondary caries, minor ceramic fractures, loss of retention, or catastrophic failure in the form of a major fracture of the veneer.[10] Thus, the role of soft tissue health in fulfilling this requirement cannot be overstated.

As mentioned in previous chapters, all of the restorative procedures performed in the process of restoring patients

Continued from chapter 5

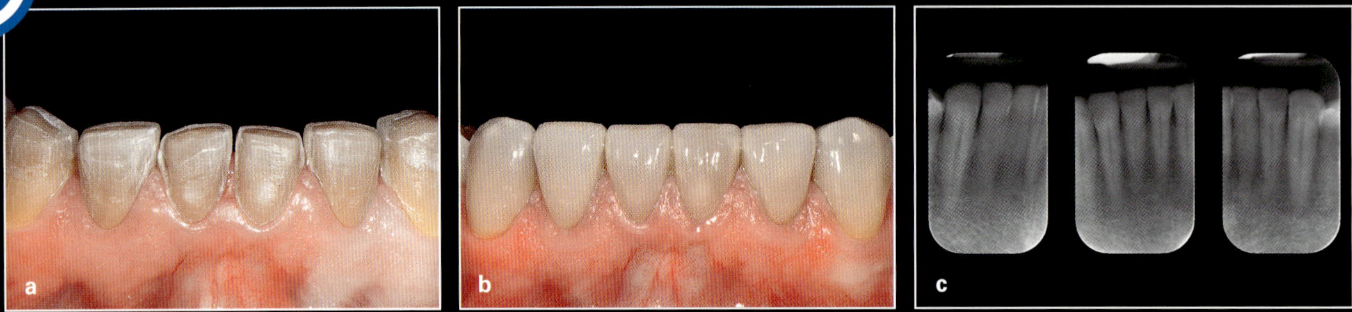

Fig 8-1 *(a)* Facial view of definitive tooth preparations for mandibular ceramic veneers. *(b)* Facial view of the definitive lithium disilicate ceramic veneers (e.max, Ivoclar Vivadent) a few weeks after delivery. Note the gingival health. *(c)* Periapical radiographs confirming residual excess cement removal at the interproximal aspects.

with ceramic veneers should be conducted with adequate soft tissue health as a principal goal. These include tooth preparation procedures with the finish line placement in relation to the free gingival margins, fabrication of provisional restorations, and impression procedures.[8] Not only will healthy soft tissues decrease any discomfort on the part of the patient, but they will also help to minimize complications associated with the delivery procedures.[11]

Although the finish line for these restorations is preferably placed supragingivally,[12] clinical findings such as dental caries, preexisting restorations, cervical discoloration, diastemata, and black triangles may all necessitate a subgingival finish line placement[13] (Figs 8-1 and 8-2). Regardless of the finish line location, proper isolation is still required to ensure that the tooth surface remains dry and free from contamination throughout delivery. Rubber dam in conjunction with the use of retraction cord is ideal for isolation. A narrow-diameter retraction cord (Ultrapak #000, Ultradent) is often sufficient[14] (see Fig 8-2p). When gently placed into the sulcus, the cord serves both to absorb any heme and gingival crevicular fluid and to limit the depth of any apical migration of cement, which facilitates the atraumatic removal of any excess cement. The narrow diameter of the cord helps to ensure adequate tissue displacement with minimal trauma.[15–17] It is the authors' experience that 000-diameter cord not impregnated with a hemostatic agent is sufficient to act as a barrier and delicate enough to ensure an atraumatic placement that minimizes the risk of gingival recession postcementation.[18–20]

The cord is cut to a length that enables it to be placed along the sulcus without the risk of any free ends interfering with the adhesive cementation procedure. To prevent any inadvertent tearing of the sulcular epithelium, the cord should be moistened with water.[19] Subsequently, it is measured and then placed in the sulcus using gentle pressure. Caution must be applied during this phase of delivery so as not to leave any stray fibers outside of the sulcus, which can become caught between the finish line of the tooth preparation and the margins of the restoration during the seating procedure.

The light-polymerized nature of the composite resin cement used in the delivery of ceramic veneers, with their high translucency and relative thinness, affords the clinician an infinite amount of working time to properly seat a restoration. This also provides an opportunity for the clinician to gently remove as much of the cement as atraumatically as possible prior to polymerization. Once the bulk of the gross cement has been removed, one may proceed with the polymerization procedure of the cement. One technique that may be used to remove excess cement prior to polymerization is the spot-cure technique. This approach utilizes a narrow-diameter tip of the curing light, which is briefly applied on the midlabial aspect of the veneer, to light-polymerize the composite resin cement. The narrow-diameter light ensures that only a small area of cement is polymerized, which stabilizes the veneer, while the cement around the margins is still not polymerized. Microbrushes and unwaxed braided floss can then be used to gently remove the excess cement at the margins prior to its polymerization.[21]

Once polymerization has been completed, cement remnants are removed with as much caution as possible so as not to traumatize the tissue. After its removal, the cord should be measured to ensure its complete removal and verify that no fragments have been left in the gingival sulcus (see Fig 8-2q). The use of a no. 12 surgical blade and interproximal strips (Sof-Lex, 3M ESPE) can help with its removal in a relatively atraumatic manner (see Figs 8-2r and 8-2s). An explorer is gently used to verify successful cement removal along the margins of the restoration and the gingival sulcus. Such a procedure should cause minimal irreversible trauma to the soft tissue (see Figs 8-2t to 8-2v). Subsequently, radiographs are taken to verify that all excess cement has been removed interproximally (see Figs 8-1c and 8-2ee).

B
Continued from chapter 3

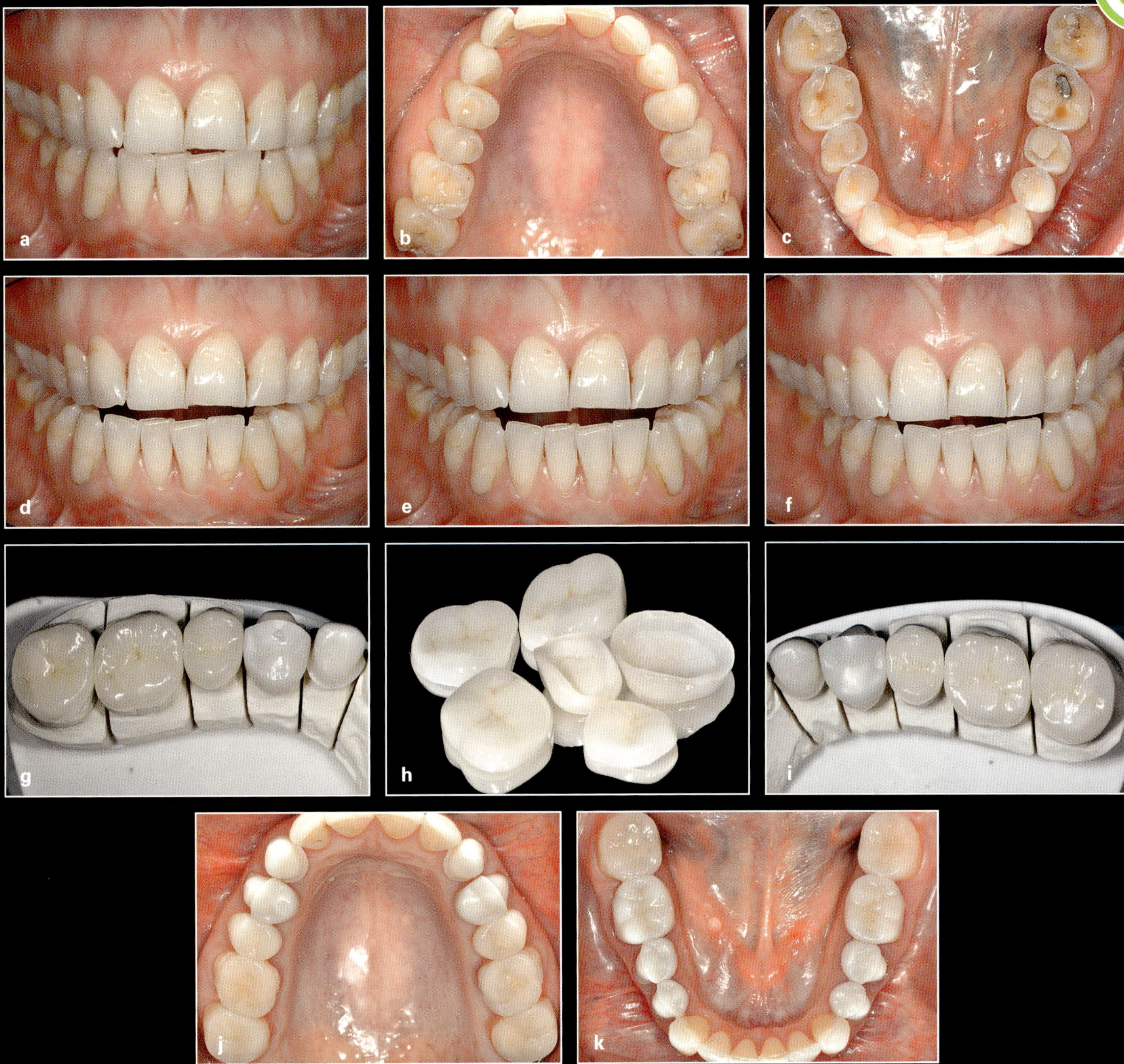

Fig 8-2 *(a)* Preoperative frontal view of a patient in maximal intercuspal position (as seen in chapter 2). *(b and c)* Maxillary and mandibular occlusal views demonstrating wear of the posterior dentition due to parafunction and erosion as well as anterior crowding and rotations. *(d to f)* Frontal views in right lateral, protrusive, and left lateral movements. Note the lack of anterior and canine guidance. *(g to i)* The definitive maxillary posterior monolithic occlusal veneers (0.5 mm) made of lithium disilicate (e.max). The zirconia copings are fabricated with a hybrid design for the maxillary first premolar, and copings designed for bilayered crowns are fabricated for the maxillary canines (Lava Plus, 3M ESPE). *(j and k)* Maxillary and mandibular occlusal views of the patient at try-in of the copings, after delivery of the monolithic posterior occlusal veneers and monolithic zirconia crowns on the mandibular first molars.

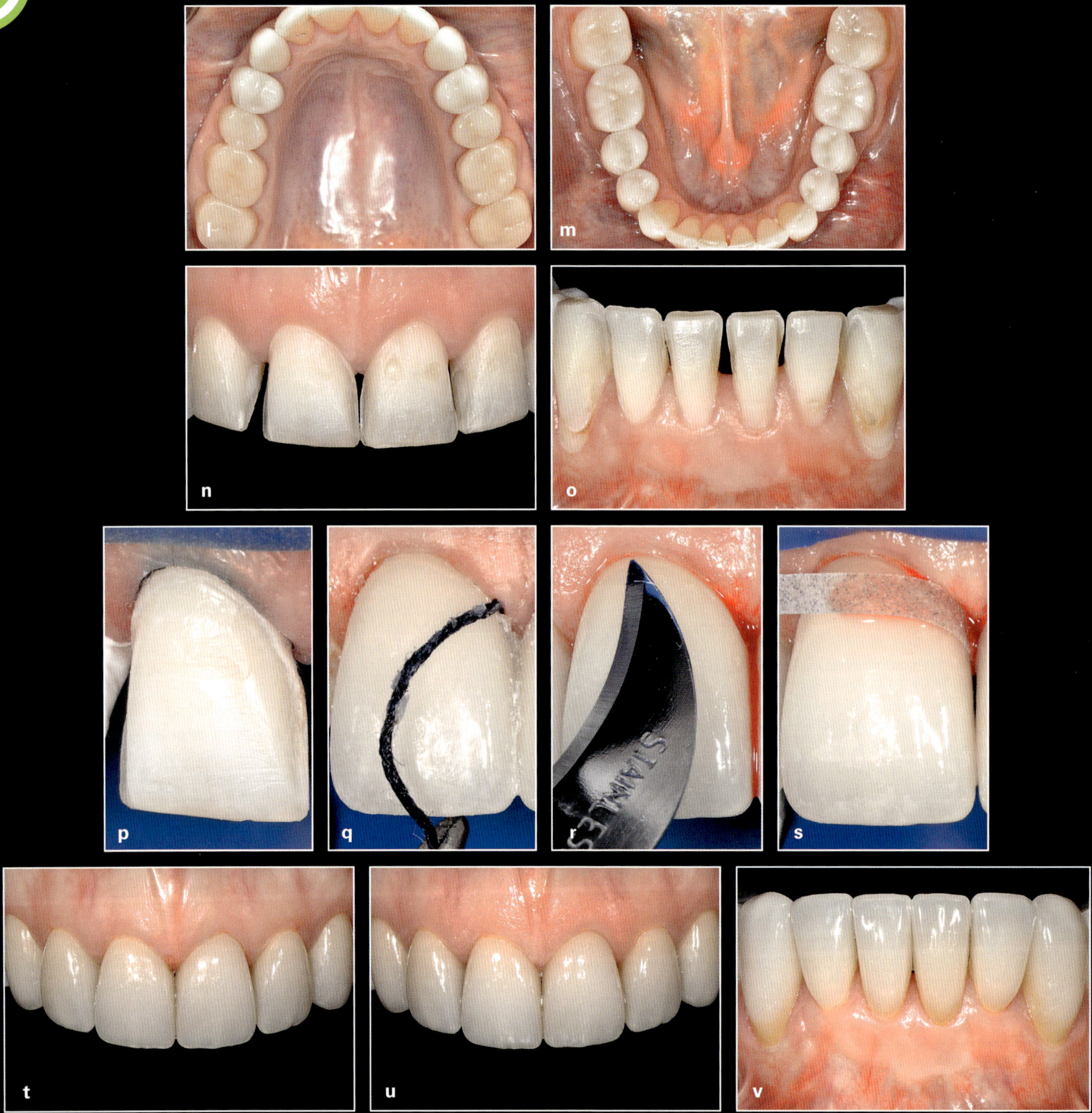

Fig 8-2 *(cont) (l and m)* Maxillary and mandibular occlusal views of the patient after delivery of all posterior restorations and maxillary canine crowns. *(n and o)* Frontal views of the definitive preparations for maxillary and mandibular anterior ceramic labial veneers. *(p)* During the delivery procedure, isolation is achieved with rubber dam and a 000 cord, which also serves as a barrier between the base of the gingival sulcus and the cement. *(q)* Once the gross excess has been removed and the cement is completely polymerized, the cord is gently removed. Note the residual excess cement particles attached to the cord. *(r)* A no. 12 blade is used to ensure complete removal of residual excess cement at the facial and palatal aspects. Care is taken so as not to cause severe trauma to the soft tissue. *(s)* An interproximal polishing strip (Sof-Lex) is used to ensure complete removal of residual excess cement at the mesial and distal interproximal aspects. *(t and u)* Facial view of the four definitive maxillary anterior veneers. Note the initial healing of the soft tissue 1 week after delivery *(t)* and the healed soft tissue 3 weeks after delivery *(u)*. *(v)* Facial view of the six definitive mandibular anterior ceramic labial veneers 3 weeks after delivery. Note the tissue health and the root simulation in terms of shade and contours.

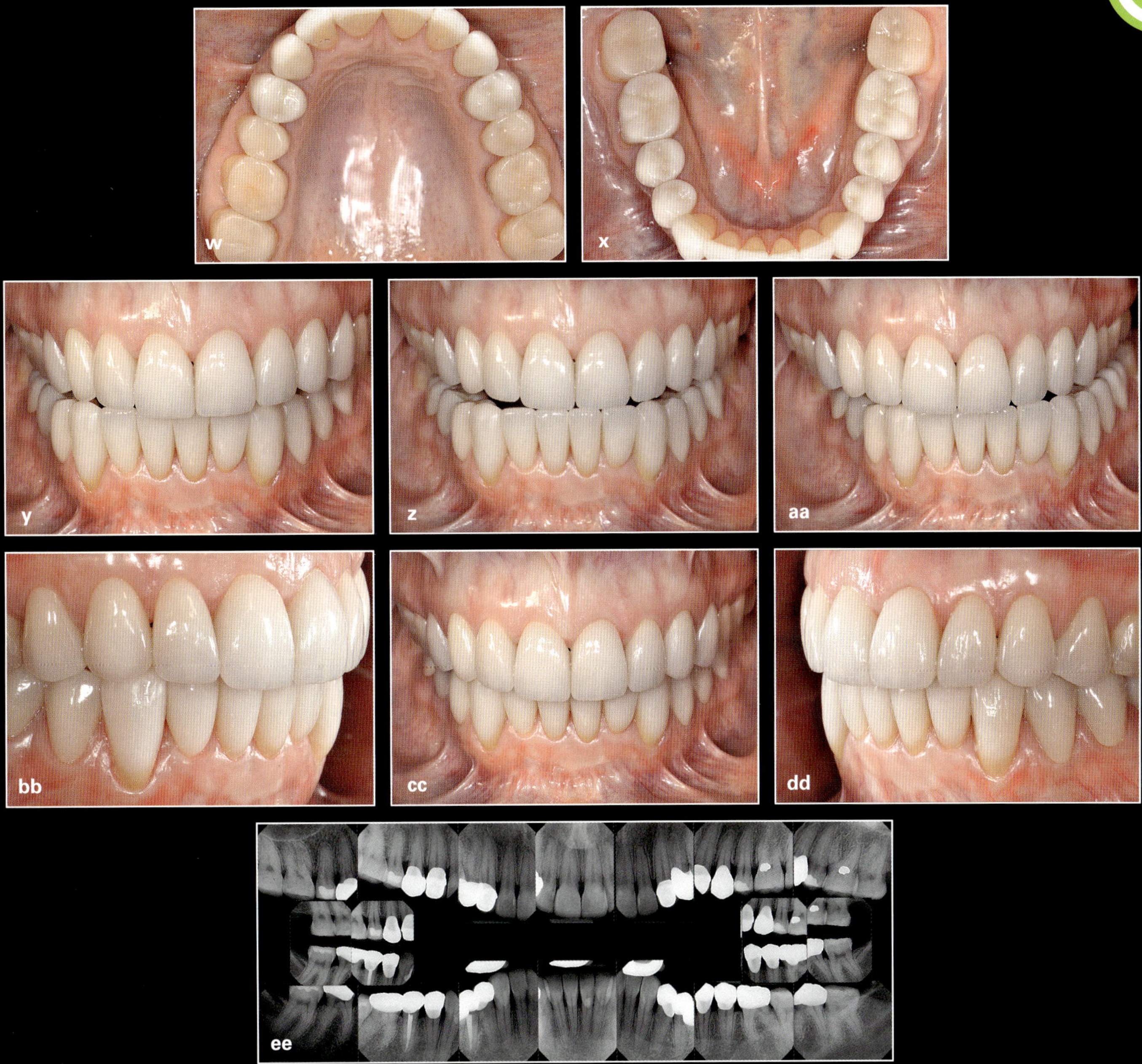

Fig 8-2 *(cont)* *(w and x)* Maxillary and mandibular occlusal views of the complete restorations. The posterior occlusal veneers were matched to the color of the foundation teeth, whereas the color of the crowns and anterior veneers was brighter at the request of the patient. *(y to aa)* Frontal views in right lateral, protrusive, and left lateral movements. Note the bilateral canine guidance in lateral excursions *(y and aa)* and the anterior guidance in protrusive movement *(z)*. *(bb to dd)* Frontal and lateral views in centric occlusion. Mutually protected occlusion has been achieved. *(ee)* Postoperative radiograph demonstrating adequate marginal integrity and no residual excess cement at the interproximal aspects. The patient has received removable Essix retainers as well as a maxillary complete-coverage occlusal guard, providing a mutually protected occlusion.

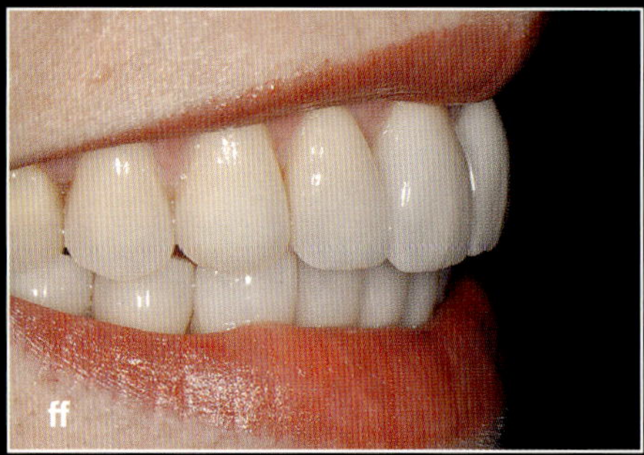

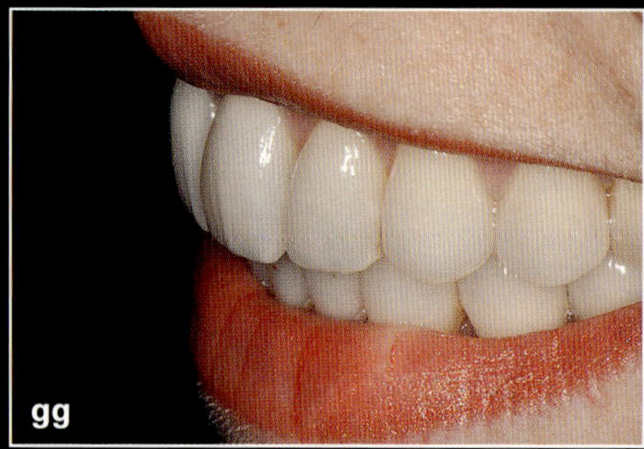

Fig 8-2 *(cont) (ff and gg)* Postoperative lateral views of the patient's new smile.

Conventional Crowns and FDPs

Similar considerations for the delivery of veneers are also applicable when delivering conventional crowns and fixed dental prostheses (FDPs) with composite resin–based cements. One major difference is that autopolymerized or dual-polymerized composite resin cements are used for crowns and FDPs rather than those polymerized solely with light. The nature of these cements necessitates a more rapid and cumbersome excess cement removal procedure that requires diligence on the part of the clinician so as not to cause trauma to the soft tissues. Another difference is that the bonding of these restorations usually occurs to a substrate of dentin, which is less predictable than bonding to enamel, even though constant development in dentin adhesion continues to improve the durability of such bonds.[13] While it is preferable to place the finish line of these restorations coronal to or at the free gingival margins to aid in soft tissue health, a slightly subgingival location is acceptable (Fig 8-3). Subgingival finish line placement should be approached with caution because the further a margin is located apically, the more difficult it is to maintain adequate isolation as well as long-term soft tissue health.[22]

An important consideration in the delivery of such restorations, where the finish line may be placed apical to the free gingival margins, is the radiopacity of the cement. The use of radiopaque cements may facilitate the benefit of a periapical digital radiograph for assessing residual excess cement removal at the interproximal areas.[23] Cements traditionally used for the delivery of complete cast metal and metal-ceramic restorations, such as zinc phosphate and polycarboxylate cements, demonstrated the highest level of radiopacity, similar to that of enamel.[24–26] Many of the composite resin cements currently available for the delivery of ceramic restorations present with radiopacity levels similar to or higher than bovine or human dentin, with some demonstrating radiopacity levels similar to bovine enamel (eg, Variolink II, Ivoclar Vivadent; RelyX Unicem, 3M ESPE).[24,26,27] Therefore, it is important for clinicians to pay consideration to the radiopacity of the cement, in addition to other cement properties, while selecting the cement.[24]

As with light-polymerized composite resin cements, isolation is required with autopolymerized and dual-polymerized composite resin cements. A 000 cord is placed circumferentially around the prepared tooth. Again, the cord should be measured prior to placement and then again after its removal. Care should be taken when placing the cord into the gingival sulcus. Excessive pressure can cause needless tearing of the sulcular epithelium, leading to increased heme and, in extreme cases, gingival recession.[28–30]

The prepared tooth surface should be gently cleaned to remove any surface contaminants to facilitate a more predictable bond between the cement and the dentin substrate[31] (Figs 8-4a to 8-4f). Once the tooth has been cleaned, the restoration is tried in, and the contacts are adjusted to ensure that the restoration is fully seated[14] (Figs 8-4g and 8-4h). Next, the cord is gently delivered into the sulcus. Care should be taken to ensure that blood and oral fluids do not contaminate the prepared dentin substrate. Such contaminants can adversely affect the bond strength between the cement and the tooth structure.[9] The use of rubber dam, cotton rolls, and gauze can help to ensure adequate moisture control. Following the manufacturer's directions for cementation, the bonding procedure is performed; subsequently, a thin coat of cement is applied to the intaglio surface and the margins of the restoration. Too much cement may hinder the seating of the restoration.[32,33] Once the restoration is placed on the prepared tooth, light finger pressure is applied to the occlusal or incisal surface to prevent any dislodgment of the restoration. Excess cement can be initially wiped away with a microbrush.

With some of the cements currently available—including RelyX Unicem 2 (3M ESPE), Multilink Automix (Ivoclar Vivadent), and Panavia SA (Kuraray Noritake)—2 to 5 seconds of tack curing (depending on the brand of cement used) immediately following seating of the restoration will facilitate gross excess cement removal because the cement is polymerized to a lesser degree of hardness and can be

Continued from page 172

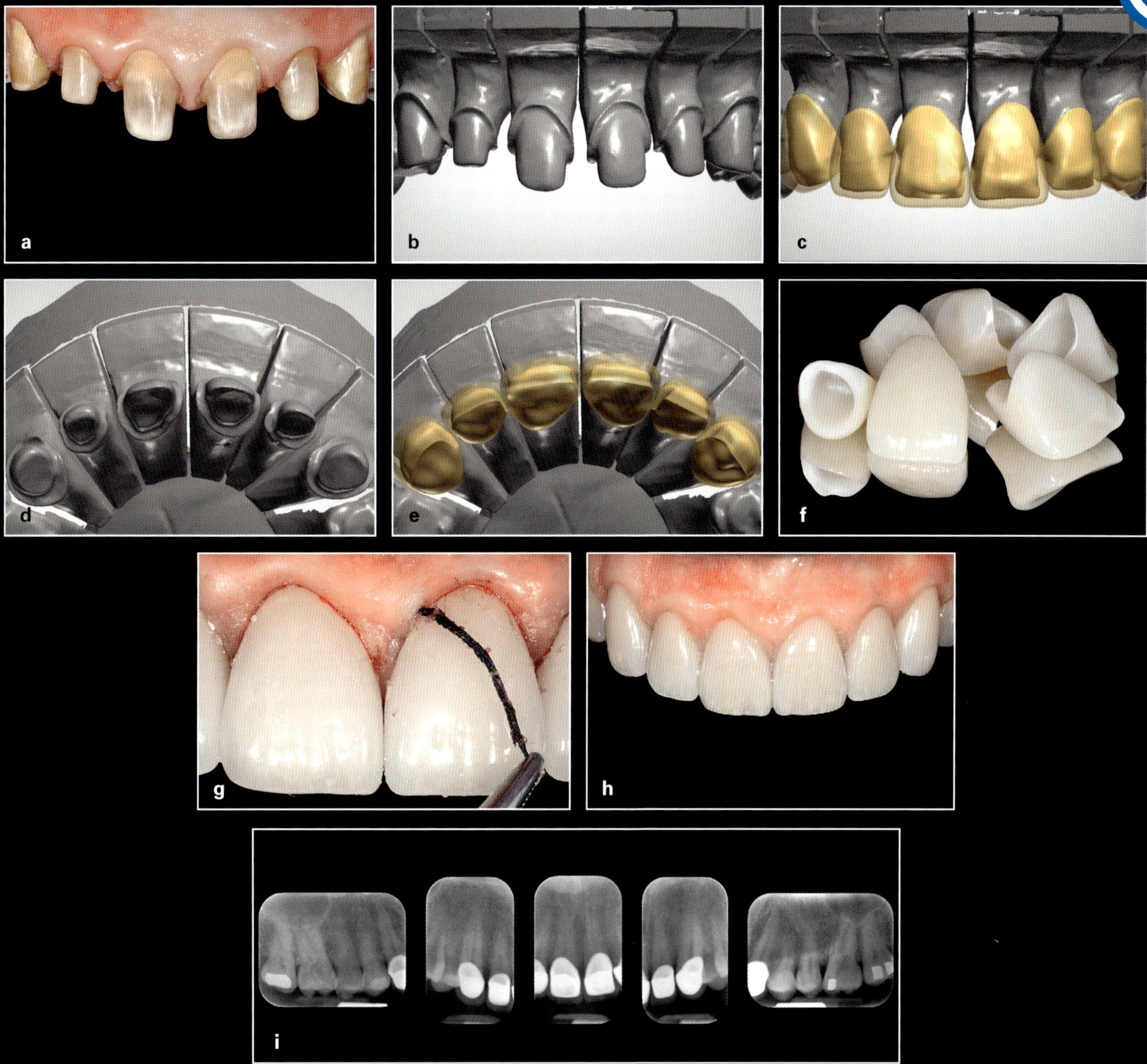

Fig 8-3 *(a)* Facial view of definitive tooth preparations for zirconia-based crowns. *(b and c)* Facial views of the computer-aided design (CAD) image of the tooth preparations *(b)* and the superimposed restorations designed based on a cast of the provisional restorations *(c)*. Note the hybrid design of the copings for zirconia-based restorations (Katana, Kuraray Noritake), simulating a tooth preparation for a ceramic veneer and the space for the veneering ceramic. *(d and e)* Occlusal views of the CAD image of the tooth preparations *(d)* and the superimposed restorations *(e)*. Note the design of the copings for monolithic zirconia on the palatal aspect of the restorations. *(f)* View of the completed zirconia-based crowns. Note the veneering ceramic on the facial and incisal aspects of the restorations. *(g)* Once the cement is completely polymerized, the cord is gently removed. Note the residual excess cement particles attached to the cord. *(h)* View of the definitive restorations a few weeks after delivery. *(i)* Periapical radiographs confirming residual excess cement removal at the interproximal aspects.

easily peeled off and removed. If the cement is completely polymerized, a greater amount of effort will be needed to remove it. Once polymerization has noticeably commenced, the tip of an explorer can be used gently in an apical to coronal direction to remove excess cement. After satisfactory removal of any visually detected excess cement, the light-polymerization procedure at the margins of the restoration is completed. Next, the cord is carefully removed, and the

Continued from chapter 5

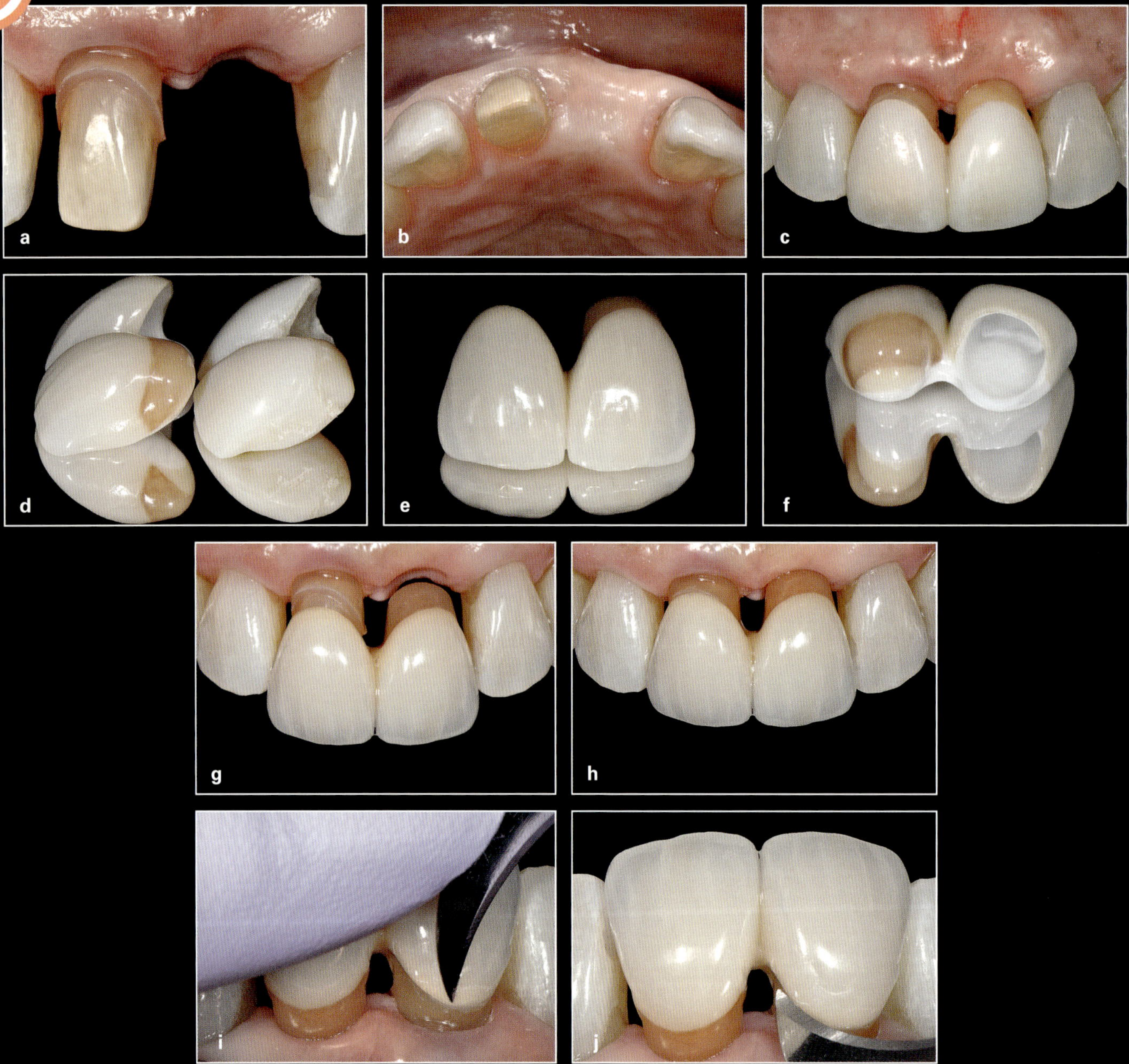

Fig 8-4 *(a and b)* Frontal and palatal views of the definitive tooth preparation for a cantilever zirconia-based FDP (Lava Plus) and the pontic site. *(c)* Frontal view of the provisional restoration approved by the patient. Note the root simulation in terms of shade and contours. *(d)* Proximal view of the provisional and definitive restorations. Note that the pontic convex contours of the definitive restoration are similar to the pontic contours of the provisional restoration. *(e and f)* Views of the definitive restoration. Note the pontic simulating the exposed root of the adjacent maxillary central incisor in terms of shade and contours. *(g and h)* Try-in of the definitive restoration demonstrates the integration of the pontic with the pontic site. *(i and j)* A no. 12 blade is used to ensure complete removal of residual excess cement at the facial and palatal aspects.

interproximal contacts are checked with floss. The cord is then measured to confirm its complete removal. A no. 12 surgical blade and interproximal strips (eg, Sof-Lex) can also be used to remove excess cement (Figs 8-4i to 8-4l). The restoration is then polished with a prophy cup and prophy paste (NUPRO extra care, Orange Polish, Dentsply) to remove any residual excess cement at the soft tissue–restorative interface (Fig 8-4m). Because of the radiopacity of many composite resin cements, a postcementation radiograph is taken to verify that the interproximal areas are clean of residual ex-

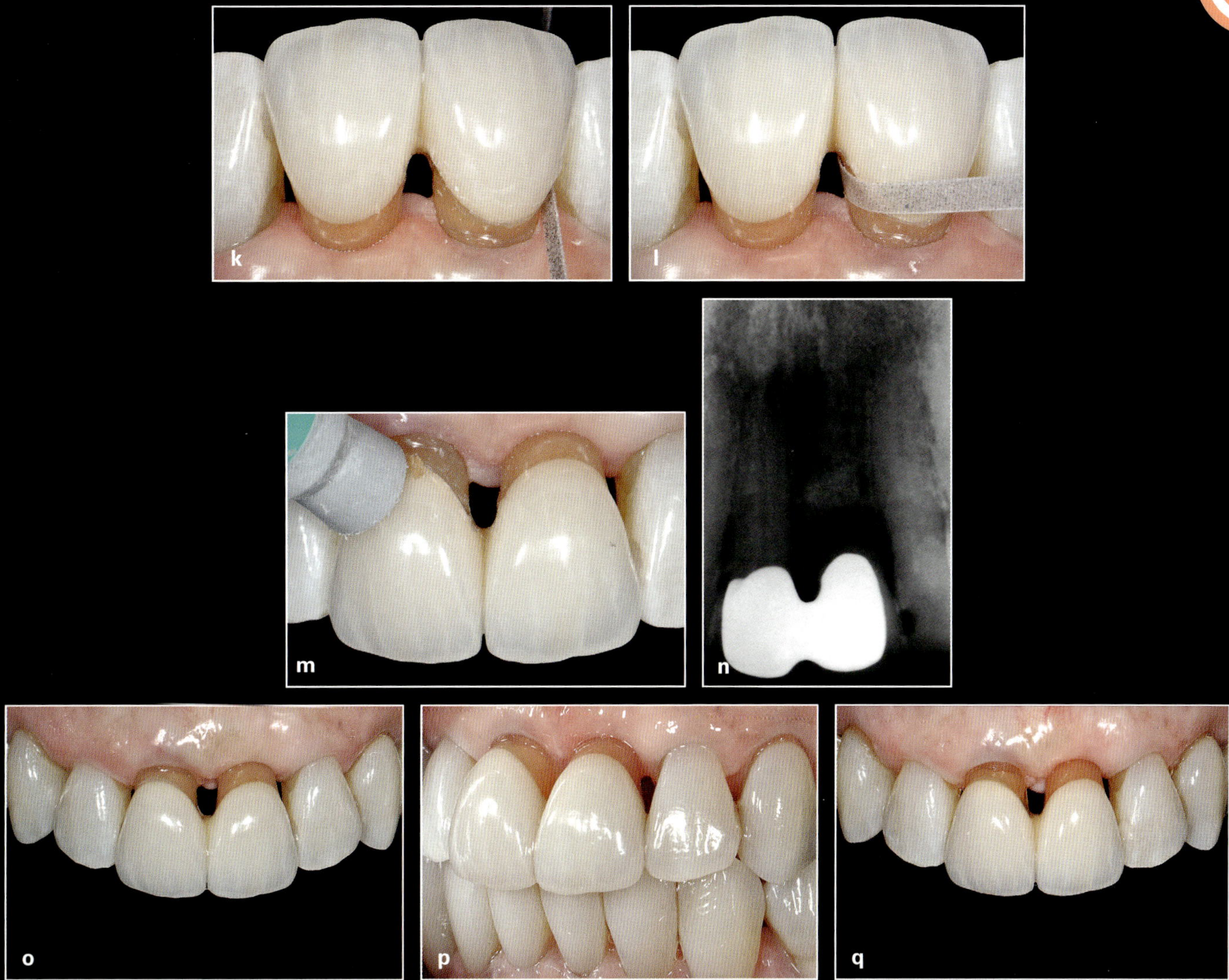

Fig 8-4 *(cont) (k and l)* An interproximal polishing strip (Sof-Lex) is used to ensure complete removal of residual excess cement at the mesial and distal interproximal aspects. *(m)* The restoration is polished with a prophy cup and prophy paste (NUPRO extra care, Orange Polish) to remove any additional excess cement. *(n)* A periapical radiograph is taken to verify adequate marginal integrity. *(o and p)* Facial views of the definitive FDP a few weeks after delivery. Note the blending with the surrounding tissues. *(q)* Facial view of the definitive FDP 2 years after delivery. Note the soft tissue stability at the pontic site.

cess cement (see Fig 8-3i), which will facilitate the health of the tissues surrounding the definitive restoration (Figs 8-4n to 8-4q).

To review, the keys for successful adhesive cementation for ceramic veneers and conventional crowns and FDPs in terms of soft tissue management are the following:

- *Achieve and maintain excellent gingival health.* Heme and gingival crevicular fluid can both adversely affect the adhesion of the cement and lead to staining around the margins of the restoration. Preventing inflammation and trauma to the gingival tissues greatly reduces these risks.
- *Adjust the restorations carefully and adequately during try-in.* Doing so will help to ensure an uneventful and more predictable cementation procedure.
- *Place a moist 000 cord into the gingival sulcus.* No excess cord should come out of the sulcus. Excess cord risks becoming trapped between the tooth preparation finish line and the margins of the restoration during cementation.
- *Gently remove the cord.* Such an approach will prevent the cord from tearing and ensure the verification of its complete removal.
- *Carefully remove all excess cement.* Verify the complete removal of cement both clinically and radiographically.

Pontic sites

An added clinical component to address with regard to adequate soft tissue contours and response during the delivery of FDPs with ovate pontics is the evaluation of the pontic's relationship with the pontic site.[34] Although the contours of the pontic site are transferred to the dental laboratory to facilitate its design (see chapter 5), sometimes the definitive pontic created may still be slightly overcontoured (Figs 8-5a and 8-5b and Figs 8-6a to 8-6c). As a result, excessive pressure of the pontic on the pontic site may generate a blanching reaction of the pontic site during try-in of the FDP (Figs 8-5c and 8-5d). Such a reaction may or may not be reversible after 10 to 15 minutes (Figs 8-5e and 8-5f and Figs 8-6d to 8-6f).

Continued from chapter 5

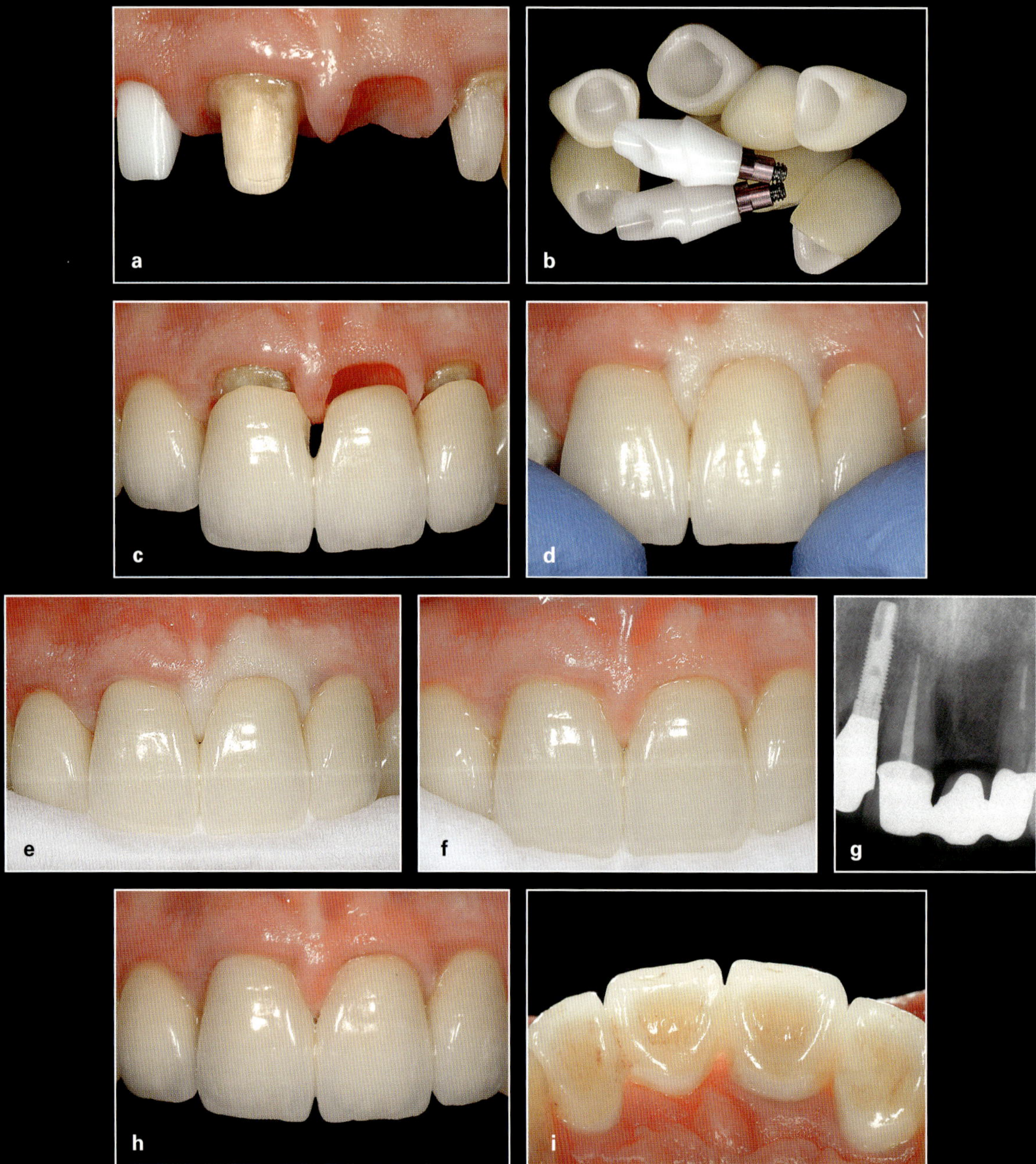

Fig 8-5 *(a)* Frontal view of the definitive custom zirconia abutment (NobelProcera Zirconia, Nobel Biocare) at the site of the maxillary right lateral incisor and the prepared teeth and pontic site for a tooth-supported FDP. *(b)* The complete zirconia-based restoration (Lava, 3M ESPE) with the custom zirconia abutment. Note the convex contours of the pontic. *(c and d)* The try-in procedure demonstrating initial blanching of the pontic site *(d)*. *(e and f)* Within 10 minutes, the blanching gradually disappeared as the patient continued to apply pressure on a cotton roll. *(g)* Periapical radiograph confirming residual excess cement removal at the interproximal aspects as well as excellent marginal integrity. *(h and i)* Frontal and occlusal views of the restoration a few weeks after delivery. Note the integration of the pontic with the soft tissue.

K

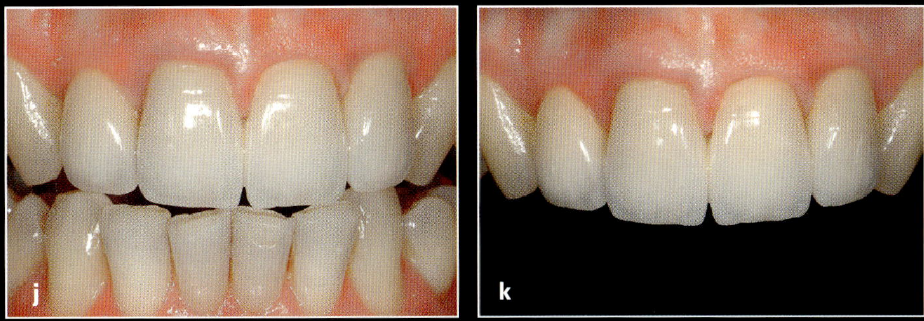

Fig 8-5 *(cont) (j and k)* Frontal views of the restoration 2 years after delivery. Note the stability of the pontic site and the integration in terms of shade matching with the opposing dentition.

C

Continued from chapter 5

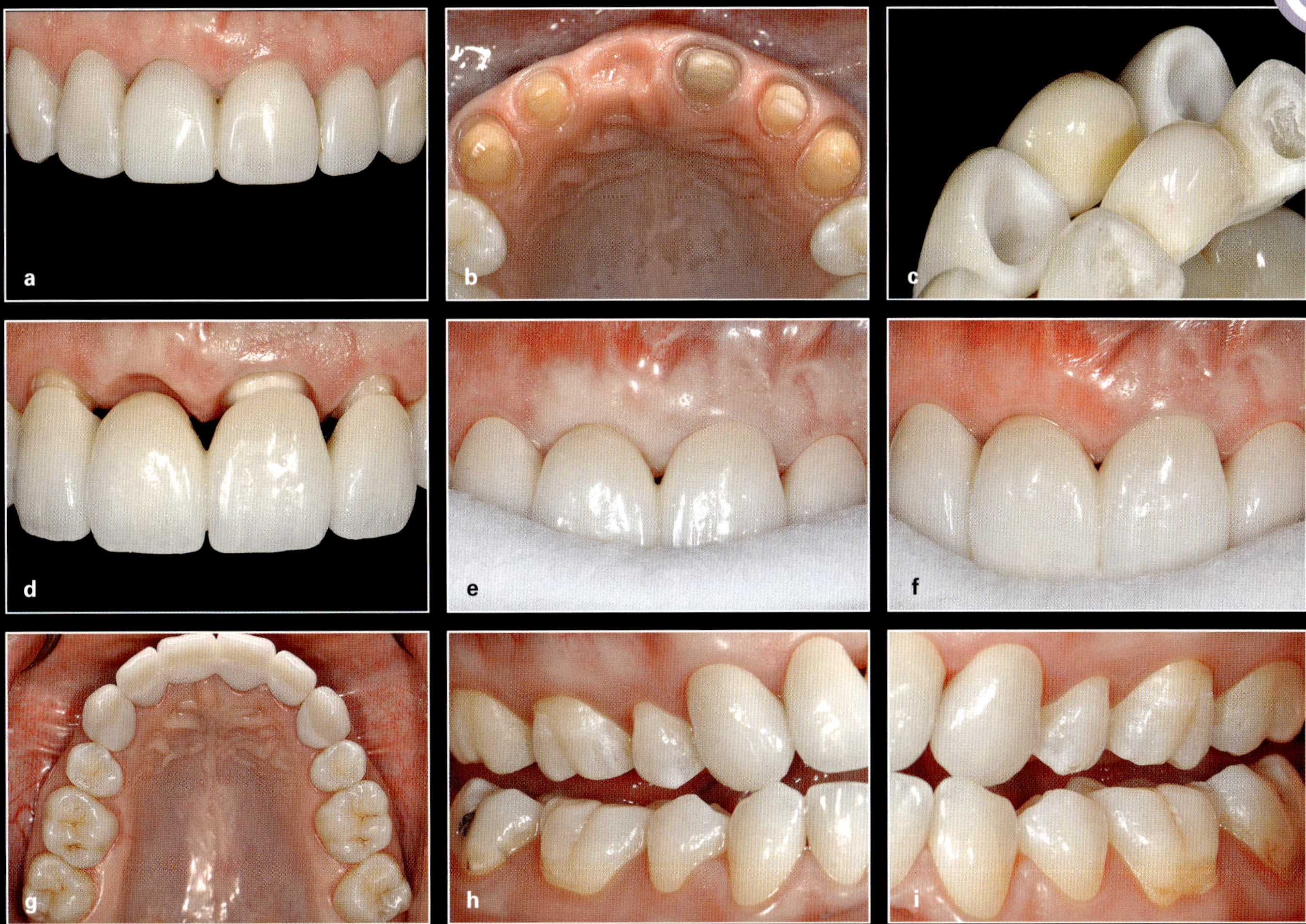

Fig 8-6 *(a)* Frontal view of the provisional restoration with the mature pontic site at the area of the maxillary right central incisor. *(b)* Occlusal view of the definitive restoration and pontic site prior to try-in of the definitive zirconia-based crowns and FDP (Lava). *(c)* Proximal view of the provisional and definitive restorations. Note that the pontic convex contours of the definitive restoration are similar to the pontic contours of the provisional restoration. *(d to f)* Frontal views of the try-in procedure *(d)*. Note the initial blanching that occurred when the patient applied pressure on a cotton roll *(e)*. The transient blanching disappeared after 10 minutes *(f)*. *(g)* Occlusal view of the definitive restoration. *(h and i)* Right and left lateral views demonstrating bilateral canine guidance in lateral excursions.

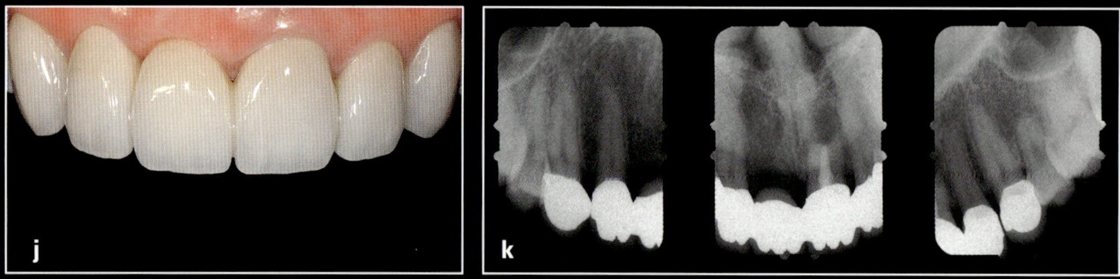

Fig 8-6 *(cont) (j)* Frontal view of the definitive restoration. *(k)* Periapical radiographs confirming residual excess cement removal at the interproximal aspects as well as excellent marginal integrity.

Because the contours of the tissue were predetermined and maintained by the provisional restoration over time, they should not be modified. Thus, the pontic should be adjusted as needed. Therefore, a disclosing agent (Fit Checker, GC America) is applied to the pontic of the FDP to determine the exact location and extent of contact between the pontic and the pontic site.[34] Once it is assessed and adjusted to the desired contours and contact with the pontic site, the pontic can be polished, and the restoration can be delivered[35] (Figs 8-5g to 8-5k and Figs 8-6g to 8-6k).

Cement-Retained Implant-Supported Restorations

In the context of implant-supported restorations, soft tissue health is vital to both maintaining bone levels around the implant body and preserving papillae levels and facial gingival architecture, which are critical factors in the overall esthetics of the definitive implant-supported restoration.[36,37] Compared with the cementation procedure for restorations on natural teeth, cement-retained implant-supported restorations require additional care and consideration. This is because the soft tissue attachment to natural teeth is different from the soft tissue attachment to implants. Therefore, the subgingival area between the implant platform, the abutment finish line, and the free gingival margins must be treated with great care.

As previously described in detail in chapter 1, the soft tissue attachment at the base of the gingival sulcus around natural teeth, commonly referred to as the *biologic width*, is characterized by a long junctional epithelium and a connective tissue attachment.[38] The long junctional epithelium is characterized by a zone of hemidesmosomal attachment, which allows the epithelial tissue to adhere to the tooth during a state of health. Below this area, the connective tissue attachment is defined by collagen fibers that, via Sharpey's fibers, insert directly into the tooth's cementum and run perpendicular to the tooth surface. These fibers act as a barrier to bacteria and foreign objects, further protecting the periodontal ligament and the alveolar crestal bone.[39]

A critical difference between peri-implant and periodontal tissues is the lack of Sharpey's fibers around implants.[40] This absence results in collagen fibers that radiate from the crestal bone and parallel the implant and its abutment. As a result of this lack of Sharpey's fibers, the histology of peri-implant tissues is defined by the presence of a long junctional epithelium.[41] Without the second zone of collagen fibers perpendicular to the sulcus, the gingival tissues around an implant are compromised in their ability to protect the supporting bone from assault.[39] This lack of resistance means that the clinician must be diligent to ensure that no delivery procedure adversely impacts the peri-implant tissue health.[42]

This issue is of particular importance with regard to cement-retained implant-supported restorations and peri-implant tissues. Without the protection of the network of interwoven periodontal fibers, the peri-implant tissues are unable to adequately prevent the apical displacement of residual excess cement. This residual cement can adhere to the implant abutment or, if it travels far enough apically, even the implant platform. After delivery of the restoration and once the cement is completely polymerized, the cement can be difficult to fully remove and can act as a locus of irritation. Retained residual excess cement has been implicated in crestal bone loss around dental implants.[43] Furthermore, a positive correlation has been shown between the presence of residual excess cement and peri-implant disease.[44]

Generally, the peri-implant tissue area is skillfully molded surgically and then further shaped and enhanced by the provisional restoration. The resulting customized shape of the soft tissue emergence profile is carefully transferred from the patient's mouth to the master cast as described in chapter 5. Based on the information supplied by this master cast, a custom abutment with a properly positioned finish line is designed and fabricated. As discussed in chapter 6, the finish line position is carefully placed supragingivally or equigingivally when possible on the lingual/palatal aspect of the implant abutment. For tooth-colored abutments, the finish line is placed 1.0 mm subgingivally apical to the free gingival margin on the facial aspect, while it is placed 1.5 mm subgingivally for non–tooth colored abutments. This facilitates the integration of function and esthetics along the interface of the restoration and soft tissue without compromising the clinician's ability to remove excess cement.

In summary, the following are key concepts for cementation of implant-supported restorations in areas where esthetics and soft tissue management are critical for a successful clinical outcome:

- *Favorable position of the abutment finish line.* When possible, supragingival placement of the finish line is preferred. This location minimizes soft tissue trauma, reduces the risk of apical migration of cement, and enables efficient and effective removal of any excess cement. However, when esthetic considerations must be taken into account, the finish line placement on custom abutments should be placed subgingivally following the scalloping of the soft tissue, not exceeding 2 mm apical to the free gingival margins so as not to increase the risk of excess cement retention.[45]
- *Isolation.* Isolation is achieved by lightly placing a cord just apical to the finish line. The cord serves as a barrier between the cement, the depth of the sulcus, and the implant platform, thus facilitating the removal of apically migrated excess cement. Care must be taken that the cord is placed just apical to the abutment's finish line and not too far apically. The stability of the soft tissue–restoration complex is enhanced by keeping any disturbance to the sulcular epithelium to a minimum.[46]
- *Meticulous excess cement removal.* Clinicians must always diligently confirm excess cement removal visually (when possible) and radiographically. Excess cement not only poses an esthetic problem, but it can also serve as a point of adhesion for bacteria and act as a locus of irritation and inflammation.[47]
- *Use clinically visible cement when possible.* This will help ensure complete removal of any excess cement. For bonding or cementing a ceramic restoration to a ceramic abutment, translucent composite resin cements are often preferred because of their esthetic properties. However, their translucent nature can make it challenging to visually confirm residual excess cement removal.
- *Use cement that can be easily removed.* Some cements such as resin-modified glass-ionomer cements, glass-ionomer cements, and some temporary cements can be used predictably with metallic abutments and metal-ceramic restorations. Temporary cements are sometimes preferred due to the relative ease of retrieving restorations luted with them. Temporary and glass ionomer–based cements can be easily cleaned during residual excess cement removal procedures. However, it may be more challenging to remove residual excess composite resin cements, which may be preferred with ceramic abutments and ceramic restorations.
- *Use radiopaque cement.* A radiopaque cement is preferred because any residual excess cement at the interproximal areas can be more easily visualized via a digital radiograph.[23–27]

Cementation protocol using composite resin cement

Case F illustrates cementation of a zirconia-based ceramic crown to a zirconia abutment with composite resin cement (Figs 8-7a to 8-7f). A very similar protocol may be used when cementing a ceramic crown to a metallic abutment. A precementation assessment of the restoration is needed before delivering the definitive restoration. After the abutment is placed in the patient's mouth and the abutment screw is hand tightened, the crown is assessed intraorally to verify that its shade and contours match and harmonize with the surrounding dentition and soft tissues. Next, the interproximal and occlusal contacts are evaluated and adjusted as needed. Once all of these parameters are addressed, the following sequence is followed: F

1. Anesthetize the patient.
2. Verify adequate seating of the abutment with a radiograph, and torque it to a value in accordance with the manufacturer's instructions (Figs 8-7g and 8-7h).
3. Seal the screw access hole. First, place a cotton pellet that has been lightly moistened in a chlorhexidine gluconate solution into the base of the screw access hole. Thread seal tape (Teflon tape) or light-body impression material can be used for that purpose as an alternative. This is done to ensure that the abutment screw is properly isolated from any cement, which will help facilitate access to the abutment screw should the crown or the abutment need to be removed in the future.
4. Next, place an interim composite resin restorative material into the screw access hole (Fermit N, Ivoclar Vivadent). The composite resin should be undercontoured, creating a concavity. This is done to ensure that the material does not interfere with the complete seating of the restoration.
5. Place a nonimpregnated 00 cord into the sulcus circumferentially. Measure, cut, and moisten the cord with water prior to placement. A 00 cord is more durable than a 000 cord, which may tear during cord removal (Fig 8-7i).
6. Ensure complete visibility of the abutment finish line. The cord should be placed subgingivally and only as far apically as necessary to just expose the finish line of the abutment. Avoid placing the cord any further apically; this will help minimize trauma to the peri-implant tissues. Ideally, the finish line on the abutment should be

Continued from chapter 6

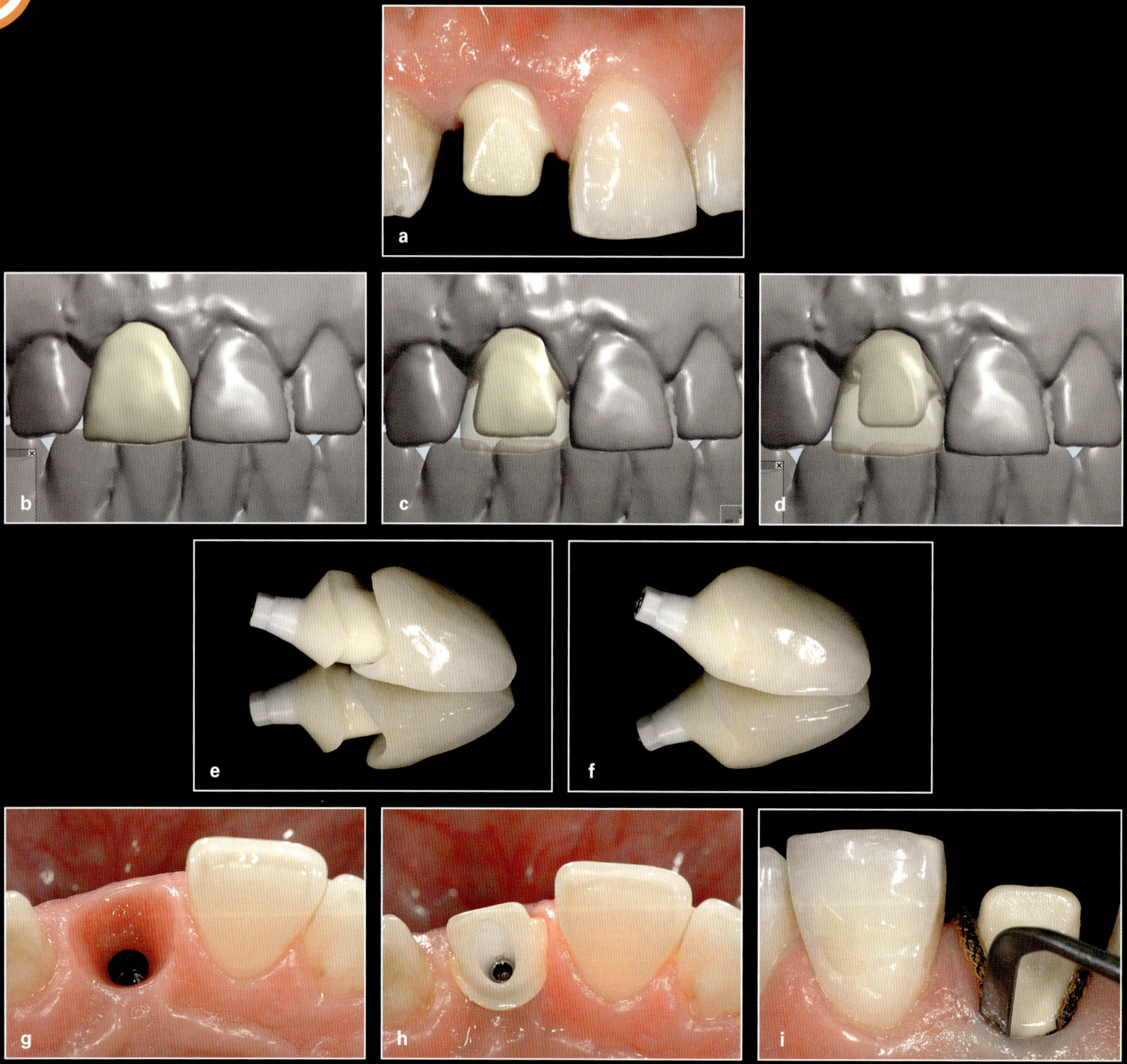

Fig 8-7 *(a)* Facial view of the definitive custom zirconia abutment (Atlantis, Astra Tech). Note that the finish line on the facial aspect is placed 1 mm below the free gingival margins following the scalloping of the soft tissue. *(b to d)* Facial views of the CAD design of the complete zirconia-based crown (Katana), demonstrating the complete contour of the restoration based on the contours of the provisional restoration *(b)*, the contours of the zirconia coping *(c)*, and the contours of the underlying zirconia abutment *(d)*. *(e and f)* Views of the definitive abutment and crown, demonstrating the customized cervical contours of the restoration. *(g and h)* Occlusal views of the implant site without and with the definitive abutment. Note the soft tissue contours and the palatal finish line of the abutment placed coronal to the free gingival margins. *(i)* A 00 cord (Ultrapak) is placed to serve as a barrier between the cement and the depth of the sulcus.

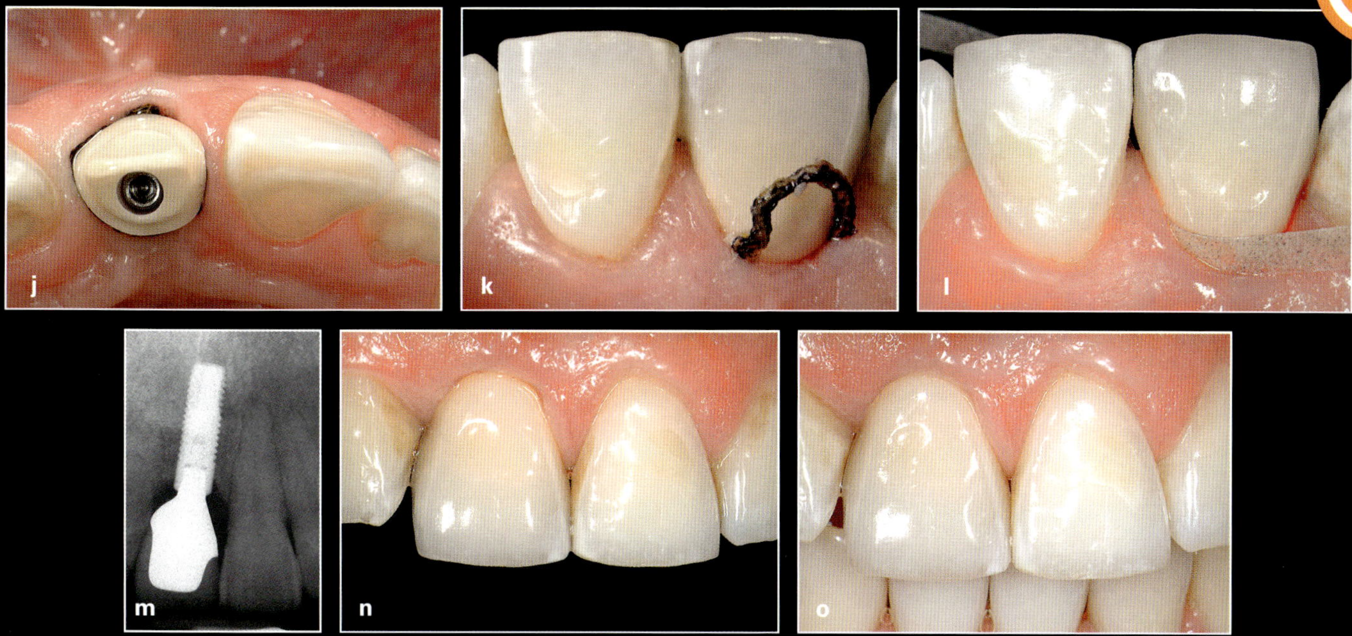

Fig 8-7 *(cont) (j)* Attention is given to ensure that any stray fibers from the cord are repositioned in the sulcus and that the finish line of the abutment is completely visible. *(k)* Once the cement is completely polymerized, the cord is gently removed. Note the residual excess cement particles attached to the cord. *(l)* An interproximal polishing strip (Sof-Lex) is used to ensure complete removal of residual excess cement at the mesial and distal interproximal aspects. *(m)* Periapical radiograph confirming residual excess cement removal at the interproximal aspects as well as excellent marginal integrity. *(n)* Frontal view of the restoration a few weeks after delivery. *(o)* Frontal view of the restoration 2 years after delivery.

relatively supragingival on the lingual aspect and slightly subgingival on the facial aspect.

7. Ensure that no residual stray fibers of the cord are covering the finish line. The use of high magnification during this step is critical to ensure that no stray fibers from the cord will become trapped between the abutment and the restoration (Fig 8-7j). If the cord's stray fibers are caught between the finish line of the abutment and the margins of the crown, it can serve as a source of local irritation, compromising the health of the peri-implant soft tissues.
8. After completing the relevant surface treatment of both the abutment and the intaglio of the crown, apply a thin coat of cement along the axial walls of the intaglio of the crown and its margins. Do not fill the crown with cement, as this may prevent full seating of the crown on the abutment. It can also result in residual excess cement being forced apically along the abutment and down toward the implant platform, making its total removal more difficult.[6,47]
9. Use a dual-polymerized composite resin cement with a relatively high radiopacity.[24–26] Attempt to remove as much excess cement as possible prior to the cement being completely polymerized. As mentioned previously, tack curing for 1 to 2 seconds immediately following seating can help facilitate gross excess cement removal with certain cements (eg, RelyX Unicem 2, Multilink Automix, Panavia SA). Once the gross excess cement is removed, complete the light-polymerization of the cement.
10. Gently remove the cord once the cement is fully polymerized. With a sharp curette or the tip of an explorer, start by teasing the cord from the mesial, distal, buccal, and lingual. Any excess cement that made contact with the cord should come out with it (Fig 8-7k). Note that without the cord, the cement adhered to it would have been displaced further apically, and its removal would have been made much more difficult. Measure the cord to confirm its complete removal.
11. Remove any residual excess cement. Because it is thin and sharp, it is preferable to use a no. 12 blade. A sharp curette can be used as well. For excess cement removal in interproximal areas, interproximal polishing strips (Sof-Lex) for composite resin can be gently used (Fig 8-7l). These strips remove composite resin cement without damaging porcelain or zirconia.
12. Verify excess cement removal at interproximal areas with a digital radiograph (Fig 8-7m).

Following these steps carefully will help to ensure successful cementation and retention of a restoration, a key factor in determining its success (Figs 8-7n and 8-7o). However, clinicians may become too focused on this one aspect of treatment while underestimating the role of the surrounding soft tissue in the delivery process and how it affects the definitive treament outcome in terms of function, health, and esthetics. The soft tissue should not be treated without regard during the various phases of treatment. Its health and condition can greatly influence the degree of complications, patient comfort, and overall procedural predictability and esthetic outcome.

Conclusion

Advances in materials science, manufacturing technologies, and surgical techniques have enabled the contemporary dentist to deliver exceptional restorations. This has elevated many patients' expectations from merely wanting practical results to wanting solutions that successfully manage the interplay between the restoration and the dentogingival complex to create a natural-appearing result. For many patients, it is no longer enough that a restoration remains in function. Discoloration at the margins, chronically inflamed gingivae, gingival recession, and loss of papillae—to name just a few complications—can greatly erode patients' satisfaction and confidence. Many of these issues can be avoided by understanding and appreciating the role of gingival health throughout the various phases of therapy. By making soft tissue health a focus and following the principles outlined in the chapters of this book, the restorative dentist can greatly increase the predictability and decrease the stress associated with these restorative procedures. Ultimately, the goal of the interdisciplinary treatment team should be to provide the highest standard of care and deliver functional and esthetic restorations that support the ongoing oral health of patients.

References

1. Thomas MS, Joseph RM, Parolia A. Nonsurgical gingival displacement in restorative dentistry. Compend Contin Educ Dent 2011; 32:26–34.
2. Magne P, Magne M, Belser UC. The esthetic width in fixed prosthodontics. J Prosthodont 1999;8:106–118.
3. Beier US, Kapferer I, Burtscher D, Dumfahrt H. Clinical performance of porcelain laminate veneers for up to 20 years. Int J Prosthodont 2012;25:79–85.
4. Layton DM, Clarke M. A systematic review and meta-analysis of the survival of non-feldspathic porcelain veneers over 5 and 10 years. Int J Prosthodont 2013;26:111–124.
5. Peumans M, Van Meerbeek B, Lambrechts P, Vanherle G. Porcelain veneers: A review of the literature. J Dent 2000;28:163–177.
6. Chee WW, Duncan J, Afshar M, Moshaverinia A. Evaluation of the amount of excess cement around the margins of cement-retained dental implant restorations: The effect of the cement application method. J Prosthet Dent 2013;109:216–221.
7. Gürel G, Sesma N, Calamita MA, Coachman C, Morimoto S. Influence of enamel preservation on failure rates of porcelain laminate veneers. Int J Periodontics Restorative Dent 2013;33:31–39.
8. Hamlett K. The art of veneer cementation. Alpha Omegan 2009;102:128–132.
9. Chung CW, Yiu CK, King NM, Hiraishi N, Tay FR. Effect of saliva contamination on bond strength of resin luting cements to dentin. J Dent 2009;37:923–931.
10. D'Arcangelo C, De Angelis F, Vadini M, D'Amario M. Clinical evaluation on porcelain laminate veneers bonded with light-cured composite: Results up to 7 years. Clin Oral Investig 2012;16:1071–1079.
11. Chang SW, Cho BH, Lim RY, et al. Effects of blood contamination on microtensile bond strength to dentin of three self-etch adhesives. Oper Dent 2010;35:330–336.
12. Lacy AM, Wada C, Du W, Watanabe I. In vitro microleakage at the gingival margin of porcelain and resin veneers. J Prosthet Dent 1992;67:7–10.
13. Liu Y, Tjäderhane L, Breschi L, et al. Limitations in bonding to dentin and experimental strategies to prevent bond degradation. J Dent Res 2011;90:953–968.
14. Kopp FR. Esthetic principles for full crown restorations. Part III: Final cementation. J Esthet Dent 1996;8:51–57.
15. de Gennaro GG, Landesman HM, Calhoun JE, Martinoff JT. A comparison of gingival inflammation related to retraction cords. J Prosthet Dent 1982;47:384–386.
16. Reiman MB. Exposure of subgingival margins by nonsurgical gingival displacement. J Prosthet Dent 1976;36:649–654.
17. Loe H, Silness J. Tissue reactions to string packs used in fixed restorations. J Prosthet Dent 1963;13:318–323.
18. Akca EA, Yildirim E, Dalkiz M, Yavuzyilmaz H, Beydemir B. Effects of different retraction medicaments on gingival tissue. Quintessence Int 2006;37:53–59.
19. Kopac I, Cvetko E, Marion L. Gingival inflammatory response induced by chemical retraction agents in beagle dogs. Int J Prosthodont 2002;15:14–19.
20. Ruel J, Schuessler PJ, Malament K, Mori D. Effect of retraction procedures on the periodontium in humans. J Prosthet Dent 1980; 44:508–515.
21. McLaren EA, Hamilton J. Tips and tricks for the adhesive cementation of ceramic inlays, onlays, and veneers. Inside Dentistry 2007;3:84–88.
22. Newcomb GM. The relationship between the location of subgingival crown margins and gingival inflammation. J Periodontol 1974; 45:151–154.
23. Antonijevic D, Obradovic-Djuricic K, Rakocevic Z, Medigovic I. In vitro radiographic detection of cement overhangs on cement-retained implant restorations. Int J Oral Maxillofac Implants 2013;28:1068–1075.
24. Tsuge T. Radiopacity of conventional, resin-modified glass ionomer, and resin-based luting materials. J Oral Sci 2009;51:223–230.
25. Antonijevic D, Jevremovic D, Jovanovic S, Obradovic-Djuricic K. An in vitro radiographic analysis of the density of dental luting cements as measured by CCD-based digital radiography. Quintessence Int 2012;43:421–428.
26. Altnitas SH, Yildirim T, Kayipmaz S, Usumez A. Evaluation of the radiopacity of luting cements by digital radiography. J Prosthodont 2013;22:282–286.
27. Pekkan G, Ozcan M. Radiopacity of different resin-based and conventional luting cements compared to human and bovine teeth. Dent Mater J 2012;31:68–75.
28. Benson BW, Bomberg TJ, Hatch RA, Hoffman W Jr. Tissue displacement methods in fixed prosthodontics. J Prosthet Dent 1986; 55:175–181.
29. Harrison JD. The effect of retraction materials on the gingival sulculus epithelium. J Prosthet Dent 1961;11:514–521.
30. Wagman SS. Tissue management for full cast veneer crowns. J Prosthet Dent 1965;15:106–117.

31. Santos MJ, Bapoo H, Rizkalla AS, Santos GC. Effect of dentin-cleaning techniques on the shear bond strength of self-adhesive resin luting cement to dentin. Oper Dent 2011;36:512–520.
32. Wilson PR. Crown behaviour during cementation. J Dent 1992; 20:156–162.
33. Wilson PR, Goodkind RJ, Delong R, Sakaguchi R. Deformation of crowns during cementation. J Prosthet Dent 1990;64:601–609.
34. Edelhoff D, Spiekermann H, Yildirim M. A review of esthetic pontic design options. Quintessence Int 2002;33:736–746.
35. Manary DG. Evaluating the pontic-tissue relationship by means of a clinical technique. J Prosthet Dent 1983;50:193–194.
36. Belser UC, Grütter L, Vailati F, Bornstein MM, Weber HP, Buser D. Outcome evaluation of early placed maxillary anterior single-tooth implants using objective esthetic criteria: A cross-sectional, retrospective study in 45 patients with a 2- to 4-year follow-up using pink and white esthetic scores. J Periodontol 2009;80:140–151.
37. Fürhauser R, Florescu D, Benesch T, Haas R, Mailath G, Watzek G. Evaluation of soft tissue around single-tooth implant crowns: The pink esthetic score. Clin Oral Implants Res 2005;16:639–644.
38. Gargiulo AW, Wentz FM, Orban B. Dimensions and relations of the dentogingival junction in humans. J Periodontol 1961;32:261–267.
39. Berglundh T, Lindhe J, Ericsson I, Marinello CP, Liljenberg B, Thomsen P. The soft tissue barrier at implants and teeth. Clin Oral Implant Res1991;2:81–90.
40. Goldberg PV, Higginbottom FL, Wilson TG. Periodontal considerations in restorative and implant therapy. Periodontol 2000 2001; 25:100–109.
41. Ericsson I, Lindhe J. Probing depth at implants and teeth. An experimental study in the dog. J Clin Periodontol 1993;20:623–627.
42. Baumann GR, Raley JW, Hallmon WW, Mills M. The peri-implant sulcus. Int J Oral Maxillofac Implants 1993;8:273–280.
43. Shapoff CA, Lahey BJ. Crestal bone loss and the consequences of retained excess cement around dental implants. Compend Contin Educ Dent 2012;33:94–101.
44. Wilson TG Jr. The positive relationship between excess cement and peri-implant disease: A prospective clinical endoscopic study. J Periodontol 2009;80:88–92.
45. Linkevicius T, Vindasiute E, Puisys A, Linkeviciene L, Maslova N, Puriene A. The influence of the cementation margin position on the amount of undetected cement. A prospective clinical study. Clin Oral Implants Res 2013;24:71–76.
46. Bennani V, Schwass D, Chandler N. Gingival retraction techniques for implants versus teeth: Current status. J Am Dent Assoc 2008; 139:1354–1363.
47. Dumbrigue HB, Abanomi AA, Cheng LL. Techniques to minimize excess luting agent in cement-retained implant restorations. J Prosthet Dent 2002;87:112–114.

Index

Page numbers followed by "f" indicate figures; those followed by "t" indicate tables; those followed by "b" indicate boxes.

A

B

C

D

E

F

R

S